# AN OVERVIEW OF TROPICAL DISEASES

Edited by **Amidou Samie**

**An Overview of Tropical Diseases**
http://dx.doi.org/10.5772/59215
Edited by Amidou Samie

**Contributors**

Rashika El Ridi, Hatem Tallima, Kevin Hadley, Amidou Samie, Ali Kamal ElBakri, Ahmed Al-Qahtani, Adeola Orogade, Satish Awasthi, Chiranjeev Sharma, José A. Oteo, Paula Santibañez, Ana M Palomar, Aránzazu Portillo, Sonia Santibáñez, Vera Scarpassa, Ronildo Alencar, Kenji Hikosaka, Keisuke Komatsuya, Shigeo Suzuki, Kiyoshi Kita, Sara Savic, Jose Mauro Peralta

**Published by InTech**

Janeza Trdine 9, 51000 Rijeka, Croatia



**Publishing Process Manager** Iva Simcic

**Technical Editor** InTech DTP team

**Cover** InTech Design team

First published December, 2015

Printed in Croatia

Additional hard copies can be obtained from orders@intechopen.com

An Overview of Tropical Diseases , Edited by Amidou Samie

p. cm.

ISBN 978-953-51-2224-1

For EU product safety concerns:
IN TECH d.o.o., Prolaz Marije Krucifikse Kozulić 3, 51000 Rijeka, Croatia,
info@intechopen.com or visit our website at intechopen.com.

# Meet the editor

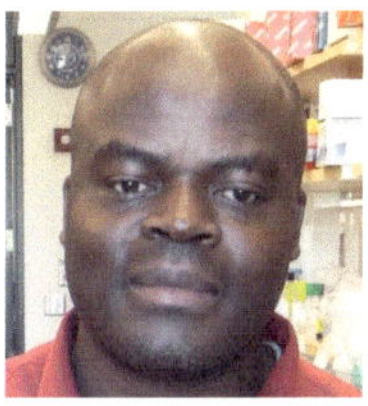

Dr. Amidou Samie is an Associate Professor of Microbiology at the University of Venda, in South Africa, where he graduated for his PhD in May 2008. He joined the Department of Microbiology the same year and has been giving lectures on topics covering parasitology, immunology, molecular biology and industrial microbiology. He is currently a rated researcher by the National Research Foundation of South Africa at category C2 and has published widely in the field of infectious diseases as well as graduated several MSc's and PhDs. His research activities mostly cover topics on infectious diseases from epidemiology to control. His particular interest lies in the study of intestinal protozoan parasites and opportunistic infections among HIV patients as well as the potential impact of childhood diarrhoea on growth and child development. He also conducts research on water-borne diseases and water quality and is involved in the evaluation of point-of-use water treatment technologies using silver and copper nanoparticles in collaboration with the University of Virginia, USA. He also studies the use of medicinal plants for the control of infectious diseases as well as antimicrobial drug resistance.

# Contents

# Preface

Changes in the eating habits as well as lifestyle of people have led to the development of non-communicable diseases in most developed countries and have set the tone for an epidemiological transition in most developing countries. However, infectious diseases still constitute an important cause of mortality, particularly in the tropical regions. There have been efforts from the international community represented by the World Health Organization (WHO) as well as from many other governmental and non-governmental organisations to control some of the common diseases in the tropical regions of the world, while many have been neglected for a long time. Therefore, an overview of the progress in our understanding of certain tropical diseases is critical.

Tuberculosis and malaria constitute two important tropical diseases, and progress has been made for the reduction of the prevalence of these infections but more importantly their control through diagnosis and treatment. The present book has identified a number of tropical diseases in order to clarify recent advances in the research pertaining to the diagnosis and treatment of these infections. Other tropical diseases such as leishmaniasis and schistosomiasis have also been discussed in the book. Of all the amoebas, *Dientamoeba fragilis* infections have not been well studied, and very little attention has been paid to this pathogen. However, recent epidemiological studies have shown an increase in the number of reported cases showing its growing impact in the society, which warrants further investigations on its role in the production of gastrointestinal symptoms among humans. Similarly, chiggers are not only confined to developing countries but are being described in some developed countries as well, where they affect both animals and humans.

This book follows in the footsteps of other books published by InTech on tropical diseases and highlights some infections that have been dealt with intensively such as tuberculosis and malaria but also some that have not been much researched on and might affect both humans and animals (chiggers) or mostly animals (dirofilariasis). The chapters have been organised in order starting from the bacterial disease (tuberculosis) followed by the protozoan diseases (malaria, *Dientamoeba fragilis, Leishmania* ), followed by the worms (dirofilariasis and schistosomiasis) and concluding with the arthropod (shiggers). Many of the chapters discuss issues related to the treatment or control of the diseases either at the level of treatment or through vector control, except for some that give a complete view of the disease from epidemiology to control. This by no means is an exhaustive list of tropical diseases, but the intention is to initiate the discussion on new ways of controlling tropical diseases and to raise awareness on certain diseases that might not have been at the forefront of research but that are progressively making an impact on the health of communities around the world.

**Prof. Amidou Samie**
Department of Microbiology
University of Venda
Limpopo, South Africa

# Chapter 1

# Emerging Public Health Issues in Drug-Resistant Tuberculosis

Adeola Orogade

Additional information is available at the end of the chapter

http://dx.doi.org/10.5772/61269

**Abstract**

Drug Resistance is a major challenge in the control of Tuberculosis which itself remains a global public health problem. Resistance is commonly encountered as MDR TB but a subset, XDR TB which has about a comparatively fivefold increase in mortality is now identified in 84 countries worldwide and increasing rates are currently reported from 65 countries. The actual burden of MDR TB is unknown though estimates have been made based on notification of cases which are usually underreported. More so there is under diagnosis in non HIV immune suppressed adults and pediatric populations largely due to lack of readily accessible diagnostic tools. In some case series, MDR TB has been found occurring mostly in newly diagnosed patients or relapse cases after previous cure and completion of treatment rather than in patients with improperly treated disease. Clinical and laboratory monitoring once therapy has been instituted have also been a daunting task both from institutional and patient points of view. The impact of these factors are highlighted and discussed as the world moves towards attainment of the 2015 global target to halve TB prevalence and death rates within the context of Millennium Development Goals (MDGs).

**Keywords:** Tuberculosis, Drug Resistant, Public Health

## 1. Introduction

*The man who moves a mountain begins by carrying away small stones* – Confucius.

Drug resistance is a major challenge in the control of Tuberculosis (TB), which itself remains a global public health problem. Resistance is commonly encountered as Multidrug-Resistant Tuberculosis (MDR TB), but a subset, Extensively Drug-Resistant Tuberculosis (XDR TB), which has about a comparatively fivefold increase in mortality, is now identified in 84 countries worldwide and increasing rates are currently reported from 65 countries. The World

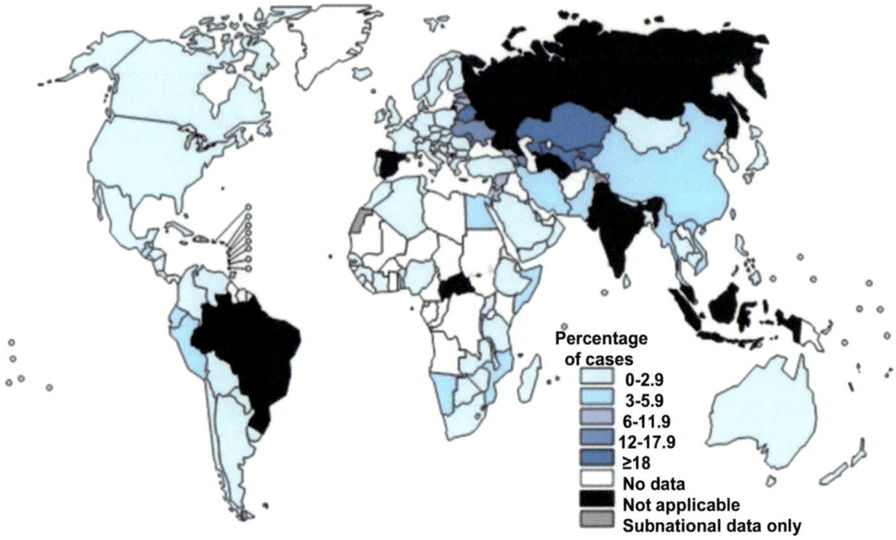


Figures are based on the most recent year for which data have been reported, which variesamong countries.

**Figure 1.** Percentage of new TB cases with MDR-TB (Adapted from WHO Global TB Report, 2014)

Health Organization (WHO) has designated 22 countries of the world as high-burden countries for Tuberculosis (HBCTB) and 27 as high-burden countries for multidrug-resistant Tuberculosis (HBC MDR TB), making a total of 36 countries in either of these categories [1]. The latter are countries where at least 4,000 cases of MDR TB are identified per year and/or at least 10% of newly registered TB cases are MDR TB.

MDR TB and XDR TB epidemics are largely driven by transmission and are mainly found in new cases and patients with TB relapse [2]. Since 1994, WHO has been receiving and analyzing data on anti-TB drug resistance from countries via its Drug Resistance Surveillance Project, which depends on continuous data based on rapid molecular diagnostics and drug sensitivity testing (DST). However, neither is widely or routinely available due to prohibitive costs involved, especially in low- and middle-income economies that are also high-burden countries. In these low- and middle-income high TB burden countries, cases of MDR TB are identified mainly through special surveys rather than continuous surveillance reporting. In 2013, only 11 of the 36 HBCTB/HBC MDRTB had up-to-date data through these drug-resistance surveys. From these surveys it is clearly understood that the MDR TB burdens attributed to these countries are only estimates based on notification of cases which in most countries is incomplete and as such may only be the tip of the iceberg (Figures 1 & 2).

Despite these shortfalls in the determination of exact incidences, especially where TB burden is highest, there have been recent global efforts to bridge the gap between diagnosis and appropriate therapy with second- and third-line drugs. Treatment after diagnosis of MDR TB and follow-up of confirmed cases is however bedeviled with unavailability of human resources, accessibility to second-line drugs in high MDR TB areas, and logistics. Global treatment

http://dx.doi.org/10.5772/61269

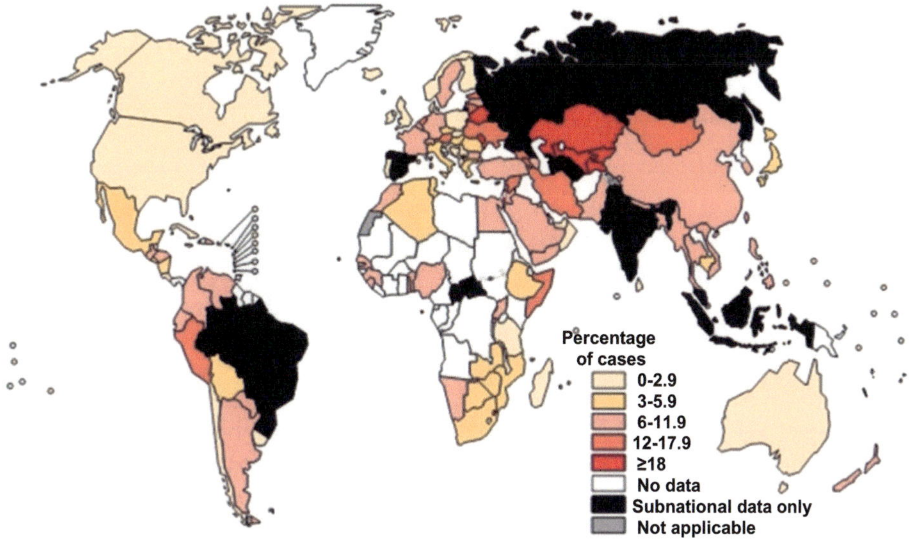


Percentages of previously treated TB cases with MDR-TB in Bahrain, Bonaire, Israel, Saint Eustatius and Saba, and Sao Tomé and Principe refer to only a small number of notified cases (range: 1-8 notified previously treated TB cases).

**Figure 2.** Percentage of previously treated TB cases with MDR-TB (Adapted from WHO Global TB Report, 2014)

targets have not been met. but there are concerted efforts to achieve them through restructuring of programs and Programmatic Management of Drug-Resistant TB (PMDT).

The key to overcoming MDR TB and XDR TB will eventually lie in the balance between prompt diagnosis and treatment of cases on one hand and prevention of transmission of drug-resistant bacilli to vulnerable populations with whom they are in contact on the other. Particular attention needs to be given to unrecognized groups: the pediatric patients in whom a high degree of clinical skill must be displayed to ensure prompt laboratory diagnosis and the health care workers whose infection can be prevented through deliberate control methods.

## 2. Epidemiology of MDR TB

It is estimated that more than 90% of new TB cases and death occur in the high TB burden developing countries [3]. Multidrug anti-tuberculous therapy had been found effective when using the Directly Observed Therapy Short Course (DOTS) strategy to improve compliance to treatment of TB. With the emergence of MDR TB, the DOTS strategy was expanded to accommodate second-line drugs in the Directly Observed Therapy short course with MDR diagnosis, management, and treatment (DOTS PLUS) strategy. Treatment failure, however, can still occur leading to relapse and development of drug-resistant TB strains to second-line drugs which is the XDR TB [4].

Multidrug-resistant Tuberculosis (MDR TB) is defined as resistance to at least both Isoniazid and Rifampicin with or without resistance to other first-line drugs. [5]. A subset of this is

Extensively Drug-Resistant Tuberculosis (XDR TB) where there is also resistance to fluoroquinolones and at least one injectable second-line drug (such as Amikacin, Kanamycin, or Capreomycin) in addition [6]. XDR TB was first noted in the late 1980s and 1990s and reported by WHO and Center for Disease Control (CDC), USA, in 2004.

In a survey of some of their National Reference laboratories, it was observed that 20% of resistant strains tested were MDR TB, while 10% were XDR TB. Asia and Eastern Europe had the highest rates [7]. From recent reports, about 60% of the global burden of Multidrug-resistant TB is in China, India and Russia occurring in 3.7% of new TB cases (CI: 2.1-5.2%) and 20% of previously treated TB cases (CI:13-26%). In countries where there are data available, 9% of MDR–TB cases have XDR (CI: 6.7-11.2%) and 14.5% have fluoroquinolone resistance (CI: 11.6-17.4%) [8].

According to the WHO, Eastern Europe's rates of MDR TB are the highest and MDR TB makes up to 20% of all new TB cases, while in The Union State, it accounts for 28% of new TB cases. In Africa, reports of MDR TB based on continuous surveillance as in South Africa [9] show progressively increasing MDR rates despite overall decreasing numbers of TB cases. This is attributed to improved notification through laboratory surveillance. In developing countries with limited access to TB drug sensitivity tests, prevalence of MDR TB is dependent on special national surveys [1] and hospital-based clinical researches as in Nigeria [10-18]. Most of the hospital-based reports in Nigeria indicate that there is some level of MDR TB, which though not documented on a regular basis show progressive increase over time. This case scenario plays out in other developing countries where continuous surveillance or monitoring of MDR TB is not available. In Nigeria, as well as in other high-burden countries such as South Africa and India, it has been noted that the increasing TB prevalence may be driven by HIV coinfection [19]. Most of these reports are, however, based on testing of adult populations.

Pediatric MDR TB has been majorly underreported in continuous surveillance and special surveys. However, in some countries like South Africa, some modest efforts have been made to document and monitor progress of disease in these populations. A recent meta-analysis [20] of WHO data between 1994 and 2011, testing associations between MDR TB and age groups <15 years, and those >15 years, revealed that MDR TB was positively associated with age <15years in Germany, Namibia, South Africa, UK, and USA. The data also revealed that similar proportions of children and adults were diagnosed with MDR TB in many settings. HIV coinfection was found to be in close association with pediatric MDR TB in South Africa invariably due to the high prevalence of HIV in this area.

### 2.1. Genesis of MDR TB

Drug-resistant TB has microbial, clinical, and programmatic causes [21]. It manifests when there is a selective growth of resistant mutants among the actively multiplying bacillary population in the presence of drugs, thus making the drug ineffective against mutant bacilli. Microbiologically, the emergence of drug resistance depends upon the frequency of drug-resistant mutants in the susceptible bacillary population, the size of the actively multiplying bacillary population in the lesions, and the antimicrobial quality of the drugs used [22]. The frequency of spontaneous mutations that can be developed to each drug are believed to be of the following magnitude: Streptomycin 1 in $10^6$, Isoniazid 1 in $10^6$, Rifampicin 1 in $10^8$, Ethambutol 1 in $10^7$, Pyrazinamide 1 in $10^6$, Fluoroquinolones 1 in $10^{6-8}$ [23]. When these drug-resistant mutants occur in large bacterial population, they have a tendency to further multiply depending on the corresponding clinical treatment regimen the patient receives. This varies from one program to the other and will depend on what drugs are available to a treatment program and the ease of access the patients have to these drugs.

Administered therapy may be inadequate in the following instances: monotherapy, poor adherence to treatment protocols, erratic or even interrupted treatment, or low drug quality. When there is inadequate treatment, resistance develops because bacilli with drug-resistant mutation proliferate and become the dominant strain in the infected individual. Inadequate treatment of susceptible TB can lead to drug resistance to first-line drugs (MDR TB), which is a marker of a failing susceptible TB treatment program. Likewise, inadequate treatment of MDR TB will lead to drug resistance to second-line drugs (XDR TB), which is a marker of failing MDR TB treatment programs.

Drug resistance of the Mycobacterium tuberculosis isolated from patients may be categorized based on length of previous anti-TB drug therapy they had received prior to the diagnosis of resistance. Acquired drug resistance is described in those who have been inadequately treated for 1 month or more; Relapse in cases previously completed treatment and reported cured; while that of patients who have never been treated previously or treated for less than 1 month is called Primary drug resistance or resistance in new case. The patients grouped as relapse or as new infections which are found to be drug resistant are grouped together as transmission cases; 82% of MDR TB are reported to be transmission cases. The other 18% are acquired cases, which are mostly adult populations. The acquired cases provoke and sustain MDR TB epidemics in both developed and undeveloped countries [24].

### 2.2. Epidemics of MDR TB

During the late 1980s and early 1990s, epidemics of MDR TB occurred in North America and Europe killing about 80% of those who were infected. Today, the greatest number of cases is in India and China [25-26], although smaller epidemics have been described due to migrations [27]. The convergence of the following were believed to precipitate MDR TB epidemics especially that of XDR TB: High TB burden, high HIV prevalence, suboptimal TB control practices, and introduction of second-line TB drugs into low- and middle-income countries [28-29]. Among the pediatric age group, there is global paucity of data on MDR TB epidemics. Most data obtained have been reported from South Africa [30]. Some of the identical issues that were identified in all these epidemics were that there was delayed diagnosis of MDR TB cases for over 6 weeks to 6 months due in turn to delayed turnaround time for mycobacterial culture and DST. This invariably led to very high mortality rates which first called attention to the need for DST. In the XDR TB epidemic reported in South Africa [29], there was prominence of associated HIV coinfection in most patients who were transmission cases. Another feature was poor observance of infection control precautions such as: inadequate patient isolation and airflow regulation within wards, which made the wards conducive for transmission between patients in contact with MDR TB cases. There was also notable direct transmission from patients to health care workers, which was evident by Tuberculin Skin Test (TST) conversion as well as later linkage mappings that correlated the strains in the patients' samples with those of the health workers [29].

### 2.3. Implications of transmission versus acquired cases

In the high-burden countries, there are reportedly 20-35.2% of new cases and 54-62% of relapse cases that develop MDR TB, accounting for 82% of all incidences of MDR TB [1]. Thus, high burdens of MDRTB and XDR TB are eventually perpetuated from direct transmission within communities. In cases where TB–HIV coinfections are also prevalent, this significantly favors direct transmissibility [31]. Direct transmission is therefore the most common way drug-resistant TB is spread and this must be stemmed to arrest the imminent global health threat from TB.

## 3. MDR TB diagnosis: Clinical versus laboratory methods

Bacteriological confirmation of TB and Drug sensitivity Testing (DST) of patients presenting with clinical features of Tuberculosis is targeted as universal standard for patient care in TB [1]. When this is incorporated into routine clinical care package and results are available for periodic analysis, it forms a strong database for information about drug resistance in that area.

### 3.1. Clinical criteria

WHO global TB report [1] revealed that only 2.8 million (58%) of the 4.9 million incident pulmonary TB patients notified in 2013 were bacteriologically confirmed (smear- or culture-positive according to a WHO-recommended rapid diagnostic such as Xpert MTB/RIF). The remaining 42% notifications were diagnosed clinically (symptoms, signs, chest X-ray abnormalities, or suggestive histology). Notifications of new cases are mainly from the high-burden countries, majority of which are low- and middle-income economies. Their capacity for confirmatory testing and DST is limited. Although almost half of notified global TB diagnosis is by clinical methods, this form of diagnosis is attended by poor specificity and false-positive diagnosis. Low laboratory rates, on the other hand, may suggest underdiagnosis of true TB cases and contribute to the gap noticed between notified and estimated incident TB cases [1]. The need for skilled health care workers who can make presumptive diagnosis to improve notification while laboratory methods are being scaled-up, especially in the high-burden countries cannot be overemphasized.

However, the drawback of clinical criteria alone to make a diagnosis in MDR TB is obvious. Detection of TB without investigating drug sensitivity potentially can lead to inadequate treatment and this could lead to spread of MDR TB.

### 3.2. Laboratory diagnosis – Screening and confirmatory tools

The field of TB diagnosis has been dynamic, changing constantly with the new challenges posed by the bacilli: from being fully susceptible to multidrug therapy to the appearance of MDR TB and now XDR TB. Whereas the need to have accurate bacteriological diagnosis and appropriate drug sensitivity has not changed, the tools to achieve these have continued to evolve as newer and hopefully equally or more effective diagnostic technologies are developed. Diagnosis of MDR TB requires culture to confirm TB and drug susceptibility testing or molecular testing. The challenges faced in achieving these include:

- Laboratory challenges with technical capacity, biosafety, cost, slow growth
- Patient challenges in access to adequately testing facilities – communication, transportation of specimen, and reporting remain critical to success
- Policy challenges in who should be tested and when to test given limited public health resources

Increasingly, molecular technologies are being incorporated into drug resistance surveys to simplify logistics. By 2009, the EXPAND –TB (Expanding Access to New Diagnostics for TB) was launched to accelerate access of MDR TB high-risk populations in high TB burden countries to sophisticated but rapid diagnostic molecular techniques and provide laboratory services. The 27 high MDR TB burden countries were equipped with 97 new or refurbished laboratories and line probe assays (DNA strip test that allows simultaneous molecular identification of TB and the most common genetic mutations causing resistance to Rifampicin and Isoniazid) in reference laboratories which can diagnose MDR TB in two days. By December 2010, the WHO issued a policy on the use of another molecular diagnostic test Xpert MTB/RIF as an initial diagnostic test for cases at risk of MDR TB with negative sputum. The Xpert test, a cartridge-based automated diagnostic test that can identify Mycobacterium tuberculosis DNA and resistance to Rifampicin by nucleic acid amplification technique was a sputum only test for pulmonary TB [32].

A review of WHO policy followed in 2013 that Xpert MTB/RIF should be used rather than conventional microscopy, culture, and DST as the initial diagnostic test in adults and children suspected of having MDR TB or HIV associated TB. It may be used for diagnosis of drug-susceptible TB, smear-negative individuals and cases of extra-pulmonary TB testing using non-respiratory specimens such as lymph nodes. By the end of June 2014, 108 countries had benefitted from procurement of Gene Xpert machines. GenoType® MTBDRplus (Hain Lifescience, Germany) was used in the national survey completed in 2012 in Nigeria and is currently being used in the national survey in Sudan. In Pakistan, Xpert® MTB/RIF (Cepheid USA) identified additional cases missed by culture in the national survey completed in 2014. In ongoing surveys in Papua New Guinea and Senegal, Xpert MTB/RIF is being used to screen specimens for rifampicin resistance and identify those requiring further testing at national or supranational TB reference laboratories. Surveys planned in 2014–2015 in Côte d'Ivoire, the Democratic Republic of the Congo, Indonesia, and Zimbabwe will adopt the same testing algorithm [1].

This approach greatly reduces the workload for laboratories and decreases the cost of national surveys. It may also result in the detection of cases that would otherwise have been missed by culture and conventional DST, particularly in settings with delays in transporting sputum samples to laboratories for testing. Although not a complete surrogate for MDR-TB, particularly in settings where levels of drug resistance are low, rifampicin resistance is the most important indicator of MDR-TB and has serious clinical implications for affected patients.

It is noteworthy that the supply of these technologically advanced diagnostics though now in more countries cannot serve the total at-risk populations, because these machines are kept strategically in reference laboratories. There is a critical need to develop within each country a framework that would address the accessibility to reference centers. In the Western Pacific and Eastern Mediterranean regions, it is reported that there was less than one reference center per 100,000 population. In Nigeria, a high TB burden country and the fourth highest African country with MDR TB, there are only 9 reference centers which are inadequate for the whole at-risk population of 170 million.

There is therefore need in the high TB burden areas to still supplement the recent high-tech diagnostic tools with sputum smear microscopy as an initial screening tool and as such be placed in such a way that these can be accessible to all. Improvements in microscopy using fluorescent light emitting diode microscopy, which is more sensitive than light microscopy, has been proposed and adopted in South Africa, and less so in Mozambique, Bangladesh, and Nigeria [1].

The other aspect that needs careful attention in laboratory diagnosis is the need for regular quality assurance of the machines. Likewise, regular capacity training for laboratory personnel to ensure optimal standards of diagnosis and DST Xpert MT/RIF Newer areas of research for improved diagnostics is the research for correlates of protective immunity and host biomarkers of TB that could help determine the potential for susceptibility or protection [33].

## 4. Unrecognised MDR TB populations

### 4.1. Pediatric MDR TB

Pediatric TB diagnosis has also been largely based on clinical criteria due to the pauci bacillary nature of their disease [3, 34-36]. In the cases of TB HIV coinfection, the diagnosis of TB disease is usually more difficult because the symptom specificity is reduced due to similarity with chronic HIV-related symptoms, and chest radiograph interpretation is complicated by HIV-related comorbidity and atypical disease presentation. In this case, diagnosis involves linking the child with an adult with confirmed pulmonary TB [37]. However, older children producing sputum can have bacteriological confirmation and where facilities are accessible DST is performed [8]. To date, there is still widespread under-diagnosis of MDR TB in younger children. Children are less likely than adults to acquire MDR TB during treatment due to the lower bacillary load and less-frequent cavity formation [38]. Acquisition of strains of MDR TB through primary transmission has been shown to be same for children as for adults [39].

The implication of this is that with increasing adult MDR TB in populations, there would be increasing incidences of pediatric MDR TB. Once a diagnosis of TB is made, MDR TB should be carefully considered by review of household source cases for drug-resistant disease [40]. Child contacts of adults with coinfection of TB HIV should particularly be screened for MDR TB. The recent efforts to improve on MDR diagnostic tests using non-respiratory specimens should be harnessed for the pediatric age populations so that rapid diagnostic tests become the first-line diagnostic tool for pediatric MDR TB. Outcomes of MDR TB in children depend on prompt diagnosis and initiation of appropriate therapy for drug-resistant strain [41].

## 5. Challenges in MDR TB therapy

The Global target of MDR TB treatment is to achieve 75% treatment success by 2015. To achieve success in treatment programs, WHO has published a document which contains the guide to Programmatic Management of Drug-resistant TB (PMDT) which covers all key policies in MDR TB care and control. The numbers of cases treated are usually reported in cohorts that commence therapy within a certain year. In this way it is hoped that treatment outcomes would be clearly understood and modifications where necessary would be implemented. WHO [1] reports increasing numbers of cases enrolled into treatment programs for MDR TB and XDR TB of 47% from 2010 to 2013. In specific terms, however, this increase has been achieved mainly in low TB burden countries. The issue of inadequate notification from weak reporting systems in most high-burden countries is also thought to contribute to only a modest increase despite all efforts made at increasing treatment coverage. Notification still plays a crucial part in the monitoring of treatment outcomes. This depends on systematic record collection, storage, and retrieval by electronic means. All these processes are not uniformly accessible in all parts of the same country and also differ significantly from country to country. Adequately trained personnel to manage this process is crucial and a vital gap.

The treatment target of 75% success outcome has only been reached by 29 out of 126 countries that have reported outcome. Only five of the 27 MDR TB high-burden countries have reached 70% treatment successes (Figure 3). The success recorded in high-burden countries is closely related to the implementation of EXPAND TB project and the scale-up of PMDT in these countries. The identified gaps to achieving treatment include unavailability of second-line TB drugs whose costs are prohibitive in many high-burden countries. This requires substantial financial and health care resources [42]. To ameliorate this, the Global Fund facility which procures TB drugs for the public sector of many countries has increased supply and dropped prices of some MDR TB drugs by 2009 [43].

### 5.1. Clinical and laboratory monitoring

Drugs used in the treatment of MDR TB are less effective, more toxic (90% experience side effects), used for longer duration (usually more than 2 years' duration), and are more costly than drugs used in susceptible TB (10-100 times more costly) [44]. In the 27 high-burden countries, the expenditure for MDR-TB treatment has increased cost of TB care from an

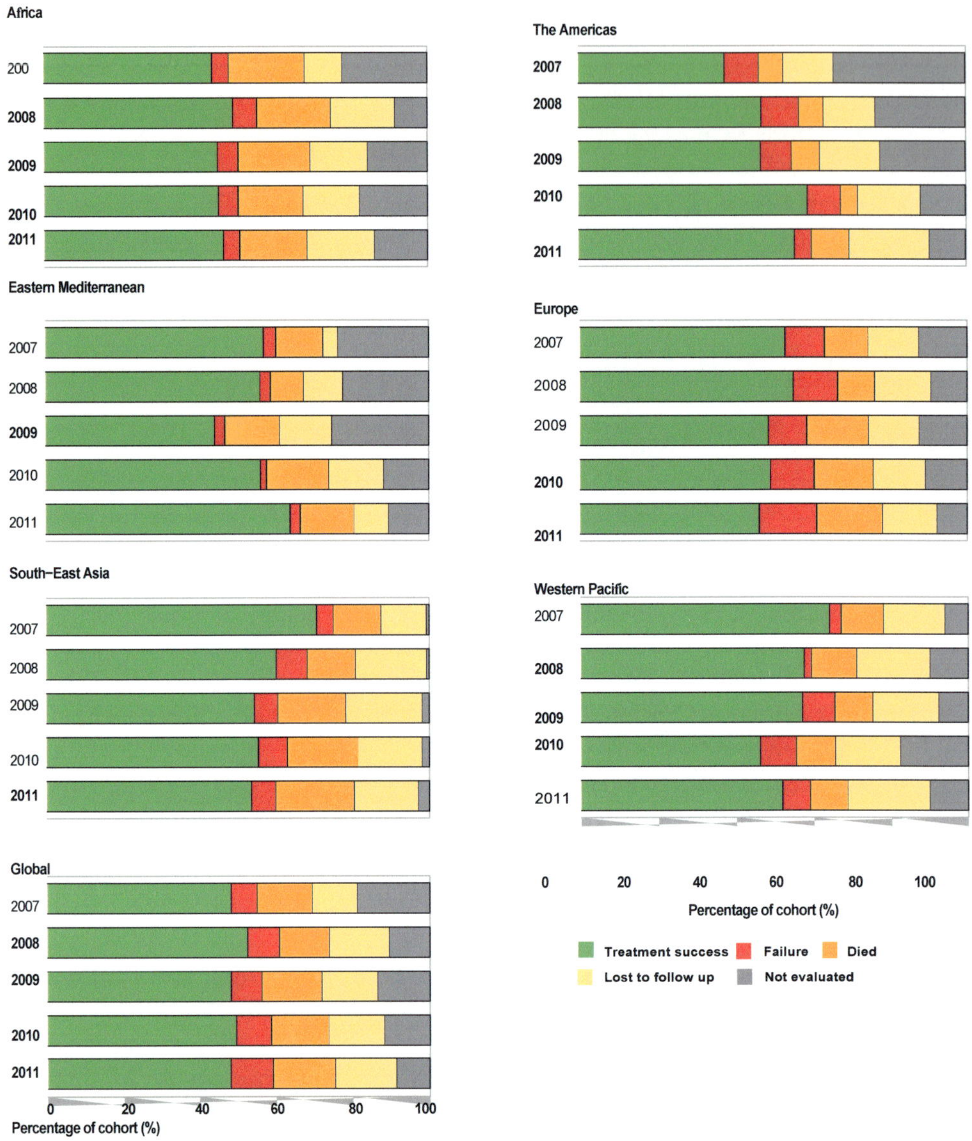


(Adapted from WHO Global TB Report, 2014)

**Figure 3.** Treatment outcomes for patients diagnosed with MDR TB by WHO region, 2007-2011 cohorts.

estimated 1.3 billion USD in 2010 to 4.4 billion USD by 2015 [45]. Some of the common adverse effects might also require monitoring such as ototoxicity and renal failure. There is also the need to document improvement by follow-up of bacteriologic cultures. In addition to these, cases need to be monitored because some MDR TB cases are in advanced stages of disease with other end-stage organ failures. MDR TB therapy is often characterized by low treatment completion rates due to death (15%), default (14-23%), and treatment failure (8-9%) [46]. To achieve increased access, compliance, effective therapy, and retention in care, there is a need for close monitoring. This is traditionally done by hospital-based care at MDR TB referral centers for the initial therapy through health care providers. The model of care involves an initial hospitalization until sputum culture conversion followed by ambulatory phase of treatment in the nearest DOTS facility. However, hospital-based care may serve as an obstacle to access. Ambulatory-based care and community-based care have been proposed in management of MDR TB cases [47]. There have been some successful experiences in some countries using these methods [1]. There would be need for collaboration between these models of care especially when dealing with patients with advanced disease who may benefit for some periods from hospital-based care but would need community- or home-based care for terminal stages. Community and Ambulatory care also serve to ensure adequate contact tracing for cases of MDR and XDR TB, which is of great importance given the role of transmission of disease in spreading the MDR TB epidemic.

When contacts are traced, there is need for DST to identify appropriate second-line drugs. Currently, the diagnostic tools recommended are molecular-based testings: Line probe Assays and Xpert MTB/RIF. There is need, however, to establish quality control measures for these tests to avoid false positives and false negatives. Such tools as would ensure international standards for reference laboratories and other peripheral centers have been developed in some countries. Laboratory monitoring also includes structured assessment tools for TB microscopy, which is shared among laboratory networks.

## 6. Prevention of MDR TB

To achieve success in the control of MDR TB, there would be a need to strengthen existing TB DOTS programs. To achieve this, some areas that should be focused on are the creation of infection control policies both within and outside institutions. Health education of how transmission of disease occurs from cases to vulnerable groups should be emphasized in communities. Community-based care should be strengthened with recruitment of staff for contact tracing of MDR cases, screening of the contacts, treatment administration, and identification of those who are defaulting on treatment or require institutionalized care. There should be expansion in the teams with involvement of all relevant health care partners to strengthen Public–Private Mix initiatives for TB care and control [48-52].

### 6.1. Infection control

This aims to prevent transmission from cases to other patients or health care workers. The following means could help to ensure the protection of health care staff: Use of N95 mask by all staff on medical and TB isolation wards and in the HIV clinics [53]; HIV testing of all staff with reallocation of those testing positive to lower-risk positions; Annual Chest Xray screening for TB for all staff [24,54].

Within health care institutions, TB control officers should be hired as well as cough officer in waiting areas who would identify those that are in hospital for other reasons but who may require TB screening. The duration of hospital admission and stay should be reduced. There should be environmental airflow control to ensure maximal ventilation (natural mechanical ventilation within the ward and the use of outdoor waiting areas for outpatients). MDR TB isolation wards should be created with attention paid to laminar airflow [55].

Infection control programs should be created with plans for intervention should transmission be proved.

## 7. Conclusions

Underdiagnoses of MDR TB and XDR TB cases pose significant challenge for TB control. The current available means for tracking and monitoring are inadequate since they are reliant on reported data which are usually incomplete. These data overlook transmission to unrecognized populations which sustain MDR TB epidemics. There is also a need to make diagnostic tools more available and accessible for cases and contacts and more reference laboratories provided. These laboratories should be monitored to assure they maintain international standards and produce reliable results. Once diagnosis has been made promptly and accurately, adequate therapy for MDR TB should be instituted. This would require clinical monitoring of cases through collaboration of hospital, community, and ambulatory care services. Control programs should also target health care givers to prevent transmission of MDR TB to them from cases. In essence, routine TB DOTS programs should be strengthened in collaboration with public–private mix initiatives to enhance MDR TB control.

## Author details

Adeola Orogade

Address all correspondence to: orogade@yahoo.com

Department of Paediatrics, Ahmadu Bello University Teaching Hospital, Shika Zaria, Nigeria

## References

[1] World Health Organization. Global Tuberculosis Report, 2014. 54-73

[2] Donald PR, van Helden PD. The global burden of tuberculosis – combating drug resistance in difficult times. *N Engl J Med* 2009; 2393-2395

[3] Tuberculosis Fact Sheet, 2012: Published by the US Embassy in Nigeria, retrieved from http://nigeria.usembassy.gov.1-3

http://dx.doi.org/10.5772/61269

[4] World Health Organization. (2005) WHO Global Task Force outlines measures to combat XDR-TB worldwide. Geneva, Switzerland. 3-5

[5] Holtz TH, Lancaster J, Laserson KF. Risk factors associated with default from multi-drug-resistant tuberculosis treatment, South Africa. *Int J Tuberc Lung Dis* 2006; 10 649-655

[6] WHO, Global Plan to stop TB 2006-2015: Progress Report 2006-2008. 25-28

[7] CDC, 2006 Centers for Disease Control and Prevention. Emergence of Mycobacterium tuberculosis with extensive resistance to second line drugs–worldwide, 2000–2004. *MMWR*; 55; 301–305.

[8] World Health Organization Global Tuberculosis Report 2012. Geneva, WHO Press, 2012. 41-51

[9] Ndjeka, N. Multi-Drug Resistant Tuberculosis. Strategic Overview on MDR TB care in SouthAfrica.2014.www.health-e.org.za/2014/03.../presentation-drug-resistant-tb-south-afri..3-25

[10] Fawcett IW, Watkins BJ. Initial resistance of Mycobacterium tuberculosis in Northern Nigeria. *Tubercle* 1976; 57, 71-73

[11] Kolo I. Bacteriological and drug sensitivity studies on Mycobacteria isolated from tuberculosis patients and their close contacts in ABUTH, Zaria, Nigeria. PhD Thesis. Ahmadu Bello University Zaria; 1991

[12] Abdullahi AA. Studies on immunological status of HIV infected patients with Tuberculosis in Kano State, Nigeria. PhD Thesis. Ahmadu Bello University, Zaria, Nigeria; 2006.

[13] Akanbi MO, Ukoli CO. Are weak health systems a brewing ground for multidrug resistant tuberculosis? *Afr J Respir Med* 2009; 21-22

[14] Lawson L, Habib AG, Okobi MI. Pilot study on multidrug resistant Tuberculosis in Nigeria. *Ann Afr Med* 2010; 9 184-187

[15] Lawson L, Yassin MA, Abdurrahman ST, Parry CM, Dacombe R et al. Resistance to first-line Tuberculosis drugs in three cities in Nigeria. *Tropic Med Int Health.* 2011; 16(8) 974-980

[16] Dim CC, Dim NR. Trends of Tuberculosis prevalence and treatment in an under-resourced setting: the case of Enugu State, South East Nigeria. *Nigeria Med J* 2013; 54(6) 392-397

[17] Olusoji D, Eltayeb O, Olanrewaju O, Olapade GD. Pre-Extensive Drug Resistant Tuberculosis (Pre-XDR-TB) among MDR-TB patients. *Global Adv Res J Microbiol* 2013 (ISSN: 2315-5116) 2(2) 22-25

[18] Nwokeukwu HI, Okafor PN, Okorie O, Ukpabi K. Paediatric Multidrug resistant Tuberculosis with HIV Co infection: a case report. *Case Reports in Medicine* 2013; Article ID 756152 1-4.

[19] Adegboyega TT, Thomas BT, Agu GC, Abiodun AT. Can Nigeria sustain the fight against Drug resistant Mycobacterium Tuberculosis? *J Microbiol Res* 2014; 4(2) 72-77

[20] Zignol M, Sismanidis C, Falzon D, Glaziou P, Dara M, et al. Multidrug resistant Tuberculosis in children: evidence from global surveillance. *Eur Respir J* 2012; 343 (3) 701-707

[21] Central TB Division, Directorate General of Health Services, Ministry of Health & Family Welfare. DOTS-Plus Guidelines 2006. Nirman Bhavan, New Delhi: Revised National Tuberculosis Control Programme; 1–46.

[22] Toman K. Tuberculosis, case finding and chemotherapy. World Health Organization. 1979. 207-211

[23] David HL. Probability distribution of drug-resistant mutants in unselected populations of *Mycobacterium tuberculosis*. *Appl Microbiol*. 1970; 20 810–814

[24] Broekmans JF. *Advanced Issues in Global TB Control: Achieving Impact*. Epi/Biostat Summer Institute Lectures, Johns Hopkins Bloomberg School of Public Health. 2014.1-6

[25] Udawadia ZF, Amale RA, Ajbani KK, Rodrigues C. Totally drug resistant Tuberculosis in India. *Clin Infect Dis* 2011. 579-581.DOI: 10.1093/cid/cir889

[26] Global Alliance for TB Drug Development. 2015. 1-3

[27] De Vries G, van Altena R, van Soolingen D, Broekmans JF, van Hest NA. An outbreak of multiresistant tuberculosis from Eastern Europe in the Netherlands. *Ned Tijdschr Geneeskd*. 2005; 149(35) 1921-1924

[28] Schecter G. Multidrug resistant Tuberculosis. Francis J Curry National Tuberculosis Center, 2008.35-42

[29] Gandhi N, Moll A, Sturm AW, Pawinski R, Govender T et al. Extensively drug-resistant tuberculosis (XDR TB) as a cause of death among TB/HIV co-infected patients in a rural area in South Africa. *Lancet* 2006; 368, 1575–1580

[30] Seddon JA, Hesseling AC, Marais BBJ, Jordaan A, Victor T, Schaaf HS. The evolving epidemic of drug resistant tuberculosis among children in Cape Town, South Africa. *Int J Tuberc Lung Dis* 2012. 16(7) 928-933. http://dx.doi.org/10.5588/ijtld. 11.0679

[31] Kwan CK, Ernst JD. HIV and Tuberculosis: a deadly human syndemic. *Clin Microbiol Rev* 2011; 24(2) 351-376

[32] [32]Xpert MTB/RIF implementation manual. Technical and operational "how-to" practical considerations.http://www.who.int/tb/labratory/en

[33] Olson S, Lebovitz y, Claiborne. The Emerging Threat of Drug Resistant Tuberculosis in Southern Africa. Global and Local Challenges and Solutions. Summary of a joint workshop. Institute of Medicine and Academy of Science of South Africa. 2011.42

[34] [34]Orogade AA, Ahmed P, Onazi S, Abubakar U. Isa H. BCG Status in children with Tuberculosis A multicentre study in Northern Nigeria. *J Med Tropic* 2013; 15(2)126-130

[35] Orogade AA., Ogala WN, Onalo R. Congenital Tuberculosis: a case report. Nigerian J Paediatri 2011; 38(2) 100-103

[36] Salazer GE, Schmitz TL, Cama R, Working group on TB in Peru. Pulmonary tuberculosis in children in a developing country. *Paediatrics* 2001; 108(2) 448-453

[37] Ugochukwu EF. HIV/TB Co infection in Nigerian Children. *Nigerian Med J* 2010; 51(3) 120-124

[38] Swanson DS, Starke JR. Drug resistant tuberculosis in paediatrics. *Paediatr Clin N Am* 1995; 42, 553-581

[39] Schaaf HS, Gie RP, Beyers N et al. Primary drug resistant tuberculosis in children. *Int J Tuberc Lung Dis* 2000; 4, 1149-1155

[40] Mukherjee J, Schaaf HS. Multidrug resistant tuberculosis in children. In: Schaaf HS, Zumla AI (eds.) *Tuberculosis. A Comprehensive Clinical Reference*: Elsevier; 2009. 532-537

[41] Ettehad D, Schaaf HS, Seddon JA. Treatment outcomes for children with multidrug resistant tuberculosis: a systemic review and meta-analysis. *Lancet Infect Dis* 2012; 12, 449-456.

[42] Pooran A, Pieterson E, Davids M, Theron G, Dheda K. What is the cost of diagnosis and management of drug resistant tuberculosis in South Africa? *PLoS One* 2013; 8(1)

[43] GDF; www.stoptb.org/gdf)

[44] The Economic Burden. Aeras. 2015. www.aeras.org/pages/beyond-a-health-crisis. 1

[45] World Health Organization. Multidrug and Extensively Drug-resistant TB (M/XDR-TB) 2010 Global Report on Surveillance and Response. 21-29

[46] Ahuja SD, Askin D, Avendano M, Banerjee R, Bauer M et al. Multidrug resistant pulmonary tuberculosis treatment regimens and patient outcomes: an individual patient data meta-analysis of 9,153 patients. *PloS* 2012; 9(9)

[47] Bassilli A, Fitzpatrick C, Qadeer E, Fatima R, Floyd K, Jaramillo E. A systematic review of the effectiveness of hospital and ambulatory based management of multidrug resistant tuberculosis. *Am J Tropic Med Hygiene* 2013; 89(2) 271-280

[48] Gidado M, Ejembi CL. Tuberculosis case management and treatment outcome: assessment of the effectiveness of public-private mix of tuberculosis programme in Kaduna state, Nigeria. *Ann Afr Med* 2009; 8(1):25-31

[49] Ahmed J, Ahmed M, Laghari A, Lohana W, Ali S, Fatmi Z. Public private mix model in enhancing tuberculosis case detection in District Thatta, Sindh, Pakistan. *J Pak Med Assoc* 2009; 59(2):82-86.

[50] Kumar MK, Dewan PK, Nair PK, Frieden TR, Sahu S, Wares F, Laserson K, Wells C, Granich R, Chauhan LS. Improved tuberculosis case detection through public-private partnership and laboratory-based surveillance, Kannur District, Kerala, India, 2001-2002. *Int J Tuberc Lung Dis* 2005; 9: 870-6

[51] Newell JN, Pande SB, Baral SC, Bam DS, Malla P. Leadership, management and technical lessons learnt from a successful public-private partnership for TB control in Nepal. *Int J Tuberc Lung Dis* 2005; 9; 1013-17

[52] Mahendradhata Y, Utarini A,Lazuardi U, Boelaert M, Stuyft P. Private practitioners and tuberculosis case detection in Jogjakarta, Indonesia: actual role and potential. *Tropic Med Int Health* 2007; 12(10)1218-1224

[53] Matlow A, Robb M Goldman C. Infection control and paediatric tuberculosis: A practical guide for the practicing paediatrician. *Paediatr Child Health* 2003; 8(10) 624-626

[54] Institute of Medicine (US) Forum on Drug Discovery, Development, and Translation; Academy of Science of South Africa. The Emerging Threat of Drug-Resistant Tuberculosis in Southern Africa: Global and Local Challenges and Solutions: Summary of a Joint Workshop. Washington (DC): National Academies Press (US); 2011. 4, Transmission and Infection Control. Available from: http://www.ncbi.nlm.nih.gov/books/NBK55584/

[55] Preventing Transmission of Tuberculosis in Healthcare facilities: An Engineering approach.www.safelab.com/DOWNLOAD/TBPaper.pdf; 10-20

Chapter 2

# Mitochondria of Malaria Parasites as a Drug Target

Kenji Hikosaka, Keisuke Komatsuya, Shigeo Suzuki and Kiyoshi Kita

Additional information is available at the end of the chapter

http://dx.doi.org/10.5772/61283

**Abstract**

Mitochondria are organelle, which is found in most eukaryotic cells, and play an important roll in production of many biosynthetic intermediates as well as energy transduction. Recently, it has been reported that mitochondria contribute to cellular stress responses such as apoptosis and autophagy. These functions of mitochondria are known to be essential for survival and maintenance of homeostasis. The mitochondria of malaria parasites are quite different from those of their vertebrate hosts. Because these differences markedly contribute to drug selectivity, we have focused on the *Plasmodium* mitochondrion to develop antimalarial drugs. Here we summarize recent advances in our knowledge of the mitochondria of malaria parasites and discuss future prospective antimalarial drugs targeting the parasite mitochondrion.

**Keywords:** malaria, *Plasmodium*, mitochondria, antimalarial drugs, atovaquone, 5-aminolevulinic acid

## 1. Introduction

Malaria is a major global health problem, shortening over 500,000 human lives annually, mainly children in tropical and subtropical regions [1]. Due to difficulties in developing antimalarial vaccine, chemotherapy is important for controlling malaria. Parasites causing malaria, however, can rapidly develop resistance against the available chemotherapies [2]. Thus, new drugs with different modes of action are urgently needed. Malaria parasites are disseminated by female *Anopheles* mosquitoes and belong to the *Plasmodium* genus. *Plasmodium* has a complicated life cycle, comprising two major cycles: asexual multiplication in humans and sexual multiplication in mosquitoes (Figure 1) [3]. The parasites invade the hepatocytes of their host and mature into merozoites. After release, the merozoites infect red blood cells (RBCs). In the RBCs, the parasites differentiate into the following stages: ring, trophozoite, and schizont. Subsequently, the infected RBCs burst and release merozoites, which invade uninfected RBCs. These stages are called the erythrocytic stages, where the parasites multiply asexually. Following the establishment of infection, some parasites differentiate to gametocytes [4]. The gametocyte stage is essential for subsequent transmission because this is the only stage where the organism undergoes sexual development in the mosquito vector. Therefore, *Plasmodium* has a complex life cycle, which seems to be an adaptation to its host environment [5]. In addition to the complex life cycle, the malaria parasites have evolved sophisticated pathways of energy transduction to adapt to their hosts.

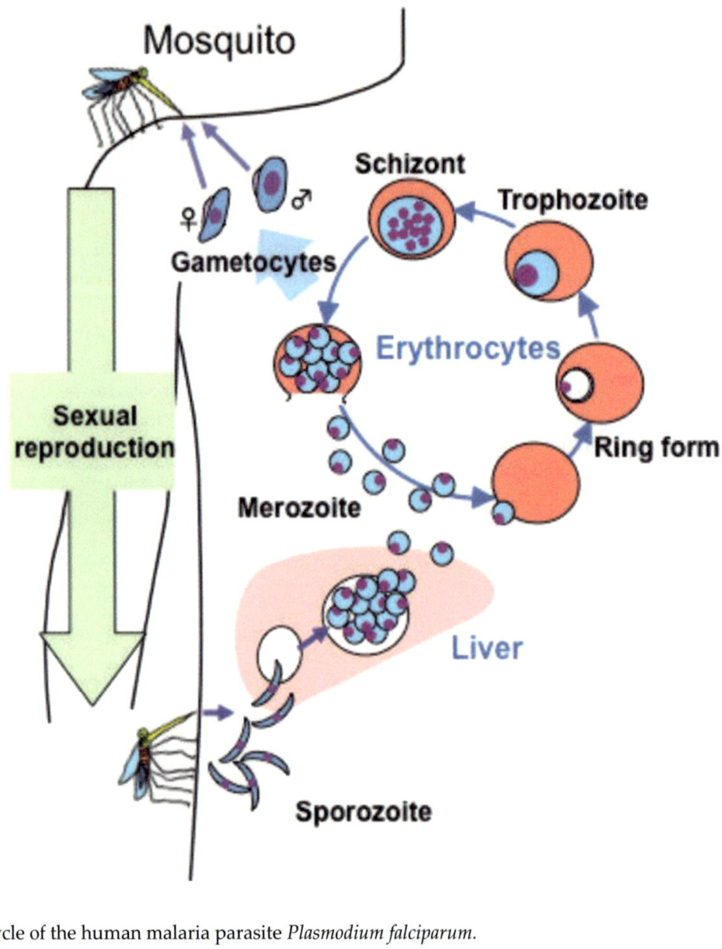


**Figure 1.** Life cycle of the human malaria parasite *Plasmodium falciparum.*

Mitochondria, an organelle arising from alpha-proteobacterium engulfed by a eukaryotic progenitor [6], play a key role in energy transduction of eukaryotic cells. In vertebrates, that can become a host for malaria parasites, mitochondria have been reported to contribute to cellular responses such as autophagy, apoptosis, and ATP production [7]. The vertebrate mitochondrion comprises two separate and functionally distinct outer and inner membranes that form cristae, and it also contains its own circular genome, the mitochondrial genome (mtDNA). With few exceptions, vertebrate mtDNA is approximately 16 kb in size, encoding

37 genes: two for ribosomal RNAs (rRNAs), 13 for proteins, and 22 for tRNAs [8]. In contrast to the vertebrate mitochondrion, the *Plasmodium* mitochondrion is a single tubular organelle structure [9] that possesses a 6-kb mtDNA, encoding only three genes for proteins and highly fragmented rRNA genes [10], and it is the smallest eukaryotic mtDNA. Furthermore, the erythrocytic stages of the parasite have been considered to mainly rely on glycolysis, with secretion of end products such as lactate and pyruvate [11, 12]. The mitochondria of malaria parasites are thus quite different from those of their vertebrate hosts. Because these differences markedly contribute to drug selectivity, we have focused on the *Plasmodium* mitochondrion to develop antimalarial drugs. Here we summarize recent advances in our knowledge of the mitochondria of malaria parasites and discuss future prospective antimalarial drugs targeting the parasite mitochondrion.

## 2. Biochemical functions of malaria parasite mitochondria

### 2.1. ATP production in canonical eukaryotes

Conventionally, a mitochondrion is the cell's powerhouse, in which energy stored in chemical bonds is turned into ATP via oxidative phosphorylation. ATP production can be divided into three pathways: glycolysis, mitochondrial tricarboxylic acid (TCA) cycle, and mitochondrial electron transport chain (mtETC). Glycolysis breaks down one molecule of glucose into two molecules of pyruvate, generating two molecules of ATP. Pyruvate then moves into the mitochondrion where it is converted to acetyl-CoA and carbon dioxide by pyruvate dehydrogenase complex (PDH). Subsequently, acetyl-CoA enters the TCA cycle. The mtETC involves the passage of electrons from TCA-cycle NADH or from succinate via mtETC complexes to oxygen, with concomitant translocation of protons into the mitochondrial intermembrane space. Generally, the mtETC comprises four integral membrane enzyme complexes in the mitochondrial inner membrane: NADH-ubiquinone oxidoreductase (complex I), succinate-ubiquinone oxidoreductase (SQR, complex II), ubiquinol-cytochrome *c* oxidoreductase (complex III or cytochrome $bc_1$), and cytochrome *c* oxidase (complex IV). Ubiquinone (Q) and cytochrome *c* (complex IV) function as electron carriers and the complexes I, III, and IV function as sites generating potential. The resultant potential across the mitochondrial inner membrane is used to drive ATP synthesis.

### 2.2. ATP production in malaria parasites

Similar to canonical eukaryotes, in the mosquito stages of malaria parasites, the organisms produce ATP in their mitochondria [13]. In the erythrocytic stages, however, the mitochondrial energy transduction system for oxidative phosphorylation is downregulated to adapt to host environments and produce ATP mainly via glycolysis using blood glucose [14, 15]. As a consequence, in malaria parasite-infected patients, plasma lactate levels tend to be high and highly variable, ranging from 2 to 26.7 mM [16, 17], compared with plasma lactate levels (0.3-1.3 mM) in normal individuals. Apart from the minor flux of carbon backbone derived from glucose, TCA metabolism of *Plasmodium* was believed to involve a branched architecture bifurcating from 2-oxoglutarate until recently [18]; however, this report was subsequently retracted [19]. More recently, the malaria parasites have been reported to use the canonical oxidative mitochondrial TCA cycle to catabolize host glucose and glutamate (Figure 2) [20], even during asexual multiplication. The TCA cycle begins with malate generated by anaplerotic reactions and 2-oxoglutarate produced from glutamine as well as conversion of acetyl-CoA to citrate by citrate synthase [20-22]. In general, pyruvate, the end product of glycolysis, is transported via the monocarboxylate transporter (MCT) family [23]. *Plasmodium* possesses two MCT genes (PF3D7_0210300 and PF3D7_0926400) identified in its genome (PlasmoDB version 11.0, website: http://plasmadb.org/plasma/). Although further evidence is required, these MCTs are considered to be associated with the transport of pyruvate across the mitochondrial membrane [24]. To convert pyruvate into acetyl-CoA, *Plasmodium* retains branched chain ketoacid dehydrogenase (BCKDH), the only enzyme implicated in branched chain amino acid degradation [22]. PDH complex, linking cytoplasmic glycolysis to the TCA cycle in canonical eukaryotes, is not localized to the mitochondrion but to a plastid, apicoplast, in *Plasmodium* [25]. The function of the *Plasmodium* PDH complex seems to include the provision of acetyl-CoA for *de novo* fatty acid synthesis within the apicoplast.

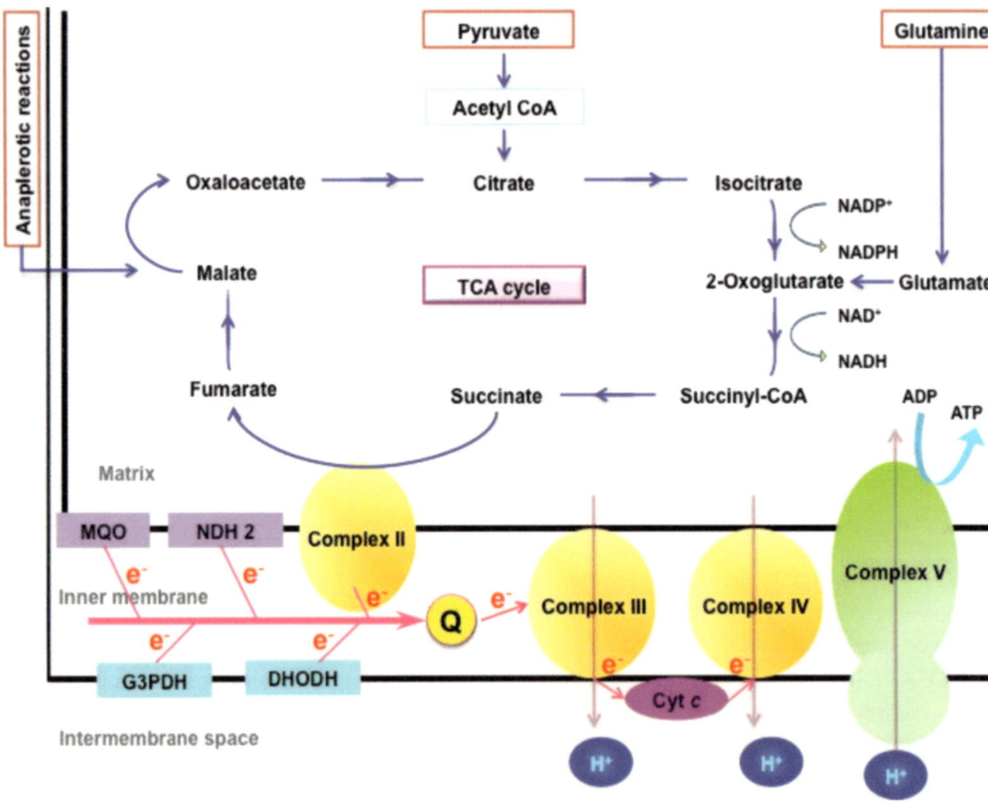


**Figure 2.** TCA cycle and oxidative phosphorylation of malaria parasites. The TCA cycle of malaria parasites begins with malate, 2-oxoglutarate, and citrate [20-22].

In the *Plasmodium* TCA cycle, succinate and malate are oxidized by SQR and malate-ubiquinone oxidoreductase (MQO), respectively, with transporting electrons to the matrix [26] (Figure 2). Similar to SQR of most eukaryotes, the *Plasmodium* SQR comprises four polypeptides: a flavoprotein (Fp) subunit, iron-sulfur (Ip) subunit [27], and two cytochrome *b* (cyt*b*) subunits (CybL and CybS) [28]. Fp and Ip form the catalytic portion of the complex. This portion acts as a succinate dehydrogenase (SDH), catalyzing the oxidation of succinate by water-soluble electron acceptors such as phenazine methosulfate in SQR, and is bound to the matrix side of the mitochondrial inner membrane via the membrane-anchoring proteins CybL and CybS. Because the mitochondria of erythrocytic stage parasites show both SQR and SDH activities [27, 29, 30], complex II has been considered to have some role in parasite survival. These activities, however, are very low, compared with those of the other eukaryotes (Table 1) [31-35]. Furthermore, our previous studies have demonstrated that disruption of the Fp subunit genes *pfsdha* and *Pbsdha* does not affect growth in the erythrocytic stages *in vitro* [36] and *in vivo* [37], respectively. These findings reveal that complex II is not essential for survival of the erythrocytic stage parasites, and this appears to be associated with relatively low activities of SQR and SDH in these developmental stages.

| Organism | SQR specific activities* (nmol/min/mg) |
|---|---|
| *Plasmodium falciparum* | 1.75 |
| *Trypanosoma cruzi* | 85 |
| *Ascaris suum* | 136 |
| Rat liver | 298 |
| Bovine heart | 111 |
| Human cell | 79.7 |

*Activity values of *P. falciparum*, *T. cruzi*, *A. suum*, rat liver, bovine heart, and human cell are obtained from references [29, 31, 32, 33, 34], and [35], respectively.

**Table 1.** Specific activities of succinate-ubiquinone oxidoreductase of various organisms

MQO is an FAD-dependent membrane-associated protein that catalyzes the oxidation of malate to oxaloacetate [38]. The electrons are donated to quinones of the mtETC, and NAD is accepted as an electron donor. The MQO has been not observed in mammals but has been found in *Plasmodium* [39] and some bacteria [40]. This implies that the *Plasmodium* MQO could be a target for drug design. In addition to SQR and MQO in the TCA cycle, *Plasmodium* possesses three oxidoreductases in its mitochondrial inner membrane: type II NADH:ubiquinone oxidoreductase (NDH2) [41], dihydroorotate dehydrogenase (DHODH) [42, 43], and glyceraldehyde-3-phosphate dehydrogenase (G3PDH) [44, 45], all of which can reduce ubiquinone (Figure 2). Unlike the large multisubunit complex I in most mitochondria, the *Plasmodium* NDH2 is a single subunit enzyme, not involved in the direct pumping of protons across the membrane [46]. The absence of NDH2 in mammalian mitochondria shows that this enzyme would be a promising target of a novel antimalarial drug. Some antimalarial activities of NDH2 inhibitors, such as HQNO [47] and 1-hydroxy-2-dodecyl-4(1H) quinolone [48], have been reported. However, a recent *in vivo* study on *Plasmodium berghei* revealed that the *Plasmodium* NDH2 could be deleted by targeted gene disruption, indicating that it is dispensable in the erythrocytic stages [49]. This disproves that NDH2 is a candidate drug target. Thus, the potential of targeting NDH2 as an antimalarial drug remains controversial.

The other dehydrogenases (DHODH and G3PDH) transfer electrons from reduced compounds in the cytosol (Figure 2). In the erythrocytic stages of the parasite, DHODH plays two roles—a generator of reduced ubiquinone and the fourth enzyme in the pyrimidine biosynthetic pathway. Since *Plasmodium* cannot salvage pyrimidine [50], DHODH is essential for its survival [42]. Therefore, in the erythrocytic stages, the mtETC appears to be essential for the pyrimidine biosynthetic pathway rather than for contributing to the ATP pool [11].

As presented above, in *Plasmodium* mitochondria, five mitochondrial dehydrogenases (SQR, MQO, NDH2, DHODH, and G3PDH) can generate reduced ubiquinone, which in turn is reoxidized by cytochrome $bc_1$ complex (complex III). Complex III is inhibited by atovaquone [51], which collapses the mitochondrial membrane potential [52]. As an antimalarial, atovaquone is very effective; however, atovaquone-resistant parasites develop easily. Mechanisms of atovaquone resistance are described in Section 4. Similar to canonical eukaryotes, *Plasmodium* utilizes cytochrome *c* (cytc) as electron carriers and complexes III and IV as sites generating potential. The resultant potential across the mitochondrial inner membrane is used to drive ATP synthesis. *Plasmodium* ATP synthase is markedly different from that of its host [53] —it is assembled as a large dimeric complex in the erythrocytic stages. In the ciliates *Tetrahymena thermophila* and *Paramecium*, the structure and arrangement of dimeric ATP synthase have been suggested to determine the tubular morphology of the mitochondrial cristae [54, 55]. This could explain how the tubular cristae found in the mitochondria of erythrocytic stages are generated.

### 2.3. Mitochondrial energy metabolism: a target of antimalarial drugs

Recently, in addition to the genetic disruptions of SDH and NDH2 described above, it has been reported that six TCA cycle enzymes can be genetically disrupted in the erythrocytic stage or sexual development stage [45]. These reports suggest that the TCA cycle would not be essential for survival in these developmental stages. Hence, to develop an antimalarial drug, promising mitochondrial targets would be DHODH, which is associated with the pyrimidine biosynthesis pathway and mtETC, and the mitochondrial complexes III, IV, and V that generate electron gradients on the mitochondrial inner membrane.

On the other hand, it has been recently demonstrated that parasites derived directly from infected patients show three distinct gene expression states. One of these states demonstrates that the expression levels of the TCA cycle- or mtETC-related genes are increased [56]. Furthermore, mice infected with *P. berghei* or *Plasmodium yoelii* perform active oxidative phosphorylation [57], suggesting that, in some physiological conditions, malaria parasites may produce ATP via the mitochondrial TCA cycle and mtETC. Thus, we cannot exclude the possibility that all the mitochondrial enzymes are potential targets for antimalarial drugs.

## 3. The mitochondrial genome of malaria parasites

Malaria parasites possess a mitochondrial genome in the form of circular and/or tandemly repeated linear elements of 6 kb, the smallest in size among eukaryotic cells [58]. Copy numbers for this element are approximately 20-fold and 150-fold of the nuclear genomes in the human malaria parasite *Plasmodium falciparum* [58] and the rodent malaria parasite *P. yoelii* [59], respectively. These differences in the copy number may reflect differences in oxidative phosphorylation activities as noted previously (see Section 2.3). The 6-kb element contains only three mitochondrial protein-coding genes in addition to the large subunit (LSU) and small subunit (SSU) rRNA genes [60, 61, 62] (Figure 3). The three protein-coding genes are cyt*c* oxidase subunit 1 (*cox1*) and subunit 3 (*cox3*), members of the cyt*c* oxidase complex (complex IV), and cyt*b* (*cob*), a member of cytochrome $bc_1$ complex. In all eukaryotic cells possessing mitochondria, *cox1* and *cob* are encoded by the mitochondrial genome. Because the organisms possessing mitochondrion-like organelles without its own DNA (e.g., hydrogenosome and mitosome) do not have *cox1* and *cob*, these two genes appear to be essential for maintenance of the mtETC.

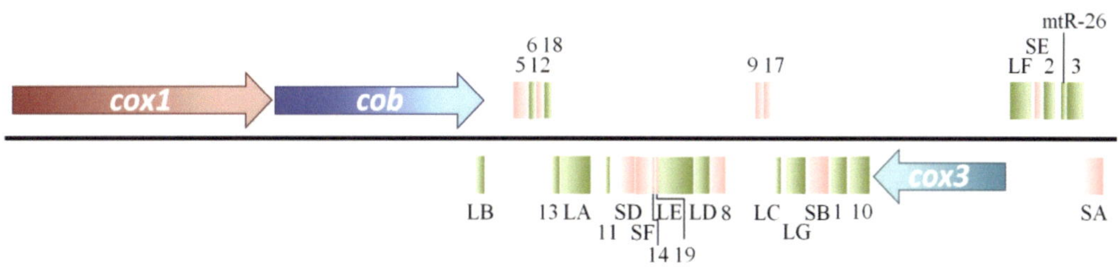


**Figure 3.** Mitochondrial (mt) genome structure of malaria parasites. Mt-genome organization is perfectly conserved among 23 *Plasmodium* species [63]. Elements within the mt genome of *Plasmodium* are tandemly repeated, so the designation of both termini is arbitrary. Light green and light magenta boxes indicate fragments of LSU and SSU rRNA genes, respectively.

The two rRNA genes of the *Plasmodium* mitochondrial genome are highly fragmented [63], and the fragmentation is the most extreme example of any described rRNA fragmentation. Recently, transcription of almost all intergenic regions of the *Plasmodium* mitochondrial genome has been demonstrated [63]. The results show that 27 small rRNA fragments (12 SSU rRNAs and 15 LSU rRNAs), ranging from 23 to 190 nt, are present in its mitochondrial genome (Figure 4). All the rRNAs are predicted to pair with at least one of the other rRNA, creating interactions that would help maintain the appropriate location and orientation of each rRNA. Notably, among the *Plasmodium* genera, the nucleotide sequences of noncoding regions, as well as fragmented rRNA gene regions, are more conserved when compared with those of the protein-coding gene regions [10]. It thus appears that these highly conserved sequence regions code for functional RNAs, including additional fragmented rRNAs.

In addition to the highly fragmented rRNAs, the mitochondria of malaria parasites have a unique property—transfer RNA (tRNA) is absent; therefore, protein translation in the

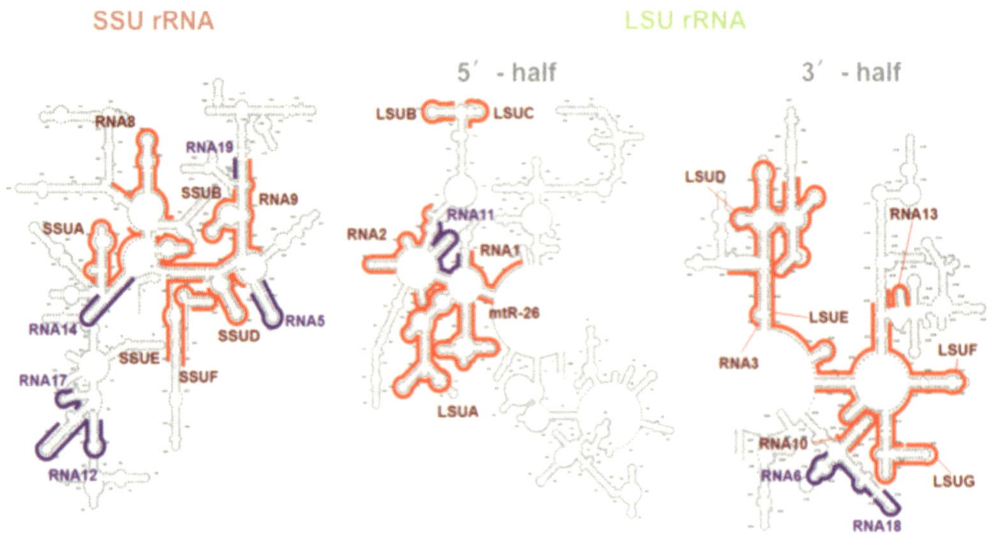


**Figure 4.** Fragmentation of the mitochondrial LSU and SSU rRNA genes of *Plasmodium falciparum*. Red line indicates rRNA regions. Purple lines indicate recently identified additional fragmented rRNA candidates[63].

mitochondrion was to date considered as being impossible. However, recently, extramitochondrial phenylalanyl-tRNA synthesis has been found in mitochondria of the erythrocytic stages, suggesting that the parasite mitochondrion can import tRNAs from the cytoplasmic tRNA pool [64]. These findings referring to the parasite rRNAs and tRNAs would make the parasite mitochondrial protein translation a desirable organelle to target as an antimalarial drug.

In malaria parasites, mtDNA is replicated via rolling circle replication to generate the linear concatemers, similar to the replication mechanism used by some bacteriophages and plasmids [58]. This replication manner is remarkably different from that of the vertebrate mtDNA, which is replicated by a theta mechanism. Furthermore, mitochondrial DNA polymerase, which has been characterized as a γ-like DNA polymerase, is strongly resistant to 2,3-dideoxythymidine-5-triphosphate and, in this aspect, differs from its vertebrate homolog [65], suggesting structural differences between the *Plasmodium* and vertebrate DNA polymerase. Further research on translation and replication mechanisms of the parasite mtDNA may help identify potential targets for drug candidates.

# 4. Atovaquone resistance in malaria parasites

## 4.1. Predicted mode of action for atovaquone

Atovaquone (a hydroxy-1,4-naphthoquinone derivative) is a broad-spectrum antiparasitic agent active against malaria, *Pneumocystis carinii* pneumonia, toxoplasmosis, and babesiosis [66]. The mode of action for atovaquone involves selective inhibition of parasite mtETC without affecting the host mitochondrial functions at effective doses, making it the first member of an entirely new class of antimalarial agents [52]. This drug shares structural similarity with ubiquinone, a coenzyme involved in mtETC and serves as a point of contact between energy metabolism and pyrimidine metabolism. Therefore, a potential molecular target of atovaquone can be the ubiquinol oxidation pocket, Qo site, of the cytochrome $bc_1$ complex [51, 67] because it may have a specific inhibitory effect on the parasite cytochrome $bc_1$ complex. Generally, the cytochrome $bc_1$ complex is a structural and functional homodimer. The catalytic core comprises three redox active subunits, cyt *b* with two *b*-type hemes, cytochrome $c_1$ (cyt$c_1$) with a *c*-type heme, and Rieske protein with a [2Fe-2S] cluster [68]. Cyt*b* catalyzes the transfer of electron from ubiquinol to cyt$c_1$, coupled to the transmembrane proton translocation across the mitochondrial membrane [69]. There are two distinct catalytic sites on the cyt*b* protein, which are involved in the proton motive Q cycle and are proposed to account for the electron transfer and proton translocating activity through the cytochrome $bc_1$ complex: center o (also designated as Qo or center P) on the cytoplasmic site of the mitochondrial inner membrane, where ubiquinol ($QH_2$) oxidation occurs, and center i (Qi or center N) on the matrix site, where ubiquinone (Q) reduction occurs. Because of its structural similarity with ubiquinone, atovaquone appears to inhibit the cytochrome $bc_1$ complex by competitive binding with coenzyme Q for one of these sites.

### 4.2. Emergence of atovaquone-resistant malaria parasites

Atovaquone is majorly used for treatment and chemoprophylaxis of falciparum malaria for international travelers [70], but the major problem is rapidity of emergence of drug resistance when it is used as a single agent. Thus far, proguanil, which inhibits the parasite dihydrofolate reductase, is combined with atovaquone to prevent the emergence. The combination drug, registered as Malarone® (GlaxoSmithKline group of companies), is approved for treating malaria in more than 30 countries and is used for chemoprophylaxis for international travelers. However, atovaquone-resistant parasites isolated from malaria patients have also been highly reported [71-73]. These studies demonstrate that atovaquone resistance is associated with point mutations of the amino acid residue at codon 268 of cyt*b* (*Pfcob*) constructing the cytochrome $bc_1$ complex. The mutations Y268S, Y268N, and Y268C have been found in atovaquone-resistant parasites.

To mimic the situation of emergence of atovaquone-resistant parasites in a clinical setting, we chose a mouse malaria model using BALB/c mice and the *P. berghei* ANKA strain. In the first trial, we administered atovaquone intraperitoneally on seven consecutive days at doses ranging from 0.4 μg/kg/day to 4.8 mg/kg/day and obtained *P. berghei* isolates with four genetic resistance variations in cyt*b* [74] (Table 2). We did not observe the mutation of the amino acid residue at codon 268, which is observed in *P. falciparum*. The two mutations, M133I and L144S, are located in $Qo_1$, and these code amino acids are critical for inhibitor resistance in yeast and mice [75, 76]. Moreover, in *Plasmodium*, the M133I and L144S amino acid changes appear to be structurally significant, altering the conformational structure of the ubiquinone-binding site and thus lowering the affinity of atovaquone to the $Qo_1$ site. The mutation V284F is located in the sixth transmembrane domain adjacent to the $Qo_2$ site, and the amino acid change by itself confers only an approximately 10-fold resistance to atovaquone. Notably, the mutation V284F has been found in all atovaquone-resistant clones [74].

| Isolate | Mutation | Reference |
|---|---|---|
| PbSK2A1Tb | M133I, L271V | [74] |
| PbSK2A1T | M133I, V284F | [74] |
| PbSK1A2 | V284F | [74] |
| PbSR-1 | L144S, V284F | [74] |
| PbLSJ1.1 | Y268N | [77] |
| PbLSJ2.1 | Y268C | [77] |
| PbLSJ3.1 | L271V, K272R | [77] |

**Table 2.** Mutations in the cytochrome *b* of *Plasmodium berghei* with atovaquone resistance

To obtain a better model for the biochemical and genetic studies of mutations found in *P. falciparum*, we performed further experiments to obtain *P. berghei* strains, resistant to atovaquone, with mutations in the $Qo_2$ region conferring high degrees of resistance [77]. The parasite-infected mice were treated intraperitoneally for 3 consecutive days at a dose of 14.4 mg/kg/day, a higher dose than in the previous experiment. The results showed three variations of the atovaquone-resistant mutation, including mutations at codon 268 (Y268N, Y268C, and L271/K272R; Table 2). All the mutations were located in the $Qo_2$ region, and these resistance levels were more than 500 times higher than those of the wild type, although the resistance levels of the previous isolates were more than 50 times higher. Administered doses of atovaquone affected the site of mutation in cyt*b* and the level of drug resistance.

As described above, our group has reported various mutations in the quinone-binding sites of the cyt*b* gene of *P. berghei*, such as M133I, L144S, L271V, K272R, Y268C, Y268S, Y268N, and V284F, using the mouse model with continuous atovaquone pressure. However, no direct evidence of a relationship between the mutations and resistance has been observed using intact mitochondria isolated from the malarial parasite, although biochemical analysis of the mutant has been reported using cell-free extract [78]. To address this point, we have further investigated the activity of dihydroorotate-cyt*c* reductase (regarding this mitochondrial pathway, see Section 2) in both atovaquone-resistant and atovaquone-sensitive *P. berghei* isolates [79]. The results showed that mutations in the quinone-binding site of the cyt*b* gene resulted in variable sensitivity to atovaquone and provided direct evidence for the atovaquone inhibitory mechanism in the parasite cytochrome $bc_1$ complex.

### 4.3. Cytochrome $bc_1$ complex as an antimalarial drug target

Recently, the X-ray crystallographic structure of the mitochondrial cytochrome $bc_1$ complex from *Saccharomyces cerevisiae* with atovaquone has been resolved, and it demonstrates atovaquone bound in the Qo site [80]. It can therefore explain the molecular basis for the broad spectrum of the antimalarial drug as well as for the species-specific differences in its effects. This would allow us to develop a drug targeting cytochrome $bc_1$ that would control the emergence of resistant parasites. Furthermore, the other group has reported cocrystallization

http://dx.doi.org/10.5772/61283

of a bovine cytochrome $bc_1$ complex with the 4(1H)-pyridone class of inhibitors [81], which are potent antimalarial agents *in vivo* [82, 83]. The X-ray structure demonstrates that these inhibitors do not bind at the Qo site but rather at the Qi site. Differences in the inhibitor-binding site to cytochrome $bc_1$ complex would aid the rational drug designing for reducing the emergence of inhibitor-resistant parasites and increasing selectivity against malaria parasites toward novel treatments. In the future, in addition to binding site analysis using modalities such as X-ray crystallography, we need to elucidate the molecular mechanisms explaining how atovaquone resistance mutation is generated in the parasite mt genome.

## 5. 5-Aminolevulinic Acid (ALA): A new antimalarial candidate targeting the mitochondrion

ALA is a precursor used in the biosynthesis of tetrapyrroles such as chlorophyll and heme. The heme is an iron-containing complex macrocycle that plays a fundamental role in several cellular processes, including oxygen transport and storage, mitochondrial respiratory chain, and detoxification [84]. Generally, in mammalian cells, heme biosynthesis begins with ALA formation by ALA synthase in the mitochondria from glycine and succinyl-CoA [85]. The next four steps and three final steps occur in the cytosol and mitochondria, respectively. In cancer cells, the uptake of a high concentration of ALA results in elevated levels of its metabolites, particularly protoporphyrin IX (PPIX), due to insufficient activity of ferrochelatase [86]. The PPIX accumulates in the mitochondria and consequently acts as a photosensitizer releasing singlet oxygen and other reactive oxygen species (ROS), resulting in induction of cell death in cancer. ALA therefore has been applied to the development of photodynamic diagnosis and photodynamic therapy (PDT) of various cancers [87, 88].

Recently, all the enzymes of *de novo* heme-biosynthetic pathway have been characterized in the human malaria parasite, *P. falciparum* [89-91]. In contrast to the mammalian enzymes of heme biosynthesis, the parasite enzymes have unique localizations (Figure 5). The first enzyme, ALA synthase, and the final two enzymes, protoporphyrinogen IX oxidase and ferrochelatase (FC), localize to the mitochondrion. The enzymes that catalyze the intermediate three steps—ALA dehydratase, porphobilinogen deaminase, and uroporphyrinogen decarboxylase (UROD)—localize to the apicoplast, a nonphotosynthetic plastid. The next enzyme, coproporphyrinogen III oxidase, is cytosolic. In addition, the catalytic efficiency of these enzymes of the erythrocytic stages differs from that of mammalian enzymes: the enzymes localizing to the apicoplast have very low catalytic efficacy [92]. Altogether, the properties of the heme-biosynthetic pathway are remarkably different between malaria parasites and their hosts. Hence, the heme-biosynthetic pathway has been recognized as a novel chemotherapeutic target in *Plasmodium*. Smith and Kain attempted PDT for human malaria parasites by adding ALA to an *in vitro* culture [93]. The growth of *Plasmodium* was completely inhibited by 0.2 mM ALA, followed by exposure to white light or by a higher concentration (2 mM) of ALA alone without light exposure. This use of PDT is, unfortunately, clinically unrealistic because white light cannot illuminate the inside of a malaria-infected patient's body and the concentration of 2 mM is extremely high to apply clinically.

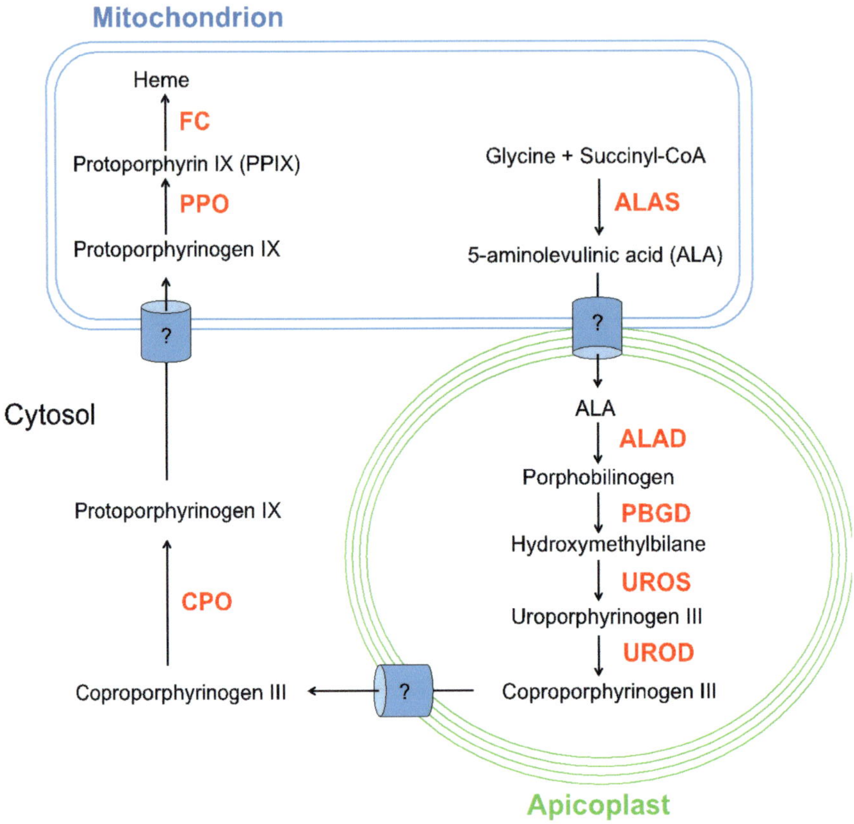


**Figure 5.** Heme biosynthesis of malaria parasites. The enzymes in the pathway are localized in the mitochondrion, apicoplast, and cytosol [89-91].

Our recent study resolved this issue: in the presence of ferrous ion, ALA efficiently inhibited the *in vitro* growth of *Plasmodium* even without light exposure [94]. Because there was a previous report on protection from malaria by elevated zinc protoporphyrin, which binds to heme crystals to inhibit further crystallization to form hemozoin [95], we first investigated effects of metal ions on growth inhibition by ALA using an *in vitro* culture system of *P. falciparum*. Our results showed that treatment with 10 μM sodium ferrous citrate (SFC) and 0.2 mM ALA increased the growth inhibition to more than 50% when compared with that of 0.2 mM ALA alone. Notably, no other metal ions (e.g., zinc, lead, and copper) had such a synergistic effect, indicating that only ferrous compounds are synergistic with ALA.

Next, to determine heme intermediate, we analyzed the cell extract of the parasite using HPLC. The extract contained three major intermediates: coproporphyrin I, coproporphyrin III (CPIII), and PPIX. Unlike in cancer cells, CPIII was majorly accumulated in the apicoplast. Although its contribution to the parasite growth inhibition remains unknown, we believe that these differences are due to the complicated heme-biosynthetic pathway (Figure 5) and life cycle of *Plasmodium* (Figure 1). Moreover, PPIX, as is the case with cancer cells, accumulated mainly in the mitochondrion. In PDT of cancer cells, PPIX acts as a photosensitizer releasing ROS, resulting in extensive cellular damage and cell death [96]. This suggests that PPIX accumulated in the parasite mitochondria is a factor contributing to the inhibition of parasite growth. Thus, the parasite heme-biosynthetic pathway in the mitochondrion and apicoplast may be a potential target of an antimalarial drug.

Recently, to confirm the efficacy of the combination of ALA and SFC (ALA/SFC) in treating malaria using an animal model, we performed a preclinical drug evaluation of orally administered ALA/SFC for the treatment of mice infected with the malaria parasite. ALA/SFC cured 50% of the Py17XL-infected mice, and the cured mice showed long-lasting humoral immune responses to the same parasite strain and protection from homologous malarial infections [97]. ALA can be safe compound because a phase I clinical study has been successfully completed. Considering the safety and mild antimalarial activities of ALA/SFC, a combination with an available antimalarial drug, such as artemisinin or chloroquine, would be applicable for the treatment of malaria.

## 6. Concluding remarks

The energy metabolism of malaria parasites has been considerably elucidated with accumulating data from several "omics" analyses. These data suggest that enzymes of the mitochondrial TCA cycle and mtETC could be attractive targets for development of antimalarial drugs. However, activity of these energy transduction pathways in the mitochondrion is considered to be very low in the erythrocytic stages of the parasite. To address these possibilities, biochemical assay data are required. However, rigorous biochemical analysis of the parasite mitochondrion, in which the TCA cycle and mtETC are present, is highly difficult because intact and pure mitochondria cannot be obtained from the parasites thus far. As a consequence, the malaria parasite mitochondrion needs to be purified to perform these future biochemical studies. Biochemical data regarding the *Plasmodium* mitochondrion would shed light on the details of mitochondrial enzyme behavior and help in the management of malaria.

## Acknowledgements

We would like to thank Y. Koyama for the helpful discussion.This work was supported by a Grant-in-aid for Scientific Research (no. 26253025) from the Japanese Society for the Promotion of Science. We also acknowledge the support of the Science and Technology Research Promotion Program for Agriculture, Forestry, Fisheries and Food Industry and JST/ JICA, SATREPS (Science and Technology Research Partnership for Sustainable Development) (no. 10000284).

## Author details

Kenji Hikosaka[1,2], Keisuke Komatsuya[3], Shigeo Suzuki[3,4] and Kiyoshi Kita[3,5*]

*Address all correspondence to: kitak@m.u-tokyo.ac.jp

1 Department of Infection and Host Defense, Graduate School of Medicine, Chiba University, Chiba, Japan

2 Department of Microbiology and Immunology, Teikyo University School of Medicine, Tokyo, Japan

3 Department of Biomedical Chemistry, Graduate School of Medicine, The University of Tokyo, Tokyo, Japan

4 SBI Pharmaceuticals Co, LTD, Izumi Garden Tower 20F, 1-6-1, Roppongi, Minato-ku, Tokyo, Japan

5 Nagasaki University, School of Tropical Medicine and Global Health, Nagasaki, Japan

## References

[1] World Health Organization (WHO). World Malaria Report 2014. Available at: http://wwwwhoint/malaria/publications/world_malaria_report_2014/en/. 2014 (Accessed January 2015).

[2] Dondorp AM, Nosten F, Yi P, Das D, Phyo AP, Tarning J, Lwin KM, Ariey F, Hanpithakpong W, Lee SJ. et al. Artemisinin resistance in *Plasmodium falciparum* malaria. New England Journal of Medicine. 2009;361(5):455-67.

[3] Cowman AF, Crabb BS. Invasion of red blood cells by malaria parasites. Cell. 2006;124(4):755-66.

[4] Dixon MW, Thompson J, Gardiner DL, Trenholme KR. Sex in *Plasmodium*: a sign of commitment. Trends in Parasitology. 2008;24(4):168-75.

[5] Seeber F, Limenitakis J, Soldati-Favre D. Apicomplexan mitochondrial metabolism: a story of gains, losses and retentions. Trends in Parasitology. 2008;24(10):468-78.

[6] Lane N, Martin W. The energetics of genome complexity. Nature. 2010;467(7318): 929-34.

[7] Nunnari J, and Suomalainen A. Mitochondria: in sickness and in health. Cell. 2012;148(6):1145-59.

[8] Boore JL. Animal mitochondrial genomes. Nucleic Acids Research. 1999;27(8): 1767-80.

[9] Das A, Syin C, Fujioka H, Zheng H, Goldman N, Aikawa M, Kumar N. Molecular characterization and ultrastructural localization of *Plasmodium falciparum* Hsp 60. Molecular and Biochemical Parasitology. 1997;88(1-2):95-104.

[10] Hikosaka K, Watanabe Y, Kobayashi F, Waki S, Kita K, Tanabe K. Highly conserved gene arrangement of the mitochondrial genomes of 23 *Plasmodium* species. Parasitology International. 2011;60(2):175-80.

[11] Painter HJ, Morrisey JM, Mather MW, Vaidya AB. Specific role of mitochondrial electron transport in blood-stage *Plasmodium falciparum*. Nature. 2007;446(7131):88-91.

[12] Jensen MD, Conley M, Helstowski LD. Culture of *Plasmodium falciparum*: the role of pH, glucose, and lactate. Journal of Parasitology. 1983;69(6):1060-7.

[13] Hall N, Karras M, Raine JD, Carlton JM, Kooij TW, Berriman M, Florens L, Janssen CS, Pain A, Christophides GK, et al. A comprehensive survey of the *Plasmodium* life cycle by genomic, transcriptomic, and proteomic analyses. Science. 2005;307(5706): 82-6.

[14] Fry M, Beesley JE. Mitochondria of mammalian *Plasmodium* spp. Parasitology. 1991;102(Pt 1):17-26.

[15] van Dooren GG, Stimmler LM, McFadden GI. Metabolic maps and functions of the *Plasmodium* mitochondrion. FEMS Microbiology Reviews. 2006;30(4):596-630.

[16] Agbenyega T, Angus BJ, Bedu-Addo G, Baffoe-Bonnie B, Guyton T, Stacpoole PW, and Krishna S. Glucose and lactate kinetics in children with severe malaria. Journal of Clinical Endocrinology and Metabolism. 2000;85(4):1569-76.

[17] Krishna S, Waller DW, ter Kuile F, Kwiatkowski D, Crawley J, Craddock CF, Nosten F, Chapman D, Brewster D, Holloway PA, et al. Lactic acidosis and hypoglycaemia in children with severe malaria: pathophysiological and prognostic significance. Transactions of the Royal Society of Tropical Medicine and Hygiene. 1994;88(1): 67-73.

[18] Olszewski KL, Mather MW, Morrisey JM, Garcia BA, Vaidya AB, Rabinowitz JD, Llinas M. Branched tricarboxylic acid metabolism in *Plasmodium falciparum*. Nature. 2010;466(7307):774-8.

[19] Olszewski KL, Mather MW, Morrisey JM, Garcia BA, Vaidya AB, Rabinowitz JD, Llinas M. Retraction: Branched tricarboxylic acid metabolism in *Plasmodium falciparum*. Nature. 2013;497(7451):652.

[20] MacRae JI, Dixon MW, Dearnley MK, Chua HH, Chambers JM, Kenny S, Bottova I, Tilley L, McConville MJ. Mitochondrial metabolism of sexual and asexual blood stages of the malaria parasite *Plasmodium falciparum*. BMC Biology. 2013;11:67.

[21] Cobbold SA, Vaughan AM, Lewis IA, Painter HJ, Camargo N, Perlman DH, Fishbaugher M, Healer J, Cowman AF, Kappe SH, et al. Kinetic flux profiling elucidates two independent acetyl-CoA biosynthetic pathways in *Plasmodium falciparum*. Journal of Biological Chemistry. 2013;288(51):36338-50.

[22] Oppenheim RD, Creek DJ, Macrae JI, Modrzynska KK, Pino P, Limenitakis J, Polonais V, Seeber F, Barrett MP, Billker O, et al. BCKDH: the missing link in apicomplexan mitochondrial metabolism is required for full virulence of *Toxoplasma gondii* and *Plasmodium berghei*. PLoS Pathogens. 2014;10(7):e1004263.

[23] Halestrap AP. The monocarboxylate transporter family—structure and functional characterization. IUBMB Life. 2012;64(1):1-9.

[24] Hikosaka K, Hirai M, Komatsuya K, Ono Y, Kita K. Lactate retards the development of erythrocytic stages of the human malaria parasite *Plasmodium falciparum*. Parasitology International. 2015;64(3):301-3.

[25] Foth BJ, Stimmler LM, Handman E, Crabb BS, Hodder AN, McFadden GI. The malaria parasite Plasmodium falciparum has only one pyruvate dehydrogenase complex, which is located in the apicoplast. Molecular Microbiology. 2005;55(1):39-53.

[26] Mogi T, Kita K. Diversity in mitochondrial metabolic pathways in parasitic protists *Plasmodium* and *Cryptosporidium*. Parasitology International. 2010;59(3):305-12.

[27] Takeo S, Kokaze A, Ng CS, Mizuchi D, Watanabe JI, Tanabe K, Kojima S, Kita K. Succinate dehydrogenase in *Plasmodium falciparum* mitochondria: molecular characterization of the SDHA and SDHB genes for the catalytic subunits, the flavoprotein (Fp) and iron-sulfur (Ip) subunits. Molecular and Biochemical Parasitology. 2000;107(2): 191-205.

[28] Kawahara K, Mogi T, Tanaka TQ, Hata M, Miyoshi H, Kita K. Mitochondrial dehydrogenases in the aerobic respiratory chain of the rodent malaria parasite *Plasmodium yoelii yoelii*. Journal of Biochemistry. 2009;145(2):229-37.

[29] Takashima E, Takamiya S, Takeo S, Mi-ichi F, Amino H, Kita K. Isolation of mitochondria from *Plasmodium falciparum* showing dihydroorotate dependent respiration. Parasitology International. 2001;50(4):273-8.

[30] Suraveratum N, Krungkrai SR, Leangaramgul P, Prapunwattana P, Krungkrai J. Purification and characterization of *Plasmodium falciparum* succinate dehydrogenase. Molecular and Biochemical Parasitology. 2000;105(2):215-22.

[31] Morales J, Mogi T, Mineki S, Takashima E, Mineki R, Hirawake H, Sakamoto K, Omura S, Kita K. Novel mitochondrial complex II isolated from *Trypanosoma cruzi* is composed of 12 peptides including a heterodimeric Ip subunit. Journal of Biological Chemistry. 2009;284:7255-63.

[32] Kita K, Takamiya S, Furushima R, Ma YC, Suzuki H, Ozawa T, Oya H. Electron-transfer complexes of *Ascaris suum* muscle mitochondria. III. Composition and fumarate reductase activity of complex II. Biochimical et Biophysica Acta. 1988;935:130-40.

[33] Mi-Ichi F, Miyadera H, Kobayashi T, Takamiya S, Waki S, Iwata S, Shibata S, Kita K. Parasite mitochondria as a target of chemotherapy: inhibitory effect of licochalcone A on the *Plasmodium falciparum* respiratory chain. Annals of the New York Academy of Science. 2005;1056:46-54.

[34] Miyadera H, Shiomi K, Ui H, Yamaguchi Y, Masuma R, Tomoda H, Miyoshi H, Osanai A, Kita K, Omura S. Atpenins, potent and specific inhibitors of mitochondrial complex II (succinate-ubiquinone oxidoreductase). Proceedings of the National Academy of Sciences of the United States of America. 2003;100:473-7.

[35] Sakai C, Tomitsuka E, Miyagishi M, Harada S, Kita K. Type II Fp of human mitochondrial respiratory complex II and its role in adaptation to hypoxia and nutrition-deprived conditions. Mitochondrion. 2013;13:602-9.

[36] Tanaka TQ, Hirai M, Watanabe Y, Kita K. Toward understanding the role of mitochondrial complex II in the intraerythrocytic stages of *Plasmodium falciparum*: gene targeting of the Fp subunit. Parasitology International. 2012;61(4):726-8.

[37] Hino A, Hirai M, Tanaka TQ, Watanabe Y, Matsuoka H, Kita K. Critical roles of the mitochondrial complex II in oocyst formation of rodent malaria parasite *Plasmodium berghei*. Journal of Biochemistry. 2012;152(3):259-68.

[38] Molenaar D, van der Rest ME, Petrovic S. Biochemical and genetic characterization of the membrane-associated malate dehydrogenase (acceptor) from *Corynebacterium glutamicum*. European Journal of Biochemistry/FEBS. 1998;254(2):395-403.

[39] Uyemura SA, Luo S, Vieira M, Moreno SN, Docampo R. Oxidative phosphorylation and rotenone-insensitive malate- and NADH-quinone oxidoreductases in *Plasmodium yoelii yoelii* mitochondria in situ. Journal of Biological Chemistry. 2004;279(1): 385-93.

[40] van der Rest ME, Frank C, Molenaar D. Functions of the membrane-associated and cytoplasmic malate dehydrogenases in the citric acid cycle of *Escherichia coli*. Journal of Bacteriology. 2000;182(24):6892-9.

[41] Fisher N, Bray PG, Ward SA, Biagini GA. The malaria parasite type II NADH:quinone oxidoreductase: an alternative enzyme for an alternative lifestyle. Trends in Parasitology. 2007;23(7):305-10.

[42] Krungkrai J. Purification, characterization and localization of mitochondrial dihydroorotate dehydrogenase in *Plasmodium falciparum*, human malaria parasite. Biochimica et Biophysica Acta. 1995;1243(3):351-60.

[43] LeBlanc SB, Wilson CM. The dihydroorotate dehydrogenase gene homologue of *Plasmodium falciparum*. Molecular and Biochemical Parasitology. 1993;60(2):349-51.

[44] Danne JC, Gornik SG, Macrae JI, McConville MJ, and Waller RF. Alveolate mitochondrial metabolic evolution: dinoflagellates force reassessment of the role of parasitism as a driver of change in apicomplexans. Molecular Biology and Evolution. 2013;30(1): 123-39.

[45] Sheiner L, Vaidya AB, McFadden GI. The metabolic roles of the endosymbiotic organelles of *Toxoplasma* and *Plasmodium* spp. Current Opinion in Microbiology. 2013;16(4):452-8.

[46] Melo AM, Bandeiras TM, Teixeira M. New insights into type II NAD(P)H:quinone oxidoreductases. Microbiology and Molecular Biology Reviews. 2004;68(4):603-16.

[47] Fry M, Webb E, Pudney M. Effect of mitochondrial inhibitors on adenosinetriphosphate levels in *Plasmodium falciparum*. Comparative Biochemistry and Physiology. B, Comparative Biochemistry. 1990;96(4):775-82.

[48] Saleh A, Friesen J, Baumeister S, Gross U, Bohne W. Growth inhibition of *Toxoplasma gondii* and *Plasmodium falciparum* by nanomolar concentrations of 1-hydroxy-2-dodecyl-4(1H)quinolone, a high-affinity inhibitor of alternative (type II) NADH dehydrogenases. Antimicrobial Agents and Chemotherapy. 2007;51(4):1217-22.

[49] Boysen KE, Matuschewski K. Arrested oocyst maturation in *Plasmodium* parasites lacking type II NADH:ubiquinone dehydrogenase. Journal of Biological Chemistry. 2011;286(37):32661-71.

[50] Gutteridge WE, Dave D, Richards WH. Conversion of dihydroorotate to orotate in parasitic protozoa. Biochimica et Biophysica Acta. 1979;582(3):390-401.

[51] Fry M, Pudney M. Site of action of the antimalarial hydroxynaphthoquinone, 2-[trans-4-(4-chlorophenyl) cyclohexyl]-3-hydroxy-1,4-naphthoquinone (566C80). Biochemical Pharmacology. 1992;43(7):1545-53.

[52] Srivastava IK, Rottenberg H, Vaidya AB. Atovaquone, a broad spectrum antiparasitic drug, collapses mitochondrial membrane potential in a malarial parasite. Journal of Biological Chemistry. 1997;272(7):3961-6.

[53] Balabaskaran Nina P, Morrisey JM, Ganesan SM, Ke H, Pershing AM, Mather MW, Vaidya AB. ATP synthase complex of *Plasmodium falciparum*: dimeric assembly in mitochondrial membranes and resistance to genetic disruption. Journal of Biological Chemistry. 2011;286(48):41312-22.

[54] Balabaskaran Nina P, Dudkina NV, Kane LA, van Eyk JE, Boekema EJ, Mather MW, Vaidya AB. Highly divergent mitochondrial ATP synthase complexes in *Tetrahymena thermophila*. PLoS Biology. 2010;8(7):e1000418.

[55] Allen RD, Schroeder CC, Fok AK. An investigation of mitochondrial inner membranes by rapid-freeze deep-etch techniques. Journal of Cell Biology. 1989;108(6): 2233-40.

[56] Daily JP, Scanfeld D, Pochet N, Le Roch K, Plouffe D, Kamal M, Sarr O, Mboup S, Ndir O, Wypij D, et al. Distinct physiological states of *Plasmodium falciparum* in malaria-infected patients. Nature. 2007;450(7172):1091-5.

[57] Uyemura SA, Luo S, Moreno SN, Docampo R. Oxidative phosphorylation, Ca(2+) transport, and fatty acid-induced uncoupling in malaria parasites mitochondria. Journal of Biological Chemistry. 2000;275(13):9709-15.

[58] Preiser PR, Wilson RJ, Moore PW, McCready S, Hajibagheri MA, Blight KJ, Strath M, and Williamson DH. Recombination associated with replication of malarial mitochondrial DNA. EMBO Journal. 1996;15(3):684-93.

[59] Vaidya AB, Arasu P. Tandemly arranged gene clusters of malarial parasites that are highly conserved and transcribed. Molecular and Biochemical Parasitology. 1987;22(2-3):249-57.

[60] Feagin JE, Gardner MJ, Williamson DH, Wilson RJ. The putative mitochondrial genome of *Plasmodium falciparum*. Journal of Protozoology. 1991;38(3):243-5.

[61] Feagin JE, Werner E, Gardner MJ, Williamson DH, Wilson RJ. Homologies between the contiguous and fragmented rRNAs of the two *Plasmodium falciparum* extrachromosomal DNAs are limited to core sequences. Nucleic Acids Research. 1992;20(4): 879-87.

[62] Feagin JE, Mericle BL, Werner E, Morris M. Identification of additional rRNA fragments encoded by the *Plasmodium falciparum* 6 kb element. Nucleic Acids Research. 1997;25(2):438-46.

[63] Feagin JE, Harrell MI, Lee JC, Coe KJ, Sands BH, Cannone JJ, Tami G, Schnare MN, Gutell RR. The fragmented mitochondrial ribosomal RNAs of *Plasmodium falciparum*. PloS One. 2012;7(6):e38320.

[64] Sharma A, Sharma A. Plasmodium falciparum mitochondria import tRNAs along with an active phenylalanyl-tRNA synthetase. Biochemical Journal. 2015;465(3): 459-69.

[65] Chavalitshewinkoon-Petmitr P, Chawprom S, Naesens L, Balzarini J, Wilairat P. Partial purification and characterization of mitochondrial DNA polymerase from *Plasmodium falciparum*. Parasitology International. 2000;49(4):279-88.

[66] Vaidya AB, Mather MW. Atovaquone resistance in malaria parasites. Drug Resistance Updates. 2000;3(5):283-7.

[67] Vaidya AB, Lashgari MS, Pologe LG, Morrisey J. Structural features of *Plasmodium* cytochrome *b* that may underlie susceptibility to 8-aminoquinolines and hydroxynaphthoquinones. Molecular and Biochemical Parasitology. 1993;58(1):33-42.

[68] Nyola A, Hunte C. A structural analysis of the transient interaction between the cytochrome *bc*$_1$ complex and its substrate cytochrome *c*. Biochemical Society Transactions. 2008;36(Pt 5):981-5.

[69] Trumpower BL, Gennis RB. Energy transduction by cytochrome complexes in mitochondrial and bacterial respiration: the enzymology of coupling electron transfer reactions to transmembrane proton translocation. Annual Review of Biochemistry. 1994;63:675-716.

[70] Sutherland CJ, Laundy M, Price N, Burke M, Fivelman QL, Pasvol G, Klein JL, Chiodini PL. Mutations in the *Plasmodium falciparum* cytochrome *b* gene are associated with delayed parasite recrudescence in malaria patients treated with atovaquone-proguanil. Malaria Journal. 2008;7(240).

[71] Fivelman QL, Butcher GA, Adagu IS, Warhurst DC, Pasvol G. Malarone treatment failure and in vitro confirmation of resistance of *Plasmodium falciparum* isolate from Lagos, Nigeria. Malaria Journal. 2002;1(1).

[72] Schwartz E, Bujanover S, Kain KC. Genetic confirmation of atovaquone-proguanil-resistant *Plasmodium falciparum* malaria acquired by a nonimmune traveler to East Africa. Clinical Infectious Diseases. 2003;37(3):450-1.

[73] Wichmann O, Muehlberger N, Jelinek T, Alifrangis M, Peyerl-Hoffmann G, Muhlen M, Grobusch MP, Gascon J, Matteelli A, Laferl H, et al. Screening for mutations related to atovaquone/proguanil resistance in treatment failures and other imported isolates of *Plasmodium falciparum* in Europe. Journal of Infectious Diseases. 2004;190(9): 1541-6.

[74] Syafruddin D, Siregar JE, Marzuki S. Mutations in the cytochrome b gene of *Plasmodium berghei* conferring resistance to atovaquone. Molecular and Biochemical Parasitology. 1999;104(2):185-94.

[75] di Rago JP, Coppee JY, Colson AM. Molecular basis for resistance to myxothiazol, mucidin (strobilurin A), and stigmatellin. Cytochrome *b* inhibitors acting at the center o of the mitochondrial ubiquinol-cytochrome *c* reductase in *Saccharomyces cerevisiae*. Journal of Biological Chemistry. 1989;264(24):14543-8.

[76] Howell N, Gilbert K. Mutational analysis of the mouse mitochondrial cytochrome *b* gene. Journal of Molecular Biology. 1988;203(3):607-18.

[77] Siregar JE, Syafruddin D, Matsuoka H, Kita K, Marzuki S. Mutation underlying resistance of *Plasmodium berghei* to atovaquone in the quinone binding domain 2 (Qo(2)) of the cytochrome b gene. Parasitology International. 2008;57(2):229-32.

[78] Fisher N, Abd Majid R, Antoine T, Al-Helal M, Warman AJ, Johnson DJ, Lawrenson AS, Ranson H, O'Neill PM, Ward SA, et al. Cytochrome *b* mutation Y268S conferring atovaquone resistance phenotype in malaria parasite results in reduced parasite *bc*$_1$

catalytic turnover and protein expression. Journal of Biological Chemistry. 2012;287(13):9731-41.

[79] Siregar JE, Kurisu G, Kobayashi T, Matsuzaki M, Sakamoto K, Mi-Ichi F, Watanabe YI, Hirai M, Matsuoka H, Syafruddin D, et al. Direct evidence for the atovaquone action on the *Plasmodium* cytochrome *bc* complex. Parasitology International. 2014. pii: S1383-5769(14)00133-0. doi: 10.1016/j.parint.2014.09.011.

[80] Birth D, Kao WC, Hunte C. Structural analysis of atovaquone-inhibited cytochrome $bc_1$ complex reveals the molecular basis of antimalarial drug action. Nature Communications. 2014;5(4029).

[81] Capper MJ, O'Neill PM, Fisher N, Strange RW, Moss D, Ward SA, Berry NG, Lawrenson AS, Hasnain SS, Biagini GA, et al. Antimalarial 4(1H)-pyridones bind to the Qi site of cytochrome $bc_1$. Proceedings of the National Academy of Sciences of the United States of America. 2015;112(3):755-60.

[82] Xiang H, McSurdy-Freed J, Moorthy GS, Hugger E, Bambal R, Han C, Ferrer S, Gargallo D, Davis CB. Preclinical drug metabolism and pharmacokinetic evaluation of GW844520, a novel anti-malarial mitochondrial electron transport inhibitor. Journal of Pharmaceutical Sciences. 2006;95(12):2657-72.

[83] Jimenez-Diaz MB, Mulet T, Viera S, Gomez V, Garuti H, Ibanez J, Alvarez-Doval A, Shultz LD, Martinez A, Gargallo-Viola D, et al. Improved murine model of malaria using *Plasmodium falciparum* competent strains and non-myelodepleted NOD-scid IL2Rgammanull mice engrafted with human erythrocytes. Antimicrobial Agents and Chemotherapy. 2009;53(10):4533-6.

[84] Heinemann IU, Jahn M, Jahn D. The biochemistry of heme biosynthesis. Archives of Biochemistry and Biophysics. 2008;474(2):238-51.

[85] Shemin D, Russell CS, and Abramsky T. The succinate-glycine cycle. I. The mechanism of pyrrole synthesis. Journal of Biological Chemistry. 1955;215(2):613-26.

[86] Ohgari Y, Nakayasu Y, Kitajima S, Sawamoto M, Mori H, Shimokawa O, Matsui H, Taketani S. Mechanisms involved in delta-aminolevulinic acid (ALA)-induced photosensitivity of tumor cells: relation of ferrochelatase and uptake of ALA to the accumulation of protoporphyrin. Biochemical Pharmacology. 2005;71(1-2):42-9.

[87] Barr H, Dix AJ, Kendall C, and Stone N. Review article: the potential role for photodynamic therapy in the management of upper gastrointestinal disease. Alimentary Pharmacology and Therapeutics. 2001;15(3):311-21.

[88] Ishizuka M, Abe F, Sano Y, Takahashi K, Inoue K, Nakajima M, Kohda T, Komatsu N, Ogura S, Tanaka T. Novel development of 5-aminolevurinic acid (ALA) in cancer diagnoses and therapy. International Immunopharmacology. 2011;11(3):358-65.

[89] Varadharajan S, Dhanasekaran S, Bonday ZQ, Rangarajan PN, Padmanaban G. Involvement of delta-aminolaevulinate synthase encoded by the parasite gene in de no-

vo haem synthesis by *Plasmodium falciparum*. Biochemical Journal. 2002;367(Pt 2): 321-7.

[90] Sato S, Clough B, Coates L, Wilson RJ. Enzymes for heme biosynthesis are found in both the mitochondrion and plastid of the malaria parasite *Plasmodium falciparum*. Protist. 2004;155(1):117-25.

[91] Nagaraj VA, Sundaram B, Varadarajan NM, Subramani PA, Kalappa DM, Ghosh SK, Padmanaban G. Malaria parasite-synthesized heme is essential in the mosquito and liver stages and complements host heme in the blood stages of infection. PLoS Pathogens. 2013;9(8):e1003522.

[92] Padmanaban G, Nagaraj VA, Rangarajan PN. An alternative model for heme biosynthesis in the malarial parasite. Trends in Biochemical Sciences. 2007;32(10):443-9.

[93] Smith TG, Kain KC. Inactivation of *Plasmodium falciparum* by photodynamic excitation of heme-cycle intermediates derived from delta-aminolevulinic acid. Journal of Infectious Diseases. 2004;190(1):184-91.

[94] Komatsuya K, Hata M, Balogun EO, Hikosaka K, Suzuki S, Takahashi K, Tanaka T, Nakajima M, Ogura S, Sato S, et al. Synergy of ferrous ion on 5-aminolevulinic acid-mediated growth inhibition of *Plasmodium falciparum*. Journal of Biochemistry. 2013;154(6):501-4.

[95] Iyer JK, Shi L, Shankar AH, Sullivan DJ, Jr. Zinc protoporphyrin IX binds heme crystals to inhibit the process of crystallization in *Plasmodium falciparum*. Molecular Medicine. 2003;9(5-8):175-82.

[96] Dougherty TJ, Gomer CJ, Henderson BW, Jori G, Kessel D, Korbelik M, Moan J, Peng Q. Photodynamic therapy. Journal of the National Cancer Institute. 1998;90(12): 889-905.

[97] Suzuki S, Hikosaka K, Balogun EO, Komatsuya K, Niikura M, Kobayashi F, Takahashi K, Tanaka T, Nakajima M, Kita K. *In vivo* curative and protective potential of orally administrated 5-aminolevulinic acid plus ferrous ion against malaria. Antimicrobial Agents and Chemotherapy. 2015. pii: AAC.01910-15.doi: 10.1128/AAC.01910-15.

Chapter 3

# Recent Advances in Antimalarial Drug Discovery — Challenges and Opportunities

Chiranjeev Sharma and Satish Kumar Awasthi

Additional information is available at the end of the chapter

http://dx.doi.org/10.5772/61191

**Abstract**

Malaria drug discovery is a challenging and difficult task due to the unavailability of the vaccine and lack of newer drugs. The most potent artemisinin and its derivatives, widely used in combination therapies for curing malaria worldwide are also now falling to resistance in some parts of the world. Thus, to combat malaria, new drugs possessing high therapeutic value, minimal toxicity, rapid efficacy and low cost are urgently needed. In this chapter, we will provide an integrated overview on the challenges and opportunities in malaria drug discovery with more emphasis on synthesis of peroxidic antimalarials.

**Keywords:** Natural Products, Quinine, Chloroquine, Artemisinin, Trioxane, Tetraoxane, Malaria, Antimalarials

## 1. Introduction

### 1.1. History

The chronicle of malaria predating humanity is as ancient as mankind.[1] Malaria continues to be a persistent menace wreaking havoc especially in tropical and subtropical regions despite tremendous efforts toward its control and eradication. The unavailability of the vaccine and the emergence of resistance in the parasite against nearly all existing antimalarial drugs have attracted attention of researchers to modify the existing antimalarial drugs with improved efficacy over older therapies and identify new compounds as appropriate clinical candidate. Mortality from malaria is increasing at an alarming rate despite various renewed efforts and eradication campaigns[2] because the parasites (*Plasmodium* strains) responsible for the majority of fatal infections have become resistant to the existing drugs. Malaria is also the cause of poverty and a major hindrance to economic development, especially in sub-Saharan countries.[3] Mostly, malaria is spread due to local transmission through female anopheles mosquitoes. Occasionally, it can also be transmitted by exposure to infected blood products (transfusion malaria) and also through congenital transmission. The major species of *Plasmodium* strains that infect humans are *P. falciparum, P. vivax, P. ovale, P. malariae,* and *P. knowlesi.* Among these, *P. falciparum* causes the most severe form of infection, which could be fatal.

The original picture of the parasitic existence and passage of malaria through historic times remains blurred. It is uncertain whether the human population settlements preceded the arrival of malaria within them.[3] The versions may vary from tentative to widely accepted or even controversial based on the general scientific evidence. However, the effect of malaria wreaking havoc to the human species is prominent, clear, and unmistakable. There was no specific treatment for malaria until the 17th century.[4] The discovery of quinine from the bark of *Cinchona calisaya* began effective treatment of malaria. Further, the synthesis of chloroquine by Hans Andersag in 1934 introduced a cheap antimalarial drug and a substitute for quinine.[5] Until the widespread resistance in 1960, quinoline-related antimalarial drugs played an important role in the treatment of malaria. Fortunately, in 1972, the Chinese discovered artemisinin from sweet wormwood plant *Artemisia annua*.[6] Artemisinin along with its derivatives artemether, arteether (artemotil), and artesunate are the main treatment for malaria that is resistant to conventional therapies.

Recent advances in the molecular genetics and biochemical technologies available for the investigation of malaria parasites within the last half century have enabled us to gain a unique perspective on the human health and health services in relation to malaria.[7]

### 1.2. Life cycle of malaria parasite

The life cycle of malaria parasites is very complex. It is completed inside two hosts, including the humans (asexual) and the mosquitoes (sexual) (Figure 1).[8, 9] Malaria infection begins when an infected female anopheles mosquito feeding on human blood bites and injects sporozoites into the bloodstream. The parasites then quickly reach liver to form merozoites by asexual multiplication. Subsequently, merozoites exit liver with the rupture of hepatic tissues and enter the bloodstream where they invade and disintegrate red blood cells. Some merozoites transform into gametocytes, which are then circulated in the bloodstream. When the second mosquito bites an infected human, it gets infected and intakes gametocytes. The sexual transformation of gametocytes into ookinetes and ookinetes into oocyst takes place inside the midgut of mosquito. Finally, sporozoites are developed from oocysts, which eventually burst, releasing sporozoites into the salivary gland. Continued infection in humans and mosquitoes alternatively propagates and spreads malaria.

A comparative study with human and rodent parasites revealed the activities of current antimalarial drugs on the life cycle stages of plasmodium.[10] 8-Aminoquinolones are known to be active for liver stage. The most currently available antimalarial drugs primarily target the human blood cell stage. In addition to the asexual blood stage, some drugs (viz., pyronar-

http://dx.doi.org/10.5772/61191

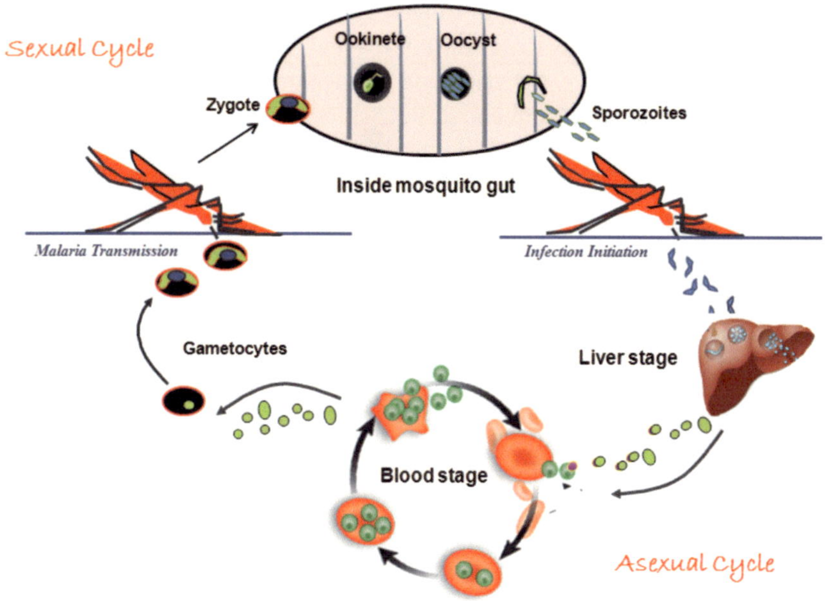


**Figure 1.** Life cycle of malaria parasite.[9]

idine and atovaquone) can also target both liver and sexual stage. Further, new stable synthetic endoperoxides can inhibit gamete formation and gametocyte maturation.[10] Furthermore, it is important to profile the currently available drugs for specific stage in parasite's life cycle to combat malaria by eradication and circumventing resistance.

### 1.3. Status quo

WHO has recommended artemisinin combination therapy (ACT) for the treatment of malaria.[11] Since 2006, artemisinin-based combination therapies remain as the first-line treatment for *P. falciparum* malaria replacing chloroquine and sulfadoxine/pyrimethamine. Combined with other drugs, its derivatives, such as artesunate and artemether, can clear symptoms of malaria in three days. However, a rise in demand has led to a shortage of artemisinin. Artemisinin-based drugs are also more expensive than conventional treatments, in part because large doses are required. Further, with recent reports on the emergence of resistance to artemisinin,[12] it can be foreseen that in the near future, new armamentarium will be required to fight against malaria. Thus, to overcome this problem, there is an urgent need to identify new chemotypes or reexamining old molecules to transform them into an appropriate clinical candidate.

## 2. Drug resistance

The greatest challenge to malaria control and eradication is the emergence of malaria parasites that are resistant to antimalarial drugs.[13] The reemergence of malaria from the areas where it was eradicated and spread of malaria to new areas is a major threat. The World Health Organization defined antimalarial drug resistance as the "ability of a parasite strain to survive and/or multiply despite the administration and absorption of a drug given in doses equal to or higher than those usually recommended but within tolerance of the subject."[14] It was modified later to specify that the drug in question must "gain access to the parasite or the infected red blood cell for the duration of the time necessary for its normal action."[15] Antimalarial drug resistance occurs through spontaneous mutations that reduces the sensitivity to a given class of drug(s).[16] Only a single point mutation is sufficient to confer resistance to some drugs, while multiple mutations appear to be required for others.

| Sl. no | Drug class | Drug | Resistance | Mechanism of action |
|---|---|---|---|---|
| 1. | 4-Aminoquinoline | Chloroquine | Since 1945 | Inhibition of hemozoin formation |
| 2. | | Amodiaquine | Yes | |
| 3. | | Piperaquine | Since 1980s | |
| 4. | 8-Aminoquinoline | Primaquine | - | Unknown |
| 5. | Aryl-amino alcohol | Quinine | Yes | Unknown |
| 6. | | Mefloquine | Since 1985 | |
| 7. | | Lumefantrine | No | |
| 8. | Antifolates | Pyrimethamine | Since 1967 | Inhibition of DHFR |
| 9. | | Trimethoprim | Yes | |
| 10. | | Proguanil | Since 2000 | |
| 11. | | Sulfonamides | Yes | |
| 12. | Napthoquinone | Atovaquone | Since 2000 | Inhibition cytochrome |
| 13. | Antibiotic | Doxycycline | No | Inhibition of protein synthesis and apicoplast |
| 14. | | Clindamycin | | |
| 15. | Artemisinin | Artesunate | Yes | Free radical mechanism Heme alkylation |
| 16. | | Artemether | Since 2001 | |
| 17. | | Dihydroartemisinin | | |

**Table 1.** Status of resistance in antimalarial drugs.

The malaria parasite has developed some level of resistance against nearly all previous generation antimalarial drugs (Table 1). Recent research has confirmed evidence of artemisinin resistance.[10] Although it is under investigation, immediate actions are needed to restrict resistance to artemisinin from spreading to new areas. It is high time that we should fight this overwhelming menace with improved tools to aim at controlling the mosquito vector and develop new armaments; otherwise, the future looks bleak and grim.

## 3. Mechanism of action

The mechanism of action of antimalarial drugs is based on the extensive studies of selected drugs. Most drugs available for the treatment were discovered based on the serendipitous identification of active compounds (natural, synthetic, and semisynthetic).[17] The progress in the understanding of the biochemistry of malarial parasite has shed light on the mechanism of action of new as well as older drugs.

It is believed that artemisinin and related drugs are transported to the food vacuole of the parasite, where they generate free radicals upon interaction with Fe(II)-heme. These free radical's interaction with heme generates oxidative stress and kills the parasite.[18] The mechanism of action of quinoline and related drugs is also well established.[19] It is shown that the drugs enter the RBC and inhabit the digestive vacuole of parasite by simple diffusion. The subsequent inhibition of hemozoin biocrystallization leads to the aggregation and accumulation of cytotoxic heme in food vacuoles resulting in parasite's death. The commercially available quinolone antimalarials target the gyrase and inhibit DNA replication. It results in the delayed death of treated parasites by formation of abnormal apicoplasts.[20]

Based on the mechanism of action, different groups of antimalarials can be classified as follows:

- Artemisinin: binds heme iron and generates oxygen radicals
- Antifolate: inhibits DNA synthesis
- Atovaquone: collapses mitrochondrial membrane potential
- Quinoline: inhibits heme crystallization
- Antibacterial: ribosome and DNA gyrase inhibition

## 4. Toxicity of the antimalarial drugs

The most important determinant of drug use and its effectiveness is the patient compliance. The toxicity of the drug must be balanced with the efficacy of the drug and the risk from malaria, i.e., the drug should cause less harm than the disease itself. The doses given to the patients should be taken into account in determining the treatment of malaria. The assessment of the tolerability of many antimalarial drugs is ongoing, but evaluating adverse drug reactions, events, side effects, and drug-related toxicity is difficult due to the unavailability of good techniques to measure the side effects.[21]

The most promising naturally occurring sesquiterpene lactone drug and its derivatives (artemether, arteether, and sodium artesunate) did not show any serious side effects. However, insufficient clinical trials to detect the toxicity stopped us from declaring artemisinin 100% safe. However, they have excellent safety profile and remarkable efficacy. The current knowledge obtained from the laboratory and clinical study is that the long-term availability of artemisinins may cause toxicity (rarely produce neurotoxicity and allergic reactions).[22] The short-term peak concentrations followed by rapid elimination of artemisinins after oral intake is relatively safe compared to administration by intramuscular injection. Evidently, the majority of animal experiments showed considerable toxicities in contrast to human studies.

Chloroquine, considered being a safe drug even at higher doses, also causes mild side effects such as reversible effect on optical accommodation, which can potentially affect eyesight. It also binds irreversibly to melanin. Hence, the patients with rheumatoid arthritis treated with the long-term use of high dose chloroquine suffer from accumulation of chloroquine in retinal melanin. Some reports also suggest that chloroquine administered to patients with light intolerant disease can aggravate psoriasis.[22] Proguanil is also assumed to be safe at a dose of 200 mg a day. However, for doses higher than 200 mg, there are reports of reversible alopecia and aphthous ulceration, nausea, and gastric irritation.[23] These side effects are common with other antimalarial agents as well. The combination of chloroquine with proguanil has good tolerability. However, gastrointestinal upset and mouth ulcers are still observed. Sulfadoxine/ pyrimethamine is also well tolerated, but it is no longer used because it causes Stevens–Johnson syndrome and toxic epidermal necrolysis. Mefloquine is another valuable drug for the treatment of malaria. Despite good tolerability to most patients, dose-related serious neuropsychiatric toxicity can occur. Cardiovascular or CNS toxicity is rare for quinine but hypoglycemia may occur. Further, due to its potential for cardiotoxicity, halofantrine is unsuitable for widespread use. Mepacrine, sulfonamides, dapsone, and amodiaquine are also withdrawn from the use because of the high frequency of adverse side effects.[24]

## 5. Malaria vaccine

Malaria vaccine development is a challenging and difficult task because of the antigenic complexity and the complex life cycle of malaria parasite. Research on the development of malaria vaccine is of prime importance because such a discovery can prevent millions of deaths worldwide. The currently available tools are insufficient for malaria eradication. Malaria vaccine could be a transformative tool to help in reduced transmission and future eradication. Extensive research has been carried out in the last two decades, and several vaccines have reached clinical trials, but there is none in the clinical practice due to insufficient immunogenicity. Although parasite vaccines are in development, there is no FDA-approved vaccine for organisms more complex than viruses and bacteria.[25]

### 5.1. Scientific challenges

The significant hurdle in the development of malaria vaccine is insufficient knowledge about the malaria parasite. Understanding the structure and antigenic variation of parasite population requires lengthy, tedious, and difficult lab and field studies. Antigenic variation and parasite polymorphism also create a major scientific barrier. Unfortunately, in nature, there are not many good examples of immunity to malaria, and many vaccine development programs are based only on naturally acquired immunity. Since the mechanism of immune protection is still unknown, it is difficult to comprehend why certain people are protected while others are not. Inadequate animal models and lack of clarity in the definition of desired outcomes create confusion in choosing the best approach to develop a malaria vaccine. Even in particular animal model systems with defined outcomes, there is always uncertainty in translating the success of protection in the model systems with success in humans.[26]

The malaria vaccine development includes recombinant proteins, gene-based (DNA or viral vector) vaccines, attenuated whole organisms, peptides, and prime-boost strategy, which involves a combination of different antigen delivery systems encoding the same epitopes or antigen using various adjuvants. Reports dating back to 1960s[26] demonstrated species-specific and strain cross-reactive protection on immunization with radiation-attenuated sporozoites in primate and experimental rodent models. Studies showed optimistic levels of protective immunity. However, the volunteers immunized against multiple strains of *P. falciparum* malaria were not protected against *P. vivax*. The target antigens were identified from the sera cells of experimental hosts immunized with attenuated sporozoite vaccine and protected volunteers. Circumsporozoite protein, the first cloned and sequenced malaria parasite in *P. knowlesi* and *P. falciparum*, is also the first antigen identified by serological screening. It plays an important role in protection. When the sporozoite was irradiated in the rodent models, antibody and cells showed different roles in malaria species and different strains. Although multifaceted cellular responses are observed, the basic mechanism of immunity is believed to target the intracellular hepatic exoerythrocytic forms by the production of interferon. The antibody eliminates most of the infectious sporozoite inoculum, when the vaccines prove a multipronged approach. The cellular responses target the rest of the intracellular exoerythrocytic forms by direct cytotoxicity or inhibitory cytokines.

The understanding of the research related to vaccine development is greatly benefitted by the lessons learned from discontinued and inactive projects. Recent findings allow us to be optimistic about the possibility of an effective malaria vaccine. Several malaria vaccine candidates have entered field trials. It is now possible to impact the host–parasite relationship using different platforms through vaccine-induced immune responses to multiple antigenic targets. The field has grown rapidly over the last two decades from the first clinical trials to the successful conduct of large-scale field studies, and substantial progress has been made in evaluating many antigens. Despite the daunting task, researchers have produced surprising progress in several areas. The malaria vaccination program has progressed to an assessment and clinical evaluation of RTS,S/AS01E in phase 3 trial.[27] The first malaria vaccine may be considered for licensure in the coming years. Further, there is a possibility of developing more efficacious second-generation vaccines. Researchers are now better equipped to establish clear product profiles. The lessons learned in terms of safety, immunogenicity, efficacy, and trial methodology from malaria vaccine research is summarized in Table 2.

| Parameters | Remarks |
|---|---|
| Safety | · It is often lower in semi-immune populations living in endemic areas than in naïve populations |
| | · Reactogenicity in young children has not been worse than in adult populations |
| Immunogenicity | · DNA alone is poorly immunogenic |
| | · Little clinically significant interference is observed between vaccine antigens and the malarial antigen |
| Efficacy | · Only RTS,S-based vaccines proved to be effective to reduce morbidity in endemic areas |
| | · Highly polymorphic blood-stage antigens have tended to lead to allele-specific efficacy, but poor efficacy against the population of circulating strains |
| Methodology | · In vitro studies and animal studies does not correlate well |
| | · For testing of new malaria vaccines, ethical and methodological issues may arise |
| | · There is a need to make formal trial design for phase trials and sample size calculations. Epidemiological studies are required to assess the effectiveness of mosquito antigen vaccines in sexual stage |

**Table 2.** Lessons from two decades of malaria vaccine development research.

## 6. Antimalarial drugs

Malaria, existing in over 100 countries, is one of the deadliest infectious diseases and major health problem worldwide. Antimalarial drugs are designed to cure malaria, many of which are in market.[28] From the 17th century onward quinine had been the drug of choice for the treatment of malaria. Later on, medication therapies heavily relied on chloroquine, primaquine, mefloquine, etc.[4] These drugs especially chloroquine have saved more lives than any other drugs in history. Recently, artemisinin and its derivatives have emerged as a new generation of antimalarials (Figure 2).

There is a critical need to develop newer synthetic and more effective drugs that could address the issues associated with the existing and traditional drug therapies. The availability of artemisinin also causes supply constraints because artemisinin and its derivatives constitute an active ingredient of many combination therapy dugs. For example, Coartem contains a fixed combination of artemether and lumefantrine. In 2012, Ranbaxy also launched a new synthetic peroxide antimalarial drug Synriam™ in the market in line with the recommendations of the WHO. It is a fixed dose combination of arterolane maleate and piperaquine phosphate. The chemical structures are shown below.

http://dx.doi.org/10.5772/61191

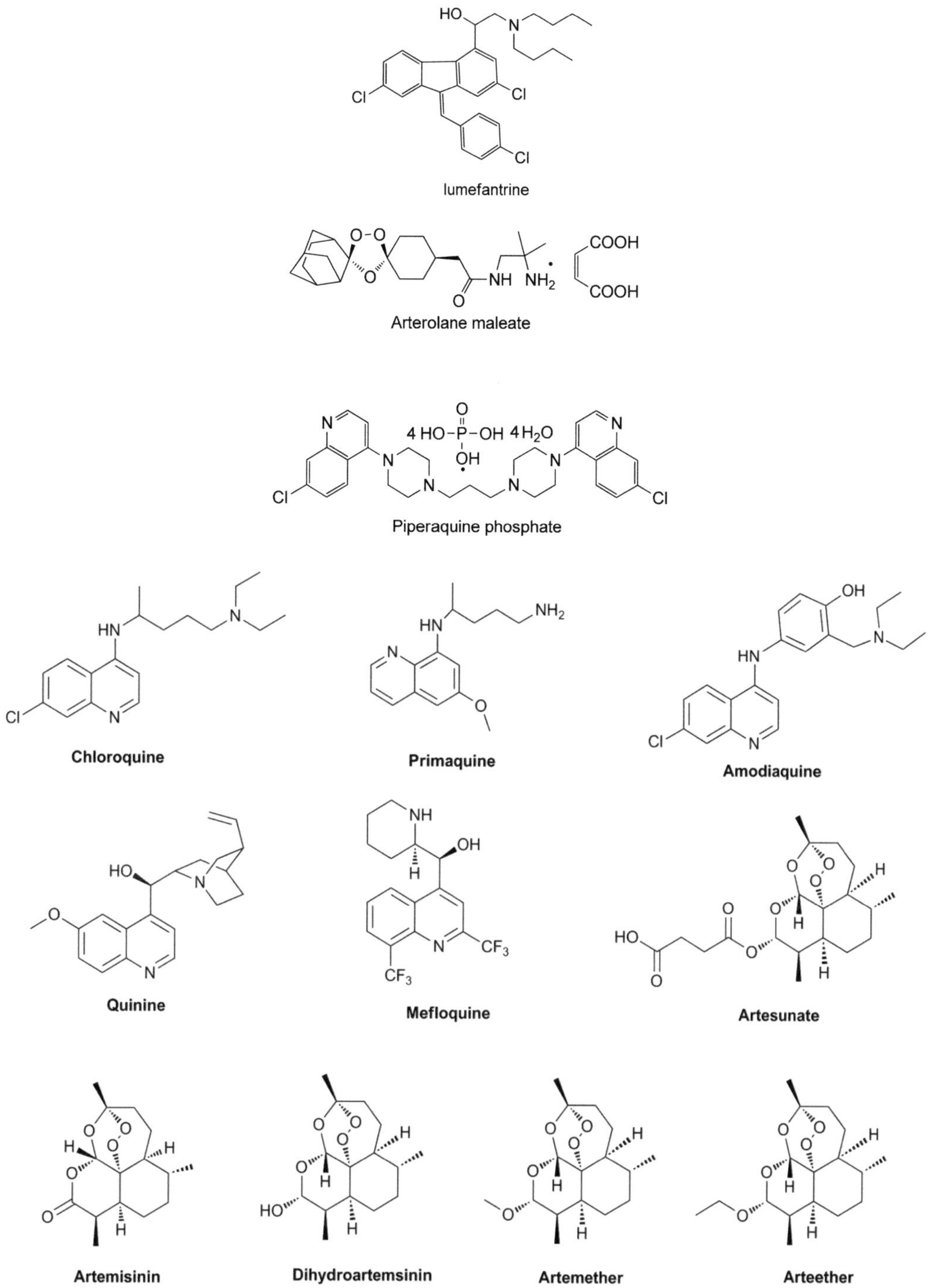


**Figure 2.** Antimalarial drugs.

Research groups across the world are united in the efforts to discover new chemicals for the treatment of malaria. Attempts to modify the established drugs are also ongoing. Long-term hopes are resting on the modification of the synthetic artemisinin-based drugs containing endoperoxide rings. The following sections will mainly focus on the development of peroxidic antimalarial agents.

### 6.1. Natural products

Natural products continue to make an immense contribution to malaria chemotherapy. The discovery of quinine and artemisinin proves that nature is a rich source of lead compounds that can provide cure and medicine for malaria. Nature has been extremely generous when it comes to search of new molecular scaffolds for good malarial activity. These scaffolds later serve as template for the development of structurally diverse analogues with more potent activity.[29] For example, quinine a bitter-tasting alkaloid, is one of the earliest natural compounds that helped man in the fight against malaria. It was isolated from the *Cinchona* bark. Later, it also served as a template for the synthesis of more potent and structurally simpler analogues such as chloroquine, primaquine, mepacrine, and mefloquine (Figure 2). Artemisinin extracted from *Artemesia annua* is another example whose diverse pharmacological potential has attracted the researchers worldwide. Artemisinin also gave rise to the development of dihydroxyartemisinin, artemether, arteether and artesunate. Thus, natural products such as quinine and artemisinin have demonstrated the enormous potential of nature in providing lead compounds, which can be further manipulated structurally for the development of more effective antimalarial agents. Many more natural products possessing various chemical structures, such as alkaloids, steroids, chalcones, terpenes, flavonoids, peptides, quinones, xanthones, coumarines, naphthopyrones, polyketides, phenols, lignans, chromenes, etc., have been tested as antimalarial drugs.[30, 33]

### 6.2. Semisynthetic drugs

The success of the most potent antimalarial drugs, quinine and artemisinin, has brought some optimism. Due to the widespread emergence of drug-resistant chloroquine, primaquine, mepacrine, and mefloquine (Figure 2) were developed. Despite the remarkable antimalarial activity, artemisinin suffers from limited availability, low solubility, high cost, metabolic stability, short half-life, poor bioavailability, and chemical stability. Thus, there is a need for new compounds more active than the parent artemisinin. To circumvent some of these problems, semisynthetic analogs were prepared. The reduction of artemisinin yields dihydroartemisinin, and the lactol group can be further converted to its ether (artemether, arteether, and artelinic acid) and ester (sodium artesunate) derivatives.[34]

### 6.3. Synthetic drugs

Artemisinin, a sesquiterpene endoperoxide, has established the role of peroxide ring for potential antimalarial activity. However, the naturally isolated artemisinin is available in short supply and expensive to synthesize. As a consequence, extensive research directed towards the discovery of peroxidic antimalarials inspired researchers to explore structurally simple peroxides. Trioxanes, tetraoxanes, and their hybrids were consequently identified as promising candidates for the development of next generation antimalarial drugs.

*6.3.1. Various synthetic procedures for the synthesis of trioxanes*

Trioxanes can be synthesized from inexpensive starting materials, and their scale-up preparations are feasible. Most methods reported for the synthesis of trioxanes starts with the reaction of singlet oxygen with carbonyls in the presence of Lewis acids. Then acid-catalyzed cyclization of hydroxyperoxides with olefins and reaction of $\alpha$-peroxy aldehydes with carbonyl compound yields trioxanes in good yields. Many synthetic strategies were developed for the synthesis 1,2,4-trioxanes, which are described below.

*6.3.1.1. Photooxygenation method*

Starting from commercially available cyclohexanediones, tricyclic 1,2,4-trioxanes can be synthesized by following simple method. Briefly, photooxygenation of the electron-rich allylic alcohols **1** using singlet oxygen gives β-hydroxyperoxide **2.** Further, β-hydroxyperoxide **2** was condensed with 1,4-cyclohexadiene followed by Lewis acid-mediated cyclization to give keto-trioxane **3.** Amino functionalized trioxanes **4** were also synthesized on reductive amination with various amines in the presence of sodium triacetoxy borohydride (Scheme 1).[35]

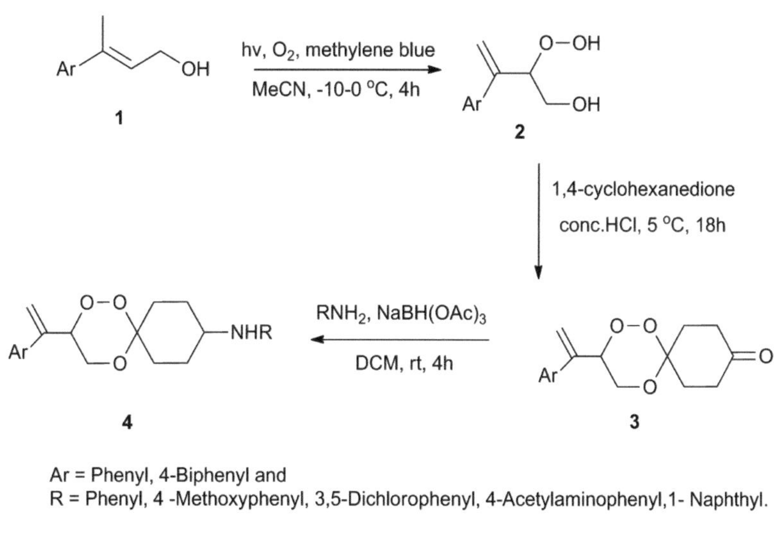


**Sheme 1.** Photooxygenation method for trioxane synthesis.

In another synthetic procedure, the geranyl acetate was transformed into aldehyde acetate **5**, which is converted into allylic alcohol **6**. Photooxygenation of **6** followed by subsequent acid catalyzed condensation of β-hydroxyhydroperoxides **7** with various ketones resulted in the formation of new 1,2,4-trioxanes **8** (Scheme 2).[36] The hydroxyl functionalized side chains can be further manipulated for the synthesize of a diverse library of compounds.

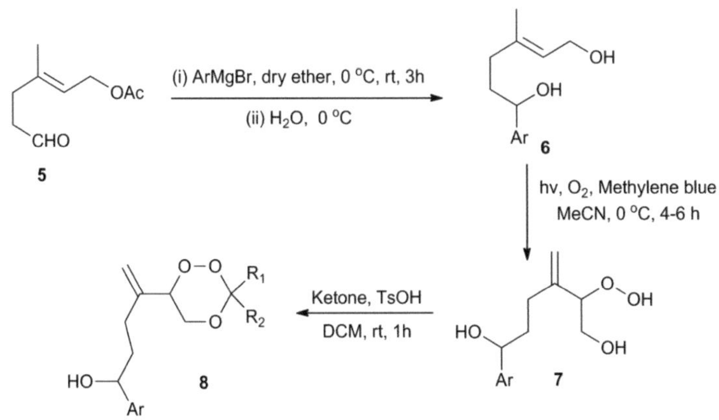


**Sheme 2.** Synthesis of Geraniol derived 1,2,4-trioxanes.

### *6.3.1.2. Epoxidation method*

The epoxidation of N-Boc piperidone **9** gives N-Boc spirooxirane **10.** Dispiro N-Boc-protected 1,2,4-trioxane can then be synthesized by $MoO_2(acac)_2$ catalyzed perhydrolysis of N-Boc spirooxirane **10**, as shown in Scheme 3.[37] Subsequent condensation of the resulting β-hydroperoxy alcohol **11** with 2-adamantanone gives N-Boc 1,2,4-trioxane **12**, which can be converted into the amine 1,2,4-trioxane hydrochloride salt **13**. Further, alkylation may result in a diversified sulfonamide trioxane derivatives **14**.

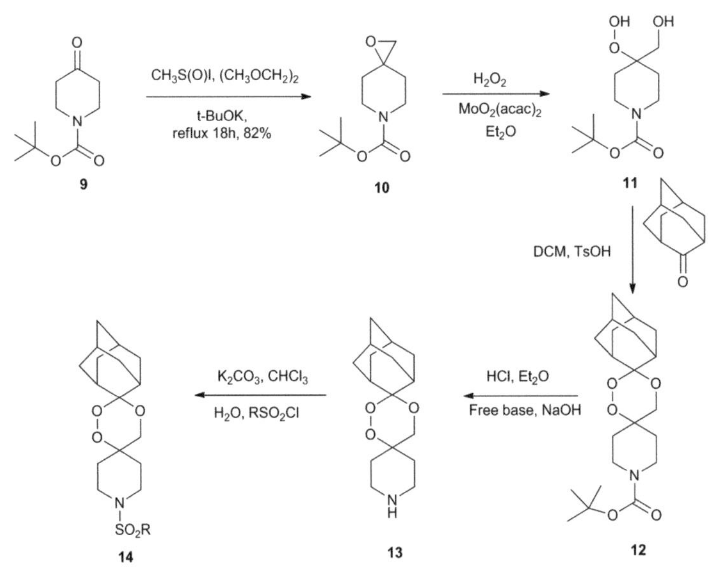


**Sheme 3.** Trioxane synthesis using epoxidation method.

http://dx.doi.org/10.5772/61191

### 6.3.1.3. *Catalytic enantioselective synthesis*

Trioxanes can also be synthesized by catalytic enantioselective synthesis. Para-cresol **15** is converted into *p*-peroxyquinols **16.** The desymmetrization of *p*-peroxyquinols **16** occurs via an acetalization/oxa-Michael cascade reaction (Scheme 4).[38] The reaction proceeds via a dynamic kinetic resolution of a peroxyhemiacetal intermediate. Various derivatized trioxanes **17** can be easily obtained by this method. The use of chiral Brønsted acid catalyst TRIP **18** gave a single diastereomer trioxane **17** in 86% ee, while using bis-(2,4,6-triisopropylphenyl)spiro-biindane phosphoric acid **19** gave 96% ee. The use of thiourea **20** as cocatalyst helped to restore the reactivity even at lower catalyst loading.

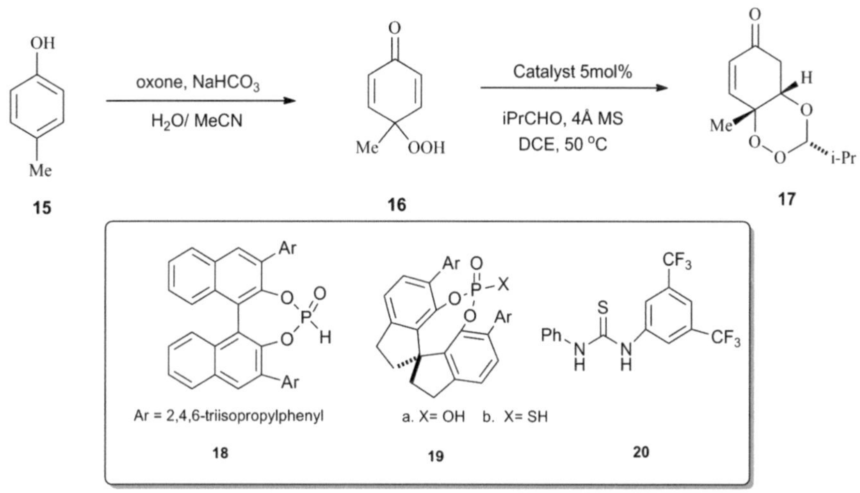


**Sheme 4.** Enantioselective synthesis of trioxanes.

### 6.3.1.4. *Solid phase synthesis*

The solid support synthesis of 1,2,4-trioxanes also needs light mediated oxygenation on polystyrene polymer support. Wang and Rink amide resins can be used as linkers. The reaction of resin-bound *p*-carboxybenzaldehydes **21** with excess of ionone derivatives **22** gave immobilized dienones **23** in the presence of LiOH in DME (Scheme 5).[39] Resin-bound trioxane **24** was obtained upon irradiation of compound **23** with UV light (354 nm) in toluene yielded. After cleavage from the solid support, the formation of **25** was confirmed by $^{13}$C NMR. Peaks at 82.4 and 94.4 ppm corresponded to the peroxy-bearing carbon and peroxyketal carbon of the trioxane ring system.

### 6.3.2. *Various synthetic procedures for the synthesis of tetraoxanes*

The chemical modification of artemisinin retaining the crucial endoperoxide ring has resulted in yet another simplified structure known as 1,2,4,5-tetraoxane. Tetraoxanes show significantly higher stability and exhibit even higher activity than natural peroxidic drugs for curing malaria

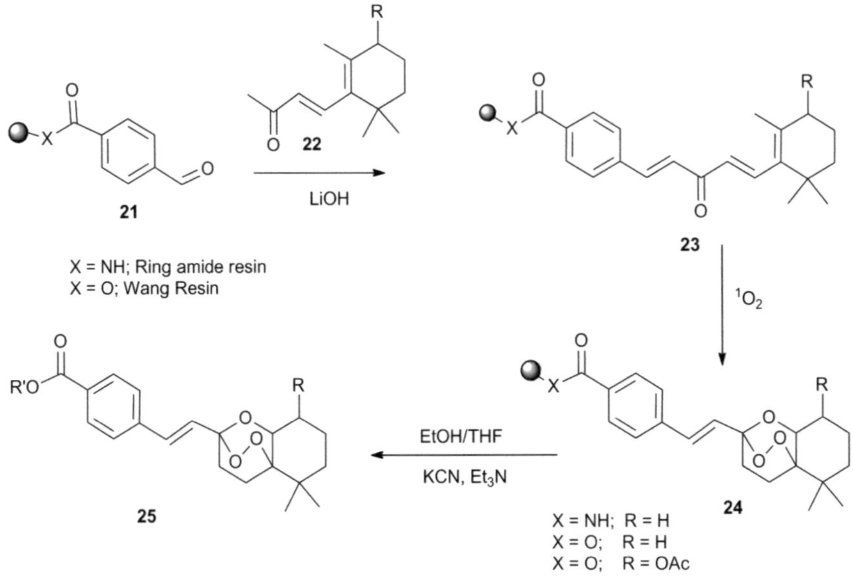


**Sheme 5.** Solid phase trioxane synthesis.

infections. In 1899, Baeyer and Villiger reported the synthesis of the first dimeric acetone peroxide upon treatment of acetone and Caro's acid in ether. Since then, the field has moved ahead significantly and newer synthetic routes and efficient methodologies were developed. The synthesis can be carried out by several methods as described below.

### *6.3.2.1. Peroxidation method*

The most commonly and widely used method for tetraoxane synthesis is known as peroxidation method. In this method, acid-catalyzed cyclocondensation of ketones or aldehydes gives the *gem*-dihydroperoxide as an important active intermediate. Generally, the acid-catalyzed addition of hydrogen peroxide to carbonyl compound **26** produce *gem*-dihydroperoxide **27**, which on subsequent cyclocondensation in the presence of strong acid such as sulfuric acid, perchloric acid, or methanesulfuric acid yield more stable symmetrical tetraoxane **28** along with side product hexaoxane **29,** as shown in Scheme 6. It is also known that the trimeric cyclic peroxide by-product hexaoxonane is formed in the presence of excess hydrogen peroxide. Dimethyl sulfide and potassium iodide can be used for the removal of hydroperoxide-related impurities. Hexaoxonanes could be removed by washing the reaction mixture with cold methanol. [40]

In our lab, we also attempted the synthesis of a new series of tetraoxane by incorporating nitrogen within the cyclohexyl ring. [41] Methyl 2-(4-oxopiperidin-1-yl)acetate **30** on reaction with *gem*-dihydroperoxide **27** may give very small amount of tetraoxane **31** and trimer **29**, as shown in Scheme 7. We characterized hexaoxonane **29** as a main side product by spectroscopy and x-ray crystallography.

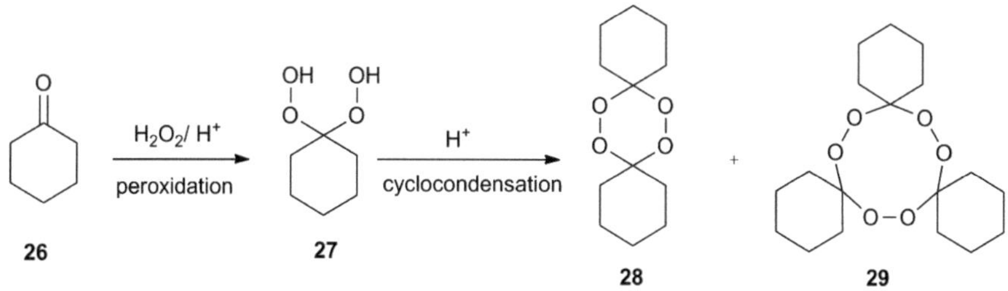


**Sheme 6.** Acid catalyzed synthesis of tetraoxanes and hexaoxonanes.

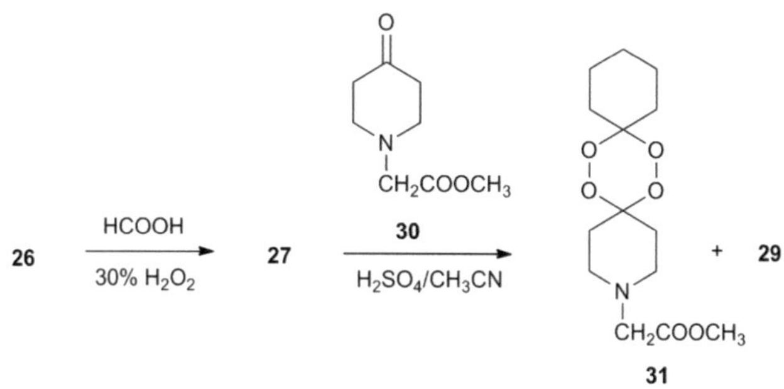


**Sheme 7.** Synthesis of piperidinetetraoxane

## *6.3.2.2. One pot synthesis*

Iskara et al.[42] developed the first one-pot synthesis of tetraoxane. Simple carbonyl compounds **32** in the presence of 30% $H_2O_2$, 0.1% MTO, and fluorous alcohols (TFE and HFIP) selectively gives tetraoxanes **33** (Scheme 8). Fluorous solvents TFE and HFIP activate both $H_2O_2$ and MTO for oxidation reactions. The one-pot synthesis of mixed tetraoxanes begins with the oxidation of the most reactive carbonyl compound, and then less oxidizable carbonyl compound is added in the presence of acid. In this reaction, no trimeric product is formed.

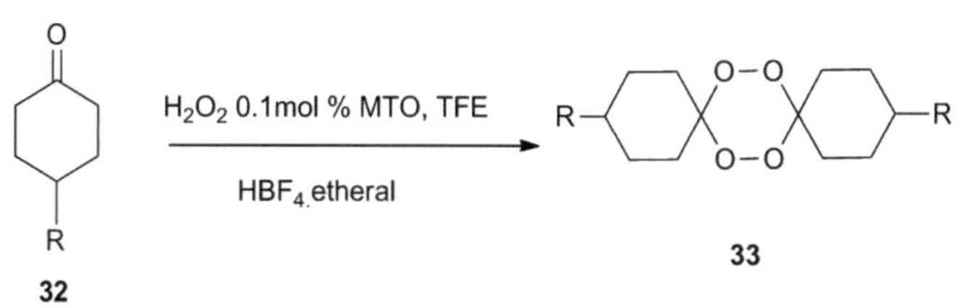


**Sheme 8.** One pot tetraoxane synthesis.

*6.3.2.3. Ozonolysis method*

The most prolific strategy for the synthesis of tetraoxanes is the ozonolysis of suitable olefins and oximes. This method has dual advantage over others: (1) the absence of hexaoxonane (a usual by-product), which is very common in acid catalyzed reactions, and (2) it is useful for the synthesis of aromatic tetraoxanes, which could not be obtained by other methods. In the 1970s, Keul et al. reported the synthesis of dimeric adamantine peroxide **35** by ozonization of methyleneadamantane **34** in pentane at –78°C. The ozonolysis of valerophenone oxime *o*-methyl ether **36** produces carbonyl oxide **38** via an intermediate ozonoid **37** to give the crystalline dimeric valerophenone peroxides **39** in the absence of carbonyl compounds or protic solvents.[43]

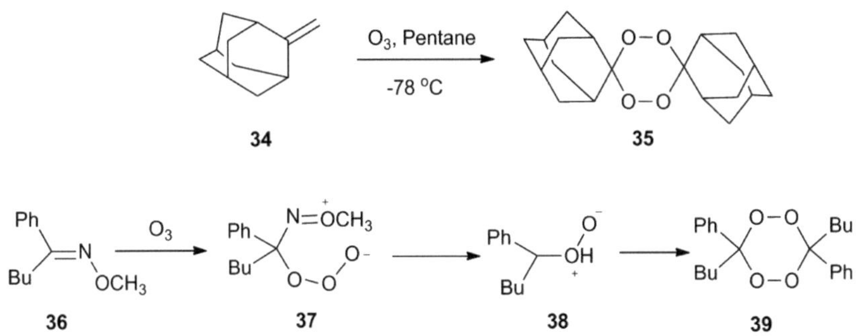


**Sheme 9.** Tetraoxane synthesis by ozonolysis method.

# 7. Prodrug and combination therapies

The search of newer drugs and the enhancement of antimalarial activity of the existing ones have led to the development of prodrug and combination therapy approaches. It presents a good platform for the usage of readily available drugs in combination with other effective drugs. The potential of drug hybrids, prodrugs, and combination therapy as new approaches are immense.[44]

Tetraoxaquine **40** contain two covalently linked pharmacophores, i.e., a tetraoxane (a radical donor) and an aminoquinoline (interferes with hematin polymerization).[45] Moreover, trioxaquine **41** contains covalently attached trioxane to a 4-aminoquinoline moiety.[46] The chimeric drug penetrates (enabled by aminoquinoline) into infected erythrocyte and targets the free heme. The hemoglobin digestion of the schizonts within infected red blood cells liberates free heme, which is alkylated by the peroxidic part. Trioxaferroquine **42** consists of a trioxane, a substituted quinoline, and an iron (II) species within a single structure.[47]

http://dx.doi.org/10.5772/61191

These new chimeric molecules containing two covalently attached moieties can be expected to possess synergistic therapeutic value, reduce resistance, and toxicity. These strategies offer a rational drug design approach for the development of next generation drug candidates. Notwithstanding few selected examples, which are discussed in this section, it explains the concept and potential applications.

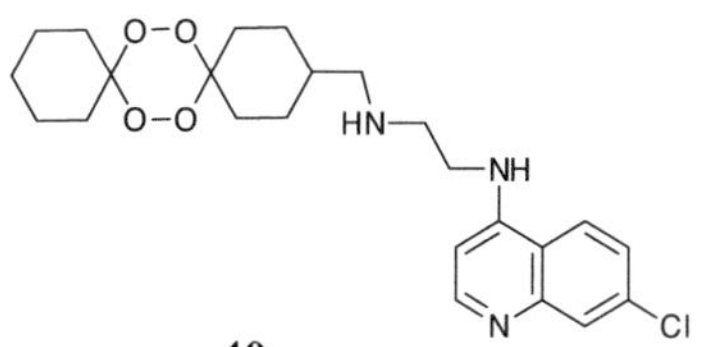

**40**

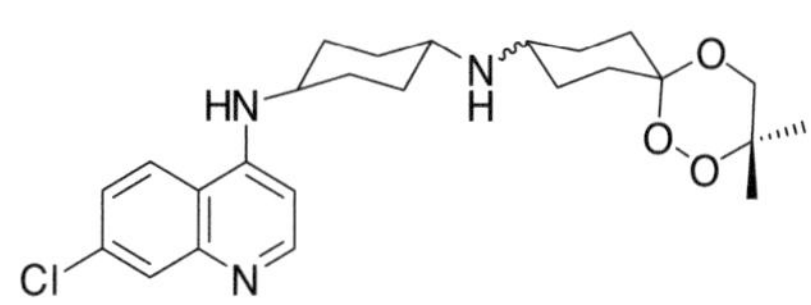

**41**

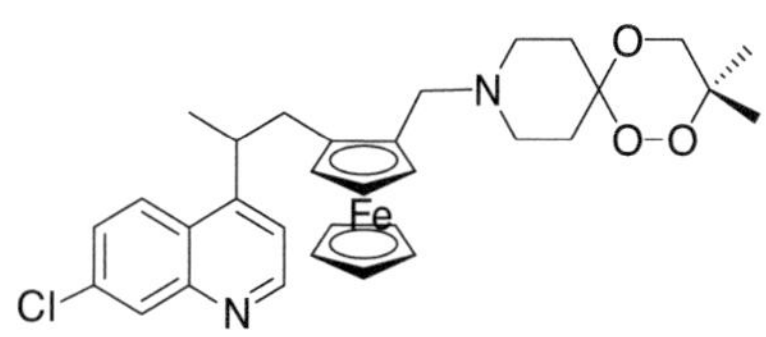

**42**

## 8. Conclusion and future prospect

The development of new drugs for malaria presents a challenging situation. Lack of alternatives and increasing ineffectiveness of the existing drugs are the main reasons for increased mortality. Traditional medicines have provided few drugs, but to combat malaria, new drugs are urgently needed. These new drugs must ideally possess minimal toxicity, rapid efficacy, and low cost. However, there is consensus among scientific community that drug combinations may create optimal control of malaria because the combination therapies are believed to be additive in potency, provide synergistic activity, and is more advantageous than monotherapies. Unfortunately, these requirements are not met by any combination at the current window of time. Besides all the challenges, failures, and setbacks, the global importance of fighting malaria is recognized. Dedicated efforts and academic engagement to discover, develop, and deliver new, effective, and affordable antimalarials have thus increased dramatically. Natural products, semisynthetic drugs, and synthetic compounds offer vast opportunity for the drug development process. Further, assessment and clinical evaluation of RTS,S/AS01E for malaria vaccination offers hope that we may soon expect some good news. Malaria drug discovery is undoubtedly challenging, but scientists are optimistic as they also have got various opportunities too. The *status quo* seems balanced. However, we believe that we have to provoke the *status quo* to gain the upper hand in the battle against this tropical scourge.

## Acknowledgements

CS is thankful to UGC, New Delhi, for SRF. SKA acknowledges the financial support from the University of Delhi, Delhi-110007, India.

## Author details

Chiranjeev Sharma and Satish Kumar Awasthi*

*Address all correspondence to: skawasthi@chemistry.du.ac.in

Chemical Biology Laboratory, Department of Chemistry, University of Delhi, Delhi, India

## References

[1] Poinar G. Plasmodium dominicana n. sp. (Plasmodiidae: Haemospororida) from Tertiary Dominican amber. *Systematic Parasitology* 2005; 61(1), 47–52

[2] World Malaria Report 2014, http://www.who.int/malaria/publications/world_malaria_report_2014/en/ (accessed 21.03.2015).

[3] Eve WE, Basu S, Hanson K. Is malaria a disease of poverty? A review of the literature. *Tropical Medicine and International Health* 2005; 10(10), 1047–1059.

[4] Greenwood D. Conflicts of interest: the genesis of synthetic antimalarial agents in peace and war. *Journal of Antimicrobial Chemotherapy* 1995; 36(5), 857–872.

[5] Krafts K, Hempelmann E, Skorska-Stania A. From methylene blue to chloroquine: a brief review of the development of an antimalarial therapy. *Parasitology Research* 2012; 111(1), 1–6.

[6] Kayman DL. Qinghaosu (artemisinin): an antimalarial drug from China. *Science* 1985; 228(4703), 1049–1055.

[7] Neafsey DE, et al. Highly evolvable malaria vectors: the genomes of 16 *Anopheles* mosquitoes. *Science* 2015; 347(6217), 1258522.

[8] Chang HH, Hartl DL. Recurrent bottlenecks in the malaria life cycle obscure signals of positive selection. *Parasitology* 2015; 142(S1): S98–S107.

[9] Neupane CS, Awasthi SK. In: Synthetic Quinolones: Emerging Antimalarial Agents. A. Pandey (eds.), Antibacterial activity in natural and synthetic compounds. 2013,443-459.

[10] Delves M, Plouffe D, Scheurer C, Meister S, Wittlin S, Winzeler EA, Sinden RE, Leroy D. The activities of current antimalarial drugs on the life cycle stages of plasmodium:

a comparative study with human and rodent parasites. *PLOS Medicine* 2012; 9(2): e1001169/1–e1001169/14.

[11] World Health Organization. Guidelines for the Treatment of Malaria. Second edition. March 2010.

[12] Carter TE, Boulter A, Existe A, Romain JR, St. Victor JY, Mulligan CJ, Okech BA. Artemisinin resistance-associated polymorphisms at the K13-propeller locus are absent in *Plasmodium falciparum* isolates from Haiti. *American Journal of Tropical Medicine and Hygiene* 2015; 92(3), 552–554.

[13] Hyde JE. Drug-resistant malaria—an insight. *FEBS Journal* 2007; 274(18), 4688–4698.

[14] Peters W. History and current status of drug resistance. In: Peters W, Richards WHG. (eds.), Antimalarial Drugs. Handbook of Experimental Pharmacology. 1984, pp. 423–445.

[15] World Health Organization. Guidelines for the Treatment of Malaria. 2006.

[16] White NJ. Antimalarial drug resistance. *Journal of Clinical Investigation* 2004; 113(8), 1084–1092.

[17] Schlesinger PH, Krogstad DJ, Herwaldt BL. Antimalarial agents: mechanism of action. *Antimicrobial Agents and Chemotherapy* 1988; 32(6), 793–798.

[18] Meshnick SR. Artemisinin: mechanisms of action, resistance and toxicity. *International Journal for Parasitology* 2002; 32(13), 1655–1660.

[19] Bray PG, Ward SA, O'Neill PM. Quinolines and artemisinin: chemistry, biology and history. *Current Topics in Microbiology and Immunology* 2005; 295, 3–38.

[20] Biagini GA, et al. Generation of quinolone antimalarials targeting the *Plasmodium falciparum* mitochondrial respiratory chain for the treatment and prophylaxis of malaria. *Proceedings of the National Academy of Sciences of the United States of America* 2012; 109(21), 8298–8303.

[21] Peto TE. Toxicity of antimalarial drugs. *Journal of the Royal Society of Medicine* 1989; 82(17), 30–33.

[22] Wesche Dl, DeCoster MA, Tortella FC, Brewer TG. Neurotoxicity of artemisinin analogs in vitro. *Antimicrobial Agents and Chemotherapy* 1994; 38(8), 1813–1819.

[23] Davidson NM. Mouth ulceration associated with proguanil. *Lancet* 1986; 327(8477), 384.

[24] Taylor WBJ, White NJ. Antimalarial drug toxicity: a review. *Drug Safety* 2004; 27(1), 25–61.

[25] Schwartz L, Brown GV, Genton B, Moorthy VS. A review of malaria vaccine clinical projects based on the WHO rainbow table. *Malaria Journal* 2012; 11, 11.

[26] Graves PM, Levine MM. Battling Malaria: Strengthening the U.S. Military Malaria Vaccine Program. 2006, pp. 26–33.

[27] Olotu A, et al. Four-year efficacy of RTS,S/AS01E and its interaction with malaria exposure. *New England Journal of Medicine* 2013; 368(12), 1111–1120.

[28] Crowther GJ, et al. Identification of inhibitors for putative malaria drug targets among novel antimalarial compounds. *Molecular and Biochemical Parasitology* 2011; 175(1), 21–29.

[29] Guantai E, Chibale K. How can natural products serve as a viable source of lead compounds for the development of new/novel anti-malarials? *Malaria Journal* 2011, 10(Suppl 1):S2.

[30] Department of International Development. Medicines For Malaria Venture (MMV) 2005–2010. MMV in natural products: harnessing the power of nature in malaria drug discovery. 2009, http://r4d.dfid.gov.uk/PDF/Outputs/MMV/MMV_in_Natural_Products.pdf (accessed 21.03.2015)

[31] Nogueira CR, Lopes LMX. Antiplasmodial natural products. *Molecules* 2011; 16, 2146–2190.

[32] Agarwal D, Sharma M, Dixit SK, Dutta RK, Singh AK, Gupta RD, Awasthi SK. In vitro synergistic effect of fluoroquinolone analogs in combination with artemisinin against *Plasmodium falciparum*; their antiplasmodial action in rodent malaria model. *Malaria Journal* 2015; 14(1), 48.

[33] Dixit SK, Yadav N, Kumar S, Good L, Awasthi SK. Synthesis and antibacterial activity of fluoroquinoone analogs. *Medicinal Chemistry Research* 2014; 23(12), 5237–5249.

[34] Yadav N, Sharma C, Awasthi SK. Diversifications in the synthesis of antimalarial trioxane and tetraxoane analogs. *RSC Advances* 2014; 4, 5469–5498.

[35] Singh C, Malik H, Puri SK. Orally active 1,2,4-trioxanes: synthesis and antimalarial assessment of a new series of 9-functionalized 3-(1-arylvinyl)-1,2,5-trioxaspiro[5.5]undecanes against multi-drug-resistant *Plasmodium yoelii nigeriensis* in mice. *Journal of Medicinal Chemistry* 2006; 49(9), 2794–2803.

[36] Singh C, Gupta N, Puri SK. Geraniol-derived 1,2,4-trioxanes with potent in-vivo antimalarial activity. *Bioorganic and Medicinal Chemistry Letters* 2003; 13(20), 3447–3450.

[37] Sabbani S, Stocks PA, Ellis GL, Davies J, Hedenstrom E, Ward SA, O'Neill PM. Piperidine dispiro-1,2,4-trioxane analogues. *Bioorganic and Medicinal Chemistry Letters* 2008; 18(21), 5804–5808.

[38] Rubush DM, Morges MA, Rose BJ, Thamm DH, Rovis T. An asymmetric synthesis of 1,2,4-trioxane anticancer agents via desymmetrization of peroxyquinols through a Brønsted acid catalysis cascade. *Journal of American Chemical Society* 2012; 134(33), 13554–13557.

[39] La-Venia A, Mata EG, Mischne MP. Photoinduced oxygen capture on immobilized dienone systems. First solid-phase synthesis of trioxane scaffolds. *Journal of Combinatorial Chemistry* 2008; 10(4), 504–506.

[40] Kumar N, Singh R, Rawat DS. Tetraoxanes: synthetic and medicinal chemistry perspective. *Medicinal Research Reviews* 2012; 32(3), 581–610.

[41] Neupane CS, Awasthi SK. Unique trifurcated hydrogen bonding in a pseudopolymorph of tricyclohexane triperoxide (TCTP) and its thermal studies. Tetrahedron letters 2012; 53(45), 6067–6070.

[42] Iskra J, Bonnet-Delpon D, Begue, JP. One-pot synthesis of non-symmetric tetraoxanes with the $H_2O_2$/MTO/fluorous alcohol system. *Tetrahedron Letters* 2003; 44(33), 6309–6312.

[43] Ito Y, Konishi M, Matsuura T. Thermal and photosensitized decomposition of dimeric valerophenone peroxide formed by ozonation of valerophenone oxime ether. *Photochemistry and Photobiology* 1979; 30(1), 53–57.

[44] Gutema GB, Hailu GS, Kidanemariam ZA, Hishe HZ. Combination therapy and its implication on clinical efficacy of artemisinins—review. *International Journal of Pharmaceutical Sciences and Research* 2011; 2(8), 1914–1921.

[45] Opsenica I, Opsenica D, Lanteri CA, Anova L, Milhous WK, Smith KS, Solaja BA. New chimeric antimalarials with 4-aminoquinoline moiety linked to a tetraoxane skeleton. *Journal of Medicinal Chemistry* 2008; 51(19), 6216–6219.

[46] Odile DC, Francoise BV, Anne R, Bernard M. Preparation and antimalarial activities of "trioxaquines," new modular molecules with a trioxane skeleton linked to a 4-aminoquinoline. *ChemBioChem* 2000; 1(4), 281–283.

[47] Francois B, Frederic C, Laure V, Jacques B, Bernard M, Anne R. Trioxaferroquines as new hybrid antimalarial drugs. Journal of Medicinal Chemistry 2010; 53(10), 4103–4109.

Chapter 4

# Advances on *Dientamoeba fragilis* Infections

Ali ElBakri, Ahmed Al-Qahtani and Amidou Samie

Additional information is available at the end of the chapter

http://dx.doi.org/10.5772/61809

**Abstract**

*Dientamoeba fragilis* is an enteric protozoan parasite that remains neglected, probably due to the misconception that it is uncommon and non-pathogenic. As more information became available and antimicrobial agents were developed with activity against this parasite, it became clear that *D. fragilis* is responsible of an active infection, associated with symptoms such as abdominal pain and diarrhea. The clinical presentation of dientamoebiasis varies from asymptomatic carriage to symptoms ranging from altered bowel motions, abdominal discomfort, nausea and diarrhea with associated eosinophilia reported in up to 50% of paediatric and 10% of adult patients. Moreover, controversy exists over the protective role of the parasite in priming the immune system in a beneficial way such as in selecting beneficial bacteria, keeping potential harmful microbial intruders at bay or producing metabolites beneficial to the host. Thus, a number of ambiguities and obscurities surrounding *D. fragilis* infections exist. Moreover, the means by which this parasite is transmitted has not been fully defined. The diagnostic recognition of this parasite in fecal examinations requires specific processing and expertise; thus, it is possible that many infections with *D. fragilis* may go undiagnosed. A number of studies conducted on small numbers of case reports have demonstrated parasite clearance, as well as resolution of clinical symptoms following treatment with various antiparasitic compounds such as paromomycin, hydroxyquinolines and the 5-nitroimidazoles, including metronidazole and tinidazole. In addition there is very little in vitro susceptibility data available for the organism making some current treatment options questionable. This chapter reviews the scientific literature relating to Dientamoeba's life cycle, prevalence, diagnosis and pathogenicity.

**Keywords:** *Dientamoeba fragilis*, epidemiology, diagnosis, treatment, tropical infections

## 1. Introduction

*Dientamoeba fragilis* is an enteric protozoan parasite that remains obscure and neglected. While many infections remain asymptomatic, it is now generally accepted that *D. fragilis* is accountable for an active infection, concomitant with abdominal symptoms, nausea, and diarrhea. Moreover, controversy exists over the protective role of the parasite in priming the immune system in a beneficial way such as in selecting beneficial bacteria, keeping potential harmful microbial intruders at bay or producing metabolites beneficial to the host. Furthermore, the parasite's transmission mode remains a mystery. The microscopic identification and diagnoses of *D. fragilis* in stool requires skill and expertise; consequently, it is likely that many infections may go unidentified. Numerous studies have reported the effectiveness of treatment regimens using compounds such as paromomycin, hydroxyquinolines, and 5-nitroimidazoles, including metronidazole and tinidazole in the parasite eradication and the resolution of clinical symptoms. In addition, there is very little *in vitro* susceptibility data available for this parasite, making some current treatment options questionable. This chapter reviews the scientific literature relating to Dientamoeba's life cycle, prevalence, diagnosis, and pathogenicity.

## 2. Recognition *D. fragilis* as a pathogen

*D. fragilis* is a ubiquitous protozoan parasite found in the gastrointestinal tract of humans. Electron microscopy [1] and molecular phylogenetic studies of the SSU rRNA gene [2,3] have recently confirmed the relationship of this parasite to trichomonads (lacking flagella). Although its pathogenic potential is still controversial, Jepps and Dobell in1918 were the first to report its pathogenicity when it was found to be the only agent detected in three patients with gastrointestinal clinical symptoms [5].

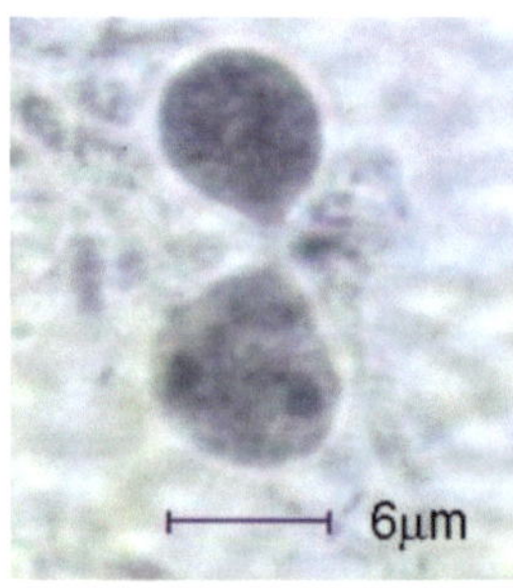


**Figure 1.** Trophozoite of *D. fragilis* stained by iron hematoxylin stain (Photo by Adnan Al-Hindi, 2005). Photo extracted from Al-Hindi and Abu Shammala, 2013 [4].

Since then, many investigators have shown that patients infected with *D. fragilis* generally presented with bowel disorders with symptoms such as diarrhea, loose stools, and epigastric abdominal pains [6–12]. Furthermore, mounting evidence is accumulating reinforcing the pathogenic potential of *D. fragilis* [13–20]. Lately, irritable bowel syndrome (IBS) has been linked to *D. fragilis* infections as a possible cause [21, 22], further underscoring its role in the causation of disease. A great deal of controversy exists on the mode of transmission of *D. fragilis*, and while *Enterobius vermicularis* nematode has been accepted to play a role in its transmission, more recently a report described the discovery of a new cyst stage in its life cycle [23].

Globally, the prevalence rates of *D. fragilis* infections vary depending on the identification tool used [6, 24, 25, 26]. Using the traditional light microscope, the rates of infections oscillate between 0.4% and 52% [26]. Nevertheless, using indirect immunoflourescent assay, Chan et al. (1996) reported a prevalence rate of 91% [27]. The application of more sensitive identification tools such as PCR and culture has the extra advantage of providing accurate prevalence data [28]. Considered as a pathogen by several researchers, numerous reports have revealed that *D. fragilis* elimination with parasitic drugs normally relieves the clinical symptoms in the absence of other pathogens. However, there is currently no consensus as to the ideal treatment regimen [20, 29, 30]. The aim of this chapter is to review the recent developments and advances made on this frequently overlooked parasite and the disease dientamoebiasis.

## 3. Biology and life cycle of *D. fragilis*

Ranging in size from 5 to 15 μm in diameter, *D. fragilis* is a single-celled pleiomorphic trophozoite containing up to four nuclei [32, 20]. A large proportion of *D. fragilis* trophozoites are typically binucleated with a large, fragmented, central karyosome without peripheral chromatin differentiated clearly in stained fecal smears [32,10]. Banik et al. (2012) have recently extensively described the surface structures and ultrasrtuctural details of *D. fragilis* populations grown in xenic culture [31]. Using the scanning electron microscope, the group reported the existence of two different trophozoite populations—smooth and ruffled cells. Whether this represents a significant difference biologically or even in terms of the parasite's pathogenicity remains to be elucidated. Using the transmission electron microscope, neither mitochondria nor peroxisomes were reported [33, 34]. Nevertheless, a conspicuous organelle detected was the hydrogenosomes. Like many other organisms living in oxygen-deprived or anaerobic environments, these hydrogenosomes most probably represent the site of anaerobic respiration and energy production [35–39]. Different activities such as amoeboid movement, phagocytosis, and bacterial adhesion to trophozoite surfaces were also reported by Banik and others (2012) [31]. Like many other parasitic protozoa such as *Trichomonas vaginalis* [40, 41, 33], *Giardia* [42], and *Leishmania* [43], virus-like particles (VLPs) have also been reported to be seen in *D. fragilis* trophozoites. Many groups have reported an association between the presence of VLPs within *T. vaginalis* and variations in protozoa phenotypes, virulence factors, and disease pathogenesis [44–46]. More details of the ultrastructure of *D. fragilis* are available in a review authored by Banik et al. (2012) [31].

The complete life cycle and the mode of transmission of *D. fragilis* remain ambiguous and equivocal. The only known stage thus far is the trophozoite (Fig. 2). Dobell (1940) was the first to predict *E. vermicularis* egg to act as a vector for the transmission of *D. fragilis* [47]. Recently, Roser et al. (2013) have detected *D. fragilis* DNA inside *E. vermicularis* eggs agreeing with the prediction of Dobell in 1940 [48]. While many reports of a higher than anticipated rate of co-infection between *D. fragilis* and E. vermicularis led researchers to postulate *E. vermicularis* as the probable vector responsible for its transmission [48, 49], other groups have proved no co-infections with *D. fragilis* and other worms, suggesting fecal-oral transmission as the possible mechanism of transmission of *D. fragilis* [9, 10]. A new study by Munasinghe et al. (2013) using

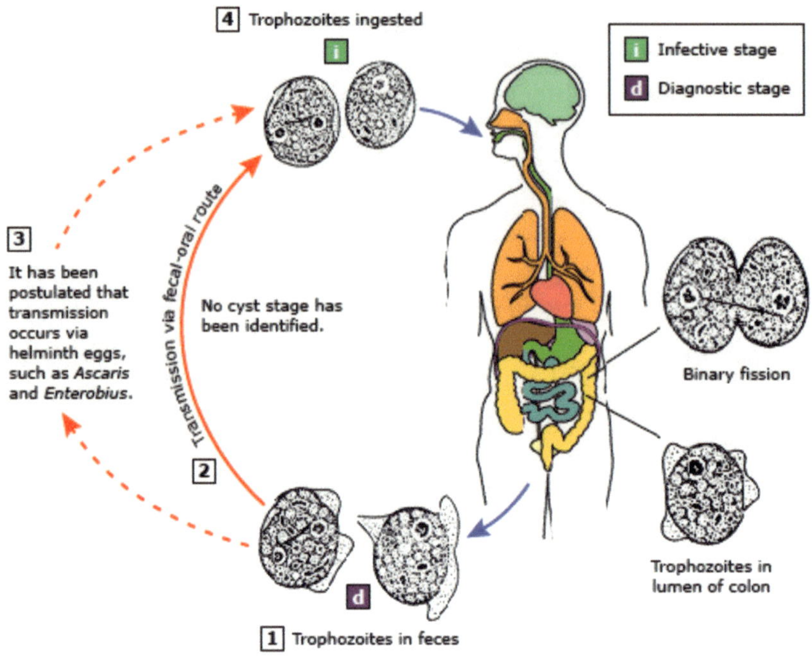


**Figure 2.** Life cycle of *D. fragilis*. Reproduced from: Centers for Disease Control and Prevention. DPDx: *Dientamoeba fragilis* infection. Available at: http://www.cdc.gov/dpdx/dientamoeba/index.html.

rodents and mice infected with human isolates reported the discovery of a new cyst stage in the life cycle of *D. fragilis* strongly suggesting oral–fecal transmission as the possible route of infection [23]. Moreover, Stark et al. (2014) have recently reported a cyst form of *D. fragilis* from human clinical samples, further supporting that cysts are likely to be the transmission forms [50]. The role of animals and zoonotic transmission of the parasite is still ambiguous despite a recent study reporting pigs and sheep as natural hosts of dientamoebiasis [51]. The reader is invited to read an excellent review on the topic written by Clark et al. (2014) [52].

## 4. Epidemiology of dientamoebiasis and its occurrence

Since its hypothetical association with IBS and other bowel disorders, probable pathogenicity, and the existence of gaps in its life cycle and mode of transmission, many investigators have become increasingly aware of the importance of *D. fragilis*. This has led to the development of more sensitive diagnostic techniques for its proper identification and determination of its accurate prevalence. It is now recognized as being more prevalent than *Giardia* [7, 11, 25, 27, 29, 53–65]. Table 1 shows the prevalence rates of *D. fragilis* ranging between 0.3% and 90% in many countries worldwide. With the exception of few studies, light microscopy was the tool used in those studies. The use of more sensitive techniques such as PCR or cultivation may result in different and more accurate prevalence rates [10, 28, 66]. Unlike many parasitic infections, *D. fragilis* has been shown to have high infection rates in developed countries than in underprivileged countries [25, 67].

| Prevalence | Sample source and type | Number of patients | Country/region | Reference |
|---|---|---|---|---|
| 36.25% | Mental asylum residents; feces | 80 | Holland | [68] |
| 2.4 | Patients; feces | 14203 | USA | [69] |
| 20.1% | Gastrointestinal tract patients; feces | 1114 | Israel | [70] |
| Not disclosed | *Ascaris lumbricoides* patients; feces | N/A | Thailand | [71] |
| About 4.2% | Fecal specimens submitted for parasitological examination | 43029 | Canada | [16] |
| 9.6% | Fecal specimens infected with *Entamoeba histolytica*/dispar | 125 | Mexico City, Mexico | [72] |
| 1.1% | School children; feces | 94 | Durban, South Africa | [73] |
| 52% | Adults; feces | 81 | Los Angeles, USA | [53] |
| 21.1% | Children attending clinics; feces | 104 | Los Angeles, USA | [74] |
| 8.6% | Children in day care centers; feces | 900 | Toronto, Canada | [65] |
| 4 | Adults in day care centers; feces | 146 | Toronto, Canada | [65] |
| 1.3% | Homosexual men; feces | 150 | San Francisco, USA | [75] |
| 16.8% | Intestinal tract patients; feces | 125 | French's Forest, Sydney, Australia | [62] |
| 1.1% | Homosexual men; diarrhea | 274 | Chicago, USA | [76] |
| 21% | Indigenous individuals; feces | 242 | Irian Jaya, Indonesia | [77] |
| 3% | Patients with bowel disorder; feces | 1350 | Christchurch, New Zealand | [78] |
| 82.9% | Children infected with other gut protozoa; feces | 123 | Germany | [64] |
| 3% | Children living in rural areas; feces | 266 | Honduras | [79] |
| 2% | Fecal specimens with light to moderate dehydration and diarrhea | 100 | Dominican Republic | [80] |
| 1.5% | Patients with diarrhea | 260 | Brisbane, Australia | [81] |
| 25.6% | HIV-positive patients with no diarrhea; feces | 82 | Buenos Aires, Argentina | [82] |
| 2.3% | Children refugees; feces | 87 | USA | [83] |
| 91% | Healthy children; sera | 189 | Canada | [27] |
| Around 8% | Patients with bowel symptoms | N/A | Netherlands | [84] |

| Prevalence | Sample source and type | Number of patients | Country/region | Reference |
|---|---|---|---|---|
| 2.1% | HIV negative patients; feces | 48 | San Pedro Sula, Honduras | [85] |
| 5.1% | Routine testing; feces | 857 | Oman | [59] |
| 5.5% | Fecal specimens submitted to a university hospital in Tunisia | 27053 | Sfax, Tunisia | [86] |
| 3% | HIV-positive patients; feces | 34 | North Brazil | [87] |
| 11.3% | Gastrointestinal tract patients; feces | 151 | Italy | [61] |
| 8.8% | Admitted patients; feces | 400 | Turkey, Celal Bayar University | [29] |
| 0.9% | Diarrhea patients; feces | 6750 | Sydney, Australia | [9] |
| 0.82% | Sanitary employees; feces | 241 | Malatya, Turkey | [88] |
| 6.3% | Patients infected with a gut parasite; feces | 448 | Brussels, Belgium | [6] |
| 3.7% | Gastrointestinal tract patients; feces | 3139 | Italy | [58] |
| 3.4% | Gastrointestinal tract patients; feces | 1141 | Italy | [57] |
| 4.1% | Gastrointestinal tract patients; feces | 1989 | Italy | [53] |
| 2% | Children and neonates patients; feces | 350 | Surt, Libya | [89] |
| 2.7% | Aborigines; feces | 112 | Salta, Argentina | [90] |
| 2.7% | Feces | 770 | Turkey | [91] |
| 8.9% | Patients infected with gut parasites; feces | 168 | Egypt | [24] |
| 29.8% | Patients infected with gut parasites; feces | 168 | Egypt | [24] |
| 0.8% | HIV negative MSM[a]; feces | 628 | Sydney, Australia | [92] |
| 0.3% | HIV-positive MSM; feces | 618 | Sydney, Australia | |
| 1.1% | Non-MSM patients; feces | 622 | Sydney, Australia | |
| 11.7% | Patients suspected of infection with gut parasites; feces | 103 | Denmark | [25] |
| 32% | Bowel complaints patients; feces | 397 | Zwolle, The Netherlands | [93] |
| 14.6%; 16.9% | Individuals attending complimentary health care practices (2002–2004 and 2005–2007); feces | 3719; 2491 | British Isles | [67] |
| 0.2% | School children; feces | 2975 | Van Province, Turkey | [94] |
| 5.2% | Bowel complaints; feces | 750 | Sydney, Australia | [11] |
| 1.6% | Digestive disorder patients; feces | 8313 | Catalonia, Spain | [95] |

| Prevalence | Sample source and type | Number of patients | Country/region | Reference |
|---|---|---|---|---|
| 21.4% | Patients suspected of infection with gut parasites; feces | 491 | Parma, Italy | [96] |
| 3.5% | Irritable bowel syndrome patients with diarrhea; feces | 171 | Karachi, Pakistan | [97] |
| 4% | Irritable bowel syndrome patients with diarrhea; feces | 171 | Karachi, Pakistan | |
| 4% | Irritable bowel syndrome patients with diarrhea; feces | 171 | Karachi, Pakistan | |
| 5.5% | Fecal samples submitted to the Department of Microbiology at St Vincent's Hospital, Sydney | 472 | Sydney, Australia | [98] |
| 8.8% | Patients with clinical symptoms, like diarrhea and abdominal pain; feces | 319 | Al-Nuseirate Refugee Camp Clinic, Gaza Strip | [4] |
| 0%<br>2.1%[b]<br>2.4% | Fecal samples from different laboratories | 1000 | Tabriz, Iran | [] |

Table adapted from Barratt et al. 2011. With kind permission from Dr. Damien Stark.

[a]MSM denotes men who have sex with men.

[b]In this Tabriz, Iran, study (Sarafraz et al., 2013), 26 samples were reported as suspicious cases in trichrome-stained smears.

**Table 1.** Global prevalence of *D. fragilis* infections in stool samples from various sources

Conflicting reports exist regarding the age-group distribution of *D. fragilis* infections. Two studies, Danish and Canadian, reported a high infection rate in subjects aged between 16 and 20 years, respectively [25, 60]. On the other hand, despite being statistically insignificant, Rayan et al. (2007) reported a higher infection rate in individuals aged between 30 and 40 years [24]. In contrast, other investigators reported a higher incidence rate in children and in less than 20 years old [8, 16, 27, 29, 63, 74, 95, 100]. In a recent study by Al-Hindi and Abu Shammala (2013) in the Gaza strip regarding age, children less than 5 years of age were reported to have a prevalence of 11.3%, while the age-group 20–26 years had 15.4% [4]. This is in contrast to findings by Girginkardesler et al. (2003), who reported that *D. fragilis* infection was higher among children than adult [29]. No plausible explanation to these variations in age distribution of *D. fragilis* incidences is proposed. Nevertheless, hygiene and modest sanitation have been suggested as likely to prejudice groups to infections with *D. fragilis* and other intestinal protozoa irrespective of age making the fecal oral route as the probable route of transmission [12, 24, 53, 101]. With respect to the association between gender and *D. fragilis* infections, numerous studies report dissimilar trends. While several investigators report more infection incidences in females than males [16, 24, 55, 57, 86, 95], other studies describe a drift towards males in certain age-groups [4, 8, 60]. For more details on the subject, the reader is advised to consult the review by Barratt et al. (2011) [12].

## 5. Pathogenicity and clinical symptoms of dientamoebiasis

Originally proposed as a pathogen in 1936 by Hakansson, there still remains some reluctance by many investigators accepting *D. fragilis* as a pathogen [102, 103]. For example, in a recent retrospective case-control study in the Netherlands elucidating the clinical importance of *D. fragilis* in children with chronic abdominal pain, De Jong et al. (2014) detected *D. fragilis* in 43.2% of patients with chronic abdominal pain and in 50.6% in the controls (without gastrointestinal symptoms) ($p = 0.255$) [104]. Thus, there are no significant differences in symptoms comparing children with and without *D. fragilis* infection. Furthermore, no relation was found between clinical and microbiological response after treatment for *D. fragilis* in the same study, suggesting that there is no association between chronic abdominal pain *D. fragilis* infection. Nevertheless, many current studies have acknowledged and confirmed the pathogenic potential of *D. fragilis*. It is often detected in the feces of patients suffering from gastrointestinal tract disorders and presenting symptoms such as loose stools, diarrhea, urgency to defecate, vomiting, nausea, anorexia, weight loss, abdominal pain, and fever [6–9, 11, 21, 29, 105, 106]. Many investigators have reported the tendency for this parasite to cause persistent diarrhea [9, 55]. An example of a study confirming the pathogenic role of *D. fragilis* is an Italian study in 2007, where Crotti and D'Annibale found that between 3.4% and 4.1% of patients with various bowel complaints carried Dientamoeba [55, 57]. Another report corroborating the pathogenic potential of the organism is an Australian study in which 5.4% (35/650) of patients with bowel disorders were reported to have Dientamoeba in their stools, with 83.3% of them suffering from diarrhea [10]. Furthermore, Dientamoeba has been linked it with irritable bowel syndrome (IBS) [22, 97, 105]. Patients carrying Dientamoeba may also experience eosinophilia [10, 63, 64, 103, 106, 107].

## 6. Treatment of *D. fragilis* infections

While still not recognized as a pathogen, the ability to resolve associated symptoms by eradicating *D. fragilis* using different drugs provides some proof for its possible pathogenic nature [6, 16, 20, 69, 102, 103, 108–110]. There is still no agreement as to the best regimen for the complete elimination of the organism. Stark et al. (2010b) and Preiss et al. (1990) reported a treatment ineffectiveness and/or relapse of dientamoebiasis following the use of metronidazole only [11, 64]. In a recent Danish randomized trial, 96 children in Denmark with *D. fragilis* infection and chronic gastrointestinal symptoms were treated with a 10-day course of metronidazole or placebo [111]. Change in gastrointestinal symptoms following treatment did not differ significantly between the groups. Eradication of *D. fragilis* was significantly greater in the metronidazole group as assessed by PCR 2 weeks after completion of therapy, although PCR positivity rebounded by 8 weeks after completion of therapy to levels comparable with those seen in placebo recipients. The eradication of *D. fragilis* was significantly greater in the metronidazole group, although it declined rapidly from 62.5% 2 weeks after end of treatment to 24.9% 8 weeks after end of treatment. The findings of the study did not provide evidence to support routine metronidazole treatment of *D. fragilis*-positive children with chronic gastro-intestinal symptoms. However, the complete resolution of symptoms and elimination of the organism were noted following the administration of either iodoquinol, paromomycin, or a combination of the two [11, 107]. Most recently, Halkjær et al. (2015) described a case history of a 16-year-old Danish patient who had suffered severe abdominal discomfort and flatulence through his lifetime following infection with *D. fragilis*. The patient was treated initially with a high dose of metronidazole, which eradicated the parasite and kept him without symptoms for 1 year [112]. However, recurrence of the symptoms and recurrence of the *D. fragilis* infection were thereafter treated successfully with paromomycin [112]. Other drugs that are also reported to effectively eradicate the parasite leading to clinical cure included oxytetracycline, doxycycline, tinidazole, secnidazole, ornidazole, and erythromycin [29, 30, 64, 102, 113]. Despite the lack of randomized controlled trial data, the literature suggests paromomycin is a more efficacious agent than metronidazole [6, 11, 114]. New potential therapeutic compounds are constantly being screened for by investigators. More recently, Stark et al. (2014) have shown that there is no therapeutic response against dientamoebiasis with benzimidazoles (such as albendazole and mebendazole) [115].

## 7. Role of genetic characteristics of the infecting strains in the pathogenesis of dientamoebiasis

The outcome of an infection may depend on several factors, among which the genetic characteristics of the specific pathogen have been identified as an important one. The virulence and disease outcome has been linked to the genotypes of few parasites such as *Entamoeba histolytica* and *Giardia lamblia* [116–124]. Despite its inability to ascertain correlation between genotype and disease outcome, evidence emerged using the ssu rRNA gene of at least two genetically distinct variants (genotypes 1 and 2) of *D. fragilis* are in existence [6, 9, 20, 125, 126]. Thus, in the case of *D. fragilis* infections, the ssu rRNA gene demonstrated inferiority as a tool for molecular epidemiological studies [127]. Accordingly, new molecular tools were employed to demonstrate the association between variants and clinical disease outcome. One such tool is the use of C-profiling in which the cysteine nucleotide pattern is compared between samples for evidence of genetic variation on the internal transcribed spacer regions (ITS1 and ITS2) of the ribosomal gene [128]. These regions are noncoding sequences reported to be suitable for molecular characterization of phylogenetically related organisms [129]. Bart et al. (2008) and Stark and his group (2009) documented the occurrence in variations of ITS1 in *D. fragilis* isolates [21, 130]. Furthermore, a correlation between certain ITS1 variants and disease outcome was reported [130]. Recently, Barratt et al. (2010) found that the growth of Dientamoeba in certain media formulations varied between different isolates, and while all Dientamoeba isolates described by Barratt and colleagues were from patients with gastrointestinal complaints, this work indicates that phenotypic diversity exists in Dientamoeba and that the variation noted is likely to have a genetic basis. Nevertheless, it is still unclear whether the two genotypes differ in their pathogenicity [131].

## 8. Diagnosis of dientamoebiasis

While it is difficult to identify the trophozoites of *D. fragilis* morphologically, the only diagnostic tool used to detect *D. fraglis* is microscopy using permanent stained smears. A large variety of stains have been used for the microscopic examination of *E. fragilis*. However, the most commonly used that also give much clearer images of the parasites are the trichrome and the iron-hematoxylin stains. The sample should be fixed immediately after staining to avoid degeneration of the trophozoites and staining should also occur sooner [107]. Trophozoites range in size from 5 to 15 μm in length, from 9 to 12 μm in width, normally with 1–2 fragmented nuclei with visible holes seen through the nucleus center. Smears may also contain trophozoites with the typical four nucleated form. No cyst stage has been recovered yet from humans despite being observed in mice [23]. Even under ideal conditions, with prompt preservation of stool and evaluation of permanent stained smears by experienced microscopists, Stark et al. (2010a and 2011) reported a sensitivity of 34% and 38%, respectively, compared to PCR (real-time and multiplex tandem—PCR) [10, 132]. Despite numerous studies reporting common occurrence of *D. fragilis* infection, no clinical antigen-based, molecular, or serologic diagnostics have been commercially developed to aid with laboratory identification to date, although current molecular based methods are used for research [133]. The culture of *D. fragilis* has been reported and is done in similar conditions as that of *E. histolytica*. Liquid or diphasic media is used that can be in xenic or axenic conditions [10]. Another diphasic medium based on the Loeffler's slope has also been demonstrated, and Earle's balanced salt solution (EBSS) has been successfully used for the growth of *D. fragilis* [23].

Molecular diagnostic methods have been very instrumental for the improvement of our understanding of different infections. There has been a significant gain in the development of molecular methods for the detection of *D. fragilis*, although compared to other organisms, this improvement has been much slower [32]. Several PCR protocols have been developed for the detection of this organism mainly for research laboratories. These protocols vary from conventional PCR to real-time PCR with increased sensitivity and specificity. Primers based on the small ribosomal RNA gene have been developed for this purpose [9]. Verweij and colleagues have developed a real-time PCR protocol using the 5.8S ribosomal RNA gene and they showed that this method was both specific and sensitive [28]. A variation of PCR based on the amplification of the internal transcribed spacer 1 region of *D. fragilis* has also been used for the molecular characterization of the parasite [130]. The actin gene has also been used as a target for the molecular characterization of this parasite [128]. Generally, the detection and/or the molecular characterization of the parasite begin with DNA purification, which is a very important and critical step in the amplification of the organism. Following DNA purification, the PCR master mixed is prepared depending on the procedure to be used. In the case of detection, the PCR protocol is generally sufficient. However, the molecular characterization often requires a sequencing step with or without the purification of the PCR amplicons. Other methods that have been used so far for the molecular characterization of *D. fragilis* include high-resolution melt curve analysis (HRM) and restriction fragment length polymorphism after amplification by PCR [9, 22].

Using HRM, Hussein and colleagues found 4 genetic profiles of which the first and most common profile and the last profile (Profile 4) were more associated with diarrhea compared to the two middle profiles [22]. However, the ITS showed two major genotypes although there were subgenotypes among those main categories. In another study, the ITS-1-5.8S rRNA gene-ITS-2 region of *D. fragilis* was found to be highly variable and pyrosequencing method identified 11 different alleles of the ITS-1 sequence showing the limitation of this gene in the molecular characterization of the parasite [130]. Briefly, the use of molecular methods has increased our knowledge on these organisms; much still remains to be discovered for the better understanding of issues related to pathogenicity, diagnosis, and prognosis.

## 9. Conclusion

Known for almost a hundred years now, *D. fragilis* still remains a mysterious organism although much has been learned. The use of molecular biology has clarified its classification not as an amoeba but as a trichomonad. However, its pathogenicity as well as its genetic diversity still remains to be clarified. Diagnosis particularly in developing areas of the world where it could be common remains difficult because microscopy is not sensitive. This is made to be even more difficult because of the uncertainty of the existence of a cyst stage, which so far has only been demonstrated in very limited studies. Real-time PCR has been proven to be more sensitive compared to all the other diagnostic methods, including conventional PCR, microscopy, and culture. Further studies are needed, and collaboration between developing and developed countries will help boost the research capacity on this infection and improve our understanding of its distribution, pathogenicity, and immunology.

## Acknowledgements

We thank Dr. Wiam Elshami from the University of Sharjah, UAE, for her help in the preparation and referencing of the chapter.

## Author details

Ali ElBakri[1], Ahmed Al-Qahtani[2] and Amidou Samie[3]

*Address all correspondence to: samieamidou@yahoo.com

1 Medical Laboratory Sciences Department, University of Sharjah, Sharjah, UAE

2 Health Sciences Department, Al Khawarizmi International College, AbuDhabi, UAE

3 Molecular parasitology and opportunistic infections program, Department of Microbiology, University of Venda, Thohoyandou, South Africa

## References


[1] Camp RR, Mattern CF, Honigberg BM. Study of *Dientamoeba fragilis* Jepps & Dobell I. Electronmicroscopic observations of the binucleate stages. II. Taxonomic position and revision of the genus. J Protozool. 1974; 21:69–82.

[2] Delgado-Viscogliosi P, Viscogliosi E, Gerbod D, Kulda J, Sogin ML, Edgcomb VP. Molecular phylogeny of parabasalids based on small subunit rRNA sequences, with emphasis on the Trichomonadinae subfamily. J Eukaryot Microbiol. 2000; 47:70–5.

[3] Gerbod D, Edgcomb VP, Noel C, Zenner L, Wintjens R, Delgado-Viscogliosi P, et al. Phylogenetic position of the trichomonad parasite of turkeys, *Histomonas meleagridis* (Smith) Tyzzer, inferred from small subunit rRNA sequence. J Eukaryot Microbiol. 2001; 48: 498–504.

[4] Al-Hindi AI, Abu-Shammala BM. *Dientamoeba fragilis* in Gaza Strip: a neglected protozoan parasite. Iran J Parasitol. 2013; 8: 249–55.

[5] Jepps MW, Dobell C. *Dientamoeba fragilis* n.g., n. sp.: a new intestinal amoeba from man. Parasitology 1918; 10:352–67.

[6] Vandenberg O, Peek R, Souayah H, Dediste A, Buset M, Scheen R, et al. Clinical and microbiological features of dientamoebiasis in patients suspected of suffering from a parasitic gastrointestinal illness: a comparison of *Dientamoeba fragilis* and *Giardia lamblia* infections. Int J Infect Dis. 2006; 10:255–61.

[7] Crotti D, D'Annibale ML, Fonzo G, Lalle M, Caccio SM, Pozio E. *Dientamoeba fragilis* is more prevalent than Giardia duodenalis in children and adults attending a day care centre in Central Italy. Parasite. 2005; 12:165–70.

[8] Norberg A, Nord CE, Evengard B. *Dientamoeba fragilis*—a protozoal infection which may cause severe bowel distress. Clin Microbiol Infect. 2003; 9:65–8.

[9] Stark D, Beebe N, Marriott D, Ellis J, Harkness J. Prospective study of the prevalence, genotyping and clinical relevance of *Dientamoeba fragilis* infections in an Australian population. J Clin Microbiol. 2005; 43:2718–23.

[10] Stark D, Barratt J, Roberts T, Marriot D, Harkness J, Ellis J. Comparison of microscopy, two xenic culture techniques, conventional and real-time PCR for the detection of *Dientamoeba fragilis* in clinical stool samples. Eur J Clin Microbiol Infect Dis. 2010a; 29:411–6.

[11] Stark D, Barratt J, Roberts T, Marriott D, Harkness J, Ellis J. A review of the clinical presentation of dientamoebiasis. Am J Trop Med Hyg. 2010b; 82:614–9.

[12] Barratt JLN, Harkness J, Marriott D, Ellis JT, Stark D. A review of *Dientamoeba fragilis* carriage in humans: several reasons why this organism should be considered in the diagnosis of gastrointestinal illness. Gut Microb. 2011; 2: 3–12.

[13] Hakansson EG. *Dientamoeba fragilis*, a cause of illness: report of a case. Am J Trop Med Hyg 1936; 16:175–8.

[14] Ottilio MJ, Luiz de Pinho A, Silva S, Rodrigues Gomes FJ. Parasitic aspects of *Dientamoeba fragilis*. Pathogenic action and therapy. Bull Soc Pathol Exot Filiales. 1968; 61:30–5.

[15] Addadi K, Le Corroller Y, Guy Y, Tabet-Derraz A. Possible pathogenicity of *Dientamoeba fragilis*. Bull Soc Pathol Exot Filiales. 1972; 65:274–5.

[16] Yang J, Scholten T. *Dientamoeba fragilis*: a review with notes on its epidemiology, pathogenicity, mode of transmission and diagnosis. Am J Trop Med Hyg. 1977; 26:16–22.

[17] Ockert G, Schulz U. Pathogenetic role of *Dientamoeba fragilis*. Dtsch Gesundheitsw. 1972; 27:1156–8.

[18] Desser SS, Yang YJ. Letter: *Dientamoeba fragilis* in idiopathic gastrointestinal disorders. Can Med Assoc J. 1976; 114:290–3.

[19] Shein R, Gelb A. Colitis due to *Dientamoeba fragilis*. Am J Gastroenterol. 1983; 78:634–6.

[20] Stark DJ, Beebe N, Marriott D, Ellis JT, Harkness J. Dientamoebiasis: clinical importance and recent advances. Trends Parasitol. 2006; 22:92–6.

[21] Windsor JJ, Macfarlane L. Irritable bowel syndrome: the need to exclude *Dientamoeba fragilis*. Am J Trop Med Hyg. 2005; 72:501–2.

[22] Hussein EM, Al-Mohammed HI, Hussein AM. Genetic diversity of *Dientamoeba fragilis* isolates of irritable bowel syndrome patients by high-resolution melting-curve (HRM) analysis. Parasitol Res. 2009; 105:1053–60.

[23] Munasinghe VS, Vella NGF, Ellis JT, Windosr P, Stark D. Cyst formation and faecal–oral transmission of *Dientamoeba fragilis*– the missing link in the life cycle of an emerging pathogen. Int J Parasitol. 2013; 43: 879–883.

[24] Rayan HZ, Ismail OA, El Gayar EK. Prevalence and clinical features of *Dientamoeba fragilis* infections in patients suspected to have intestinal parasitic infection. J Egypt Soc Parasitol. 2007; 37:599–608.

[25] Stensvold CR, Arendrup MC, Molbak K, Nielsen HV. The prevalence of *Dientamoeba fragilis* in patients with suspected enteroparasitic disease in a metropolitan area in Denmark. Clin Microbiol Infect. 2007; 13:839–42.

[26] Barratt J, Harkness J, Marriott D, Ellis J, Stark D. The ambiguous life of *Dientamoeba fragilis*: the need to investigate current hypotheses on transmission. Parasitology. 2011a; 138: 557–572.

[27] Chan F, Stewart N, Guan M, Robb I, Fuite L, Chan I, et al. Prevalence of *Dientamoeba fragilis* antibodies in children and recognition of a 39 kDa immunodominant protein antigen of the organism. Eur J Clin Microbiol Infect Dis. 1996; 15:950–4.

[28] Verweij JJ, Mulder B, Poell B, van Middelkoop D, Brienen EA, van Lieshout L. Real-time PCR for the detection of *Dientamoeba fragilis* in fecal samples. Mol Cell Probes. 2007; 21:400–4.

[29] Girginkardesler N, Coskun S, Cuneyt Balcioglu I, Ertan P, Ok UZ. *Dientamoeba fragilis*, a neglected cause of diarrhea, successfully treated with secnidazole. Clin Microbiol Infect. 2003; 9:110–3.

[30] Kurt O, Girginkardesler N, Balcioglu IC, Ozbilgin A, Ok UZ. A comparison of metronidazole and singledose ornidazole for the treatment of dientamoebiasis. Clin Microbiol Infect. 2008; 14:601–4.

[31] Banik et al. A microscopic description and ultrastructural characterisation of *Dientamoeba fragilis*: an emerging cause of human enteric disease. International Journal for Parasitology. 2012; 42: 139–53.

[32] Johnson EH, Windsor JJ, Clark CG. Emerging from obscurity: biological, clinical and diagnostic aspects of *Dientamoeba fragilis*. Clin Microbiol Rev. 2004; 17:553–70.

[33] Benchimol M. Trichomonads under microscopy. Microsc Microanal. 2004a; 10: 528–550.

[34] Carlton JM, Hirt RP, Silva JC, Delcher AL, Schatz M, Zhao Q, Wortman JR, Bidwell SL, Alsmark UCM, Besteiro SB, Sicheritz-Ponten T, Noel CJ, Dacks JB, Foster PG et al. Draft genome sequence of the sexually transmitted pathogen *Trichomonas vaginalis*. Science. 2007; 315: 207–212.

[35] Benchimol M, Kachar B, de Souza W. The structural organization of the pathogenic protozoan *Tritrichomonas foetus* as seen in replicas of quick frozen, freeze-fractured and deep etched cells. Biol Cell. 1993; 77: 289–295.

[36] Benchimol M, Engelke F. Hydrogenosome behavior during the cell cycle in *Tritrichomonas foetus*. Biol Cell. 2003; 95: 283–293.

[37] Benchimol M. Hydrogenosomes under microscopy. Tissue Cell. 2009; 41: 151–168.

[38] Shiflett AM, Johnson PJ. Mitochondrion-related organelles in eukaryotic protists. Annu Rev Microbiol. 2010; 64:409–429.

[39] Stairs CW, Roger AJ, Hampl V. Eukaryotic pyruvate formate lyase and its activating enzyme were acquired laterally from a firmicute. Mol Biol Evol. 2011; 28: 2087–2099.

[40] Wang AL, Wang CC. A linear double-stranded RNA in *Trichomonas vaginalis*. J Biol Chem. 1985; 260: 3697–3702.

[41] Wang AL, Wang CC. The double-stranded RNA in *Trichomonas vaginalis* may originate from virus-like particles. Proc Natl Acad Sci USA. 1986a; 83: 7956–7960.

[42] Wang AL, Wang CC. Discovery of a specific double-stranded RNA virus in *Giardia lamblia.* Mol Biochem Parasitol. 1986b; 21: 269–276.

[43] Tarr PI, Aline Jr. RF, Smiley BL, Scholler J, Keithly J, Stuart K. LR1: a candidate RNA virus of *Leishmania.* Proc Natl Acad Sci USA. 1988; 85: 9572–9575.

[44] Gerhold RW, Allison AB, Sellers H, Linnemann E, Chang TH, Alderete JF. Examination for double-stranded RNA viruses in Trichomonas gallinae and identification of a novel sequence of a *Trichomonas vaginalis* virus. Parasitol Res. 2009; 105: 775–779.

[45] Fraga J, Rojas L, Sariego I, Fernández-Calienes A. Double-stranded RNA viral infection of *Trichomonas vaginalis* and correlation with genetic polymorphism of isolates. Exp Parasitol. 2011; 127: 593–599.

[46] Malla N, Kaul P, Sehgal R, Gupta I. The presence of dsRNA virus in *Trichomonas vaginalis* isolates from symptomatic and asymptomatic Indian women and its correlation with in vitro metronidazole sensitivity. Indian J Med Microbiol. 2011; 29: 152–157.

[47] Dobell C. Researches on intestinal protozoa in monkeys and man. X. The life history of *Dientamoeba fragilis*: observations, experiments and speculations. Parasitology. 1940; 32:417–61.

[48] Roser D, Nejsum P, Carlsgart AJ, Nielsen HV, Stensvold CR. DNA of *Dientamoeba fragilis* detected within surface-sterilized eggs of *Enterobius vermicularis*. Exp Parasitol. 2013; 133: 57–61.

[49] Girginkardesler N, Kurt O, Kilimcioglu AA, Ok UZ. Transmission of *Dientamoeba fragilis*: evaluation of the role of *Enterobius vermicularis.* Parasitol Int. 2008; 57: 72–75.

[50] Stark D, Garcia LS, Barratt JLN, Phillips O, Roberts T, Marriott D, harkness D, Ellis JT. Description of *Dientamoeba fragilis* cyst and precystic forms from human samples. J Clin Microbiol. 2014; 52: 2680–3.

[51] Caccio SM, Sannella AR, Manuali E, Tosini F, Sensi M, Crotti D, Pozio E. Pigs as natural hosts of *Dientamoeba fragilis* genotypes found in humans. Emerg Infect Dis. 2012; 18: 838–841.

[52] Clark CG, Röser D, Stensvold CR. Transmission of *Dientamoeba fragilis*: pinworm or cysts? Trends Parasitol. 2014; 30: 136–40.

[53] Millet V, Spencer MJ, Chapin M, Stewart M, Yatabe JA, Brewer T, et al. *Dientamoeba fragilis*, a protozoan parasite in adult members of a semicommunal group. Dig Dis Sci. 1983; 28:335–9.

[54] Spencer E, Araya M, Sandino AM, Pacheco I, Brunser O. Faecal excretion of rotavirus and other enteropathogens in newborns of the high and low socio-economic stratum in Santiago, Chile. Epidemiol Infect. 1988; 101:425–36.

[55] Crotti D, D'Annibale ML. Intestinal infections caused by *Dientamoeba fragilis* and Giardia duodenalis in our experience. Recenti Prog Med. 2007a; 98:361–6.

[56] Hamze M, Naja M, Mallat H. Biological analysis of workers in the food sector in north Lebanon. East Mediterr Health J. 2008; 14:1425–34.

[57] Crotti D, D'Annibale ML. Role of *Dientamoeba fragilis* in human bowel infections. Infez Med. 2007b; 15:30–9.

[58] Crotti D, D'Annibale ML. Human intestinal parasitosis: role of *Dientamoeba fragilis* in human infections. Ann Ig. 2007c; 19:27–34.

[59] Windsor JJ, Rafay AM, Shenoy AK, Johnson EH. Incidence of *Dientamoeba fragilis* in faecal samples submitted for routine microbiological analysis. Br J Biomed Sci. 1998; 55:172–5.

[60] Lagace-Wiens PR, VanCaeseele PG, Koschik C. *Dientamoeba fragilis*: an emerging role in intestinal disease. CMAJ. 2006; 175:468–9.

[61] Crotti D, D'Annibale ML. *Dientamoeba fragilis* and dientamoebiasis: aspects of clinical parasitology and laboratory diagnosis. Parassitologia. 2001; 43:135–8.

[62] Walker JC, Bahr G, Ehl AS. Gastrointestinal parasites in Sydney. Med J Aust. 1985; 143:480.

[63] Preiss U, Ockert G, Broemme S, Otto A. On the clinical importance of *Dientamoeba fragilis* infections in childhood. J Hyg Epidemiol Microbiol Immunol. 1991; 35:27–34.

[64] Preiss U, Ockert G, Bromme S, Otto A. *Dientamoeba fragilis* infection, a cause of gastrointestinal symptoms in childhood. Klin Padiatr. 1990; 202:120–3.

[65] Keystone JS, Yang J, Grisdale D, Harrington M, Pillon L, Andreychuk R. Intestinal parasites in metropolitan Toronto day-care centres. Can Med Assoc J. 1984; 131:733–5.

[66] Windsor JJ, Macfarlane L, Hughes-Thapa G, Jones SK, Whiteside TM. Detection of *Dientamoeba fragilis* by culture. Br J Biomed Sci. 2003; 60: 79–83.

[67] Schuster H, Jackson RS. Prevalence of *Dientamoeba fragilis* among patients consulting complementary medicine practitioners in the British Isles. J Clin Pathol. 2008; 62:182–4.

[68] Brug SL. Observations on *Dientamoeba fragilis*. Ann Trop Med Parasitol. 1938; 30:441–52.

[69] Kean BH, Malloch CL. The neglected ameba: *Dientamoeba fragilis*. A report of 100 "pure" infections. Am J Dig Dis. 1966; 11:735–46.

[70] Steinitz H, Talis B, Stein B. *Entamoeba histolytica* and *Dientamoeba fragilis* and the syndrome of chronic recurrent intestinal amoebiasis in Israel. Digestion. 1970; 3:146–53.

[71] Sukanahakeru S. The presence of *Dientamoeba fragilis* in the Ascaris lumbricoides ova: the first report from Thailand. J Med Assoc Thai. 1977; 60:256–8.

[72] Sargeaunt PG, Williams JE, Kumate J, Jimenez E. The epidemiology of *Entamoeba histolytica* in Mexico City. A pilot survey I. Trans R Soc Trop Med Hyg. 1980; 74:653–6.

[73] Sargeaunt PG, Williams JE, Jackson TF, Simjee AE. A zymodeme study of *Entamoeba histolytica* in a group of South African schoolchildren. Trans R Soc Trop Med Hyg. 1982; 76:401–2.

[74] Spencer MJ, Millet VE, Garcia LS, Rhee L, Masterson L. Parasitic infections in a pediatric population. Pediatr Infect Dis. 1983; 2:110–3.

[75] Ortega HB, Borchardt KA, Hamilton R, Ortega P, Mahood J. Enteric pathogenic protozoa in homosexual men from San Francisco. Sex Transm Dis. 1984; 11:59–63.

[76] Peters CS, Sable R, Janda WM, Chittom AL, Kocka FE. Prevalence of enteric parasites in homosexual patients attending an outpatient clinic. J Clin Microbiol. 1986; 24:684–5.

[77] Muller R, Lillywhite J, Bending JJ, Catford JC. Human cysticercosis and intestinal parasitism amongst the Ekari people of Irian Jaya. J Trop Med Hyg. 1987; 90:291–6.

[78] Oxner RB, Paltridge GP, Chapman BA, Cook HB, Sheppard PF. *Dientamoeba fragilis*: a bowel pathogen? N Z Med J. 1987; 100:64–5.

[79] Kaminsky RG. Parasitism and diarrhoea in children from two rural communities and marginal barrio in Honduras. Trans R Soc Trop Med Hyg. 1991; 85:70–3.

[80] Tavarez LA, Pena F, Placencia F, Mendoza HR, Polanco D. Prevalence of protozoans in children with acute diarrheal disease. Arch Domin Pediatr. 1991; 27:43–7.

[81] Sawangjaroen N, Luke R, Prociv P. Diagnosis by faecal culture of *Dientamoeba fragilis* infections in Australian patients with diarrhoea. Trans R Soc Trop Med Hyg. 1993; 87:163–5.

[82] Mendez OC, Szmulewicz G, Menghi C, Torres S, Gonzalez G, Gatta C. Comparison of intestinal parasite infestation indexes among HIV positive and negative populations. Medicina (B Aires). 1994; 54:307–10.

[83] Meropol SB. Health status of pediatric refugees in Buffalo NY. Arch Pediatr Adolesc Med. 1995; 149:887–92.

[84] van Gool T, Dankert J. 3 emerging protozoal infections in the Netherlands: Cyclospora, Dientamoeba and Microspora infections. Ned Tijdschr Geneeskd. 1996; 140:155–60.

[85] Lindo JF, Dubon JM, Ager AL, De Gourville EM, Solo-Gabriele H, Klaskala WI, et al. Intestinal parasitic infections in human immunodeficiency virus (HIV)-positive and

HIV-negative individuals in San Pedro Sula, Honduras. Am J Trop Med Hyg. 1998; 58:431–5.

[86] Ayadi A, Bahri I. *Dientamoeba fragilis*: pathogenic flagellate? Bulletin de la Societe de Pathologie Exotique. 1999; 92:299–301.

[87] Lainson R, da Silva BA. Intestinal parasites of some diarrhoeic HIV-seropositive individuals in North Brazil, with particular reference to Isospora belli Wenyon, 1923 and *Dientamoeba fragilis* Jepps & Dobell 1918. Mem Inst Oswaldo Cruz. 1999; 94:611–3.

[88] Karaman U, Atambay M, Aycan O, Yologlu S, Daldal N. Incidence of intestinal parasites in municipal sanitary workers in Malatya. Turkiye Parazitol Derg. 2006; 30:181–3.

[89] Kassem HH, Zaed HA, Sadaga GA. Intestinal parasitic infection among children and neonatus admitted to Ibn-Sina Hospital, Sirt, Libya. J Egypt Soc Parasitol. 2007; 37:371–80.

[90] Menghi CI, Iuvaro FR, Dellacasa MA, Gatta CL. Survey of intestinal parasites among an aboriginal community in Salta. Medicina (B Aires). 2007; 67:705–8.

[91] Ozcakir O, Gureser S, Erguven S, Yilmaz YA, Topaloglu R, Hascelik G. Characteristics of *Blastocystis hominis* infection in a Turkish university hospital. Turkiye Parazitol Derg. 2007; 31:277–82.

[92] Stark D, Fotedar R, van Hal S, Beebe N, Marriott D, Ellis JT, et al. Prevalence of enteric protozoa in human immunodeficiency virus (HIV)-positive and HIV-negative men who have sex with men from Sydney, Australia. Am J Trop Med Hyg. 2007; 76:549–52.

[93] Bruijnesteijn van Coppenraet LE, Wallinga JA, Ruijs GJ, Bruins MJ, Verweij JJ. Parasitological diagnosis combining an internally controlled real-time PCR assay for the detection of four protozoa in stool samples with a testing algorithm for microscopy. Clin Microbiol Infect. 2009; 15:869–74.

[94] Cengiz ZT, Akbayram S, Cicek M, Yilmaz H. Intestinal parasitoses detected in primary schoolchildren in the Van province. Turkiye Parazitol Derg. 2009; 33:289–93.

[95] Gonzalez-Moreno O, Domingo L, Teixidor J, Gracenea M. Prevalence and associated factors of intestinal parasitisation: a cross-sectional study among outpatients with gastrointestinal symptoms in Catalonia, Spain. Parasitol Res. 2011; 108: 87–93.

[96] Calderaro A, Gorrini C, Montecchini S, Peruzzi S, Piccolo G, Rossi S, et al. Evaluation of a real-time polymerase chain reaction assay for the detection of *Dientamoeba fragilis*. Diagn Microbiol Infect Dis. 2010; 67:239–45.

[97] Yakoob J, Jafri W, Beg MA, Abbas Z, Naz S, Islam M, et al. *Blastocystis hominis* and *Dientamoeba fragilis* in patients fulfilling irritable bowel syndrome criteria. Parasitol Res. 2010; 107:679–84.

[98] Stark D, Al-Qassab SE, Barratt JL, Stanley K, Roberts T, Marriott D, et al. An evaluation of a multiplex tandem real-time PCR for the detection of Cryptosporidium spp, *Dientamoeba fragilis*, *Entamoeba histolytica* and *Giardia intestinalis* from clinical stool samples. J Clin Microbiol. 2010c; 49:257–62.

[99] Sarafraz S, Farajnia S, Jamali J, Khodabakhsh F, Khanipour F. Detection of *Dientamoeba fragilis* among diarrheal patients referred to Tabriz health care centers by nested PCR. Tropical Biomedicine. 2013; 30: 113–118.

[100] de Wit MA, Koopmans MP, Kortbeek LM, van Leeuwen NJ, Vinje J, van Duynhoven YT. Etiology of gastroenteritis in sentinel general practices in the Netherlands. Clin Infect Dis. 2001; 33:280–8.

[101] El-Taweel GE, Shaban AM. Microbiological quality of drinking water at eight water treatment plants. Int J Environ Health Res. 2001; 11:285–90.

[102] Bosman DK, Benninga MA, van de Berg P, Kooijman GC, van Gool T. *Dientamoeba fragilis*: possibly an important cause of persistent abdominal pain in children. Ned Tijdschr Geneeskd. 2004; 148:575–9.

[103] Spencer MJ, Garcia LS, Chapin MR. *Dientamoeba fragilis*. An intestinal pathogen in children? Am J Dis Child. 1979; 133:390–3.

[104] De Jong MJ, Korterink JJ, Benninga Ma, Hilbink M, Widdershoven J, Deckers-Kocken JM. *Dientamoeba fragilis* and chronic abdominal pain in children: a case-control study. Arch Dis Child. 2014; 99: 1109–13. doi: 10.1136/archdischild-2014-305942.

[105] Stark D, Barratt J, Ellis J, Harkness J, Marriott D. Repeated *Dientamoeba fragilis* infections: a case report of two families from Sydney, Australia. Infect Dis Rep. 2009; 1:7–9.

[106] Cuffari C, Oligny L, Seidman EG. *Dientamoeba fragilis* masquerading as allergic colitis. J Pediatr Gastroenterol Nutr. 1998; 26:16–20.

[107] Windsor JJ, Johnson EH. *Dientamoeba fragilis*: the unflagellated human flagellate. Br J Biomed Sci. 1999; 56:293–306.

[108] Borody TJ, Warren EF, Wettstein A, Robertson G, Recabarren P, Fontela A, et al. Eradication of *Dientamoeba fragilis* can resolve IBS-like symptoms. J Gastroenterol Hepatol. 2002; 17:103.

[109] Chan FT, Guan MX, Mackenzie AM, Diaz-Mitoma F. Susceptibility testing of *Dientamoeba fragilis* ATCC 30948 with iodoquinol, paromomycin, tetracycline and metronidazole. Antimicrob Agents Chemother. 1994; 38:1157–60.

[110] Spencer MJ, Chapin MR, Garcia LS. *Dientamoeba fragilis*: a gastrointestinal protozoan infection in adults. Am J Gastroenterol. 1982; 77:565–9.

[111] Röser D, Simonsen J, Stensvold CR, Olsen KE, Bytzer P, Nielsen HV, Mølbak K. Metronidazole therapy for treating dientamoebiasis in children is not associated with

better clinical outcomes: a randomized, double-blinded and placebo-controlled clinical trial. Clin Infect Dis. 2014; 58: 1692–9. DOI: 10.1093/cid/ciu188.

[112] Halkjær S, Stensvold CR, Petersen AM. *Dientamoeba fragilis* infection as cause of severe abdominal discomfort and flatulence. Ugeskr Laeger. 2015; 177:2A.

[113] Butler WP. *Dientamoeba fragilis*. An unusual intestinal pathogen. Dig Dis Sci. 1996; 41:1811–3.

[114] van Hellemond JJ, Molhoek N, Koelewijn R, Wismans PJ, van Genderen PJ. Is paromomycin the drug of choice for eradication of *Dientamoeba fragilis* in adults? Int J Parasitol Drugs Drug Resist. 2012; 14:162–5. doi: 10.1016/j.ijpddr.2012.03.002.

[115] Stark D, Barratt JL, Roberts T, Marriott D, Harkness JT, Ellis J. Activity of benzimidazoles against *Dientamoeba fragilis* (Trichomonadida, Monocercomonadidae) in vitro and correlation of beta-tubulin sequences as an indicator of resistance. Parasite. 2014;21:41. doi: 10.1051/parasite/2014043. Epub 2014 Aug 25.

[116] Ali IKM, Mondal U, Roy S, Haque R, Petri WA, Jr, Clark CG. Evidence for a link between parasite genotype and outcome of infection with *Entamoeba histolytica*. J Clin Microbiol. 2007; 45: 285–289.

[117] Paul J, Srivastava S, Bhattacharya S. Molecular methods for diagnosis of *Entamoeba histolytica* in a clinical setting: an overview. Exp Parasitol. 2007; 116: 35–43.

[118] 118. Clark CG. Methods for the investigation of diversity in *Entamoeba histolytica*. Arch Med Res. 2006; 37:258–262.

[119] Aydin AF, Besibellioglu BA, Avci IY et al. Classification of *Giardia duodenalis* parasites in Turkey into groups A and B using restriction fragment length polymorphism. Diagn Microbiol Infect Dis. 2004;50:147–51.

[120] Haque R, Roy S, Kabir M et al. *Giardia* assemblage A infection and diarrhea in Bangladesh. J Infect Dis. 2005;192:2171–3.

[121] Homan WL, Mank TG. Human giardiasis: genotype linked differences in clinical symptomatology. Int J Parasitol. 2001;31:822–6.

[122] Paintlia AS, Mahajan RC, Chakraborti A et al. Characterization of *Giardia lamblia* groups A and B from North India by isoenzyme and random amplified polymorphic DNA analysis. Parasitol Res. 1999;85:510–2.

[123] Mohammed Mahdy AK, Surin J, Wan KL et al. *Giardia intestinalis* genotypes: risk factors and correlation with clinical symptoms. Acta Trop. 2009;112:67–70.

[124] Al-Mohammed HI. Genotypes of *Giardia intestinalis* clinical isolates of gastrointestinal symptomatic and asymptomatic Saudi children. Parasitol Res. 2011;108:1375–81. doi: 10.1007/s00436-010-2033-5.

[125] Johnson JA, Clark CG. Cryptic genetic diversity in *Dientamoeba fragilis*. J Clin Microbiol. 2000; 38:4653–4.

[126] Clark CG. Cryptic genetic variation in parasitic protozoa. J Med Microbiol. 2000; 49:489–91.

[127] Peek R, Reedeker FR, van Gool T. Direct amplification and genotyping of *Dientamoeba fragilis* from human stool specimens. J Clin Microbiol. 2004; 42: 631–5.

[128] Stensvold CR, Clark CG, Roser D. Limited intra-genetic diversity in *Dientamoeba fragilis* housekeeping genes. Infect Genet Evol. 2013; 18: 284–6. doi:10.1016/j.meegid.2013.05.003

[129] Hillis, D. M., and M. T. Dixon. Ribosomal DNA: molecular evolution and phylogenetic inference. Quar Rev Bio. 1991; 66:411–53.

[130] Bart A, van der Heijden HM, Greve S, Speijer D, Landman WJ, van Gool T. Intragenomic variation in the internal transcribed spacer 1 region of *Dientamoeba fragilis* as a molecular epidemiological marker. J Clin Microbiol. 2008; 46:3270–5.

[131] Barratt JL, Banik GR, Harkness J, Marriott D, Ellis JT, Stark D. Newly defined conditions for the in vitro cultivation and cryopreservation of *Dientamoeba fragilis*: new techniques set to fast track molecular studies on this organism. Parasitology. 2010; 137:1867–78.

[132] Stark D, Al-Qassab SE, Barratt JL, Stanley K, Roberts T, Marriott D, Harkness J, Ellis JT. Evaluation of multiplex tandem real-time PCR for detection of *Cryptosporidium* spp., *Dientamoeba fragilis*, *Entamoeba histolytica*, and *Giardia intestinalis* in clinical stool samples. J Clin Microbiol. 2011; 49:257–62.

[133] McHardy IH, Wu M, Shimizu-Cohen R, Couturier MR, Humphries RM. Detection of intestinal protozoa in the clinical laboratory. J Clin Microbiol. 2014; 52: 712–20.

Chapter 5

# Speciation in the *Leishmania guyanensis* Vector *Lutzomyia umbratilis* (Diptera: Psychodidae) from Northern Brazil — Implications for Epidemiology and Vector Control

Vera Margarete Scarpassa and
Ronildo Baiatone Alencar

Additional information is available at the end of the chapter

http://dx.doi.org/10.5772/60921

**Abstract**

This chapter starts with a brief mention of the *Leishmania* species and sandflies vectors that occur in the Neotropical region, especially in the Brazilian Amazon. The main focus of this chapter is a review of the taxonomic, biologic and epidemiologic studies conducted in *Lutzomyia umbratilis*, the main vector of *Leishmania guyanensis* in the northern region of Brazil. We associated these data with the population genetics studies carried out in this sandfly vector by our research team. The genetic studies were made with six samples of *L. umbratilis* from the central region of the Brazilian Amazon, using a large fragment (1,181 bp) of the mitochondrial DNA *COI* gene. Also, another study was conducted in these samples using the DNA barcode region. The results revealed rather high levels of genetic variability for all samples analyzed and a pronounced genetic differentiation between samples from both banks of the Negro and Amazon rivers. The degree of differentiation found may reflect the presence of distinct species within *L. umbratilis*, suggesting that the Amazon and Negro rivers may be acting as effective barriers, preventing gene flow between populations living on the two sides. These findings have important implications for epidemiology, especially regarding vector competence, which is vital information for surveillance and vector control strategies. Furthermore, this diversification process of *L. umbratilis* represents an interesting example for speciation studies.

**Keywords:** Sandflies, Brazilian Amazon, Population genetics, Speciation, Cryptic species

## 1. Introduction

Phlebotomine sandflies (Diptera: Psychodidae) are insects of medical and veterinary importance since they are involved in transmission of various pathogens (bacteria, virus and protozoa) that cause diseases such as Bartonellosis, Arboviruses and Leishmaniasis. The latter is caused by trypanosomatids of the genus *Leishmania*, the pathogenic agent of human leishmaniasis. *Leishmania* infection is characterized by a species-specific pathology, varying from cutaneous lesions to the potentially fatal visceral form [1-3]. The distribution of this disease encompasses the tropical, subtropical and Mediterranean regions of the world and its global burden has been estimated to be approximately 500,000 cases of visceral leishmaniasis (VL) and approximately 1.1-1.5 million cases of cutaneous leishmaniasis (CL) per year (4,5]. Despite its widespread distribution, most of the leishmaniasis cases occur in only a few countries: more than 90% of the VL cases occur in Bangladesh, Brazil, Ethiopia, India, South Sudan and Sudan, and most of the CL cases occur in Afghanistan, Algeria, Brazil, Colombia, Iran, Pakistan, Peru, Saudi Arabia and Syria [5].

In the Americas, CL occurs from southern USA to northern Argentina, but its main focus is concentrated in South America, especially in Bolivia, Brazil and Peru, with approximately 90% of the recorded cases of the muco-cutaneous type [5,6]. Yet, in spite of its importance, leishmaniasis is one of the most neglected tropical diseases in the world [5].

In Brazil, there has been an expansion of this disease since 1950 [7,8]. Currently, CL has been reported in all Brazilian states, causing outbreaks in several regions of country [9], especially in the Brazilian Amazon. This situation has been correlated to several factors, such as deforestation, the construction of highways and dams, implementation of agricultural poles, migrations of human populations, new mining ventures, the emergence of villages and cities, the use of forest locations for military training, among other factors [6-8,10-16].

*Leishmania* displays two main morphological forms, the amastigote and the promastigote, which are found in close association with vertebrate (mammals) and invertebrate (phlebotomine sandflies) hosts, respectively, comprising the link of several transmission cycles [13,17,18]. The vertebrate hosts include a large variety of mammals, such as rodents, xenarthrans (armadillo, anteater and sloth), marsupials (opossum), canids and primates, including humans [19-21].

There are approximately 30 species of *Leishmania* described in the World and, of these, at least 20 are pathogenic in mammals [22]. In the Neotropical region 22 species were recorded; of these, 12 were reported in Brazil [23] and seven were found infecting humans in the Brazilian Amazon region [24]. The studies conducted in Brazil have found a large number of dermotropic *Leishmania* species that are proved to infect humans, such as *Leishmania amazonensis, Le. braziliensis, Le. guyanensis, Le. lainsoni, Le. naiffi, Le. shawi* and *Le. lindenbergi*. There are others species too, but they have been found only in their natural reservoir hosts, as follows: *Le. enriettii, Le. forattinii, Le. deanei* and *Le. utingensis* [18,20,23,25-27]. With the exception of the two species (*Le. enriettii* and *Le.forattinii*), all those listed above were reported in the Brazilian Amazon, including *Leishmania chagasi* that causes visceral leishmaniasis and whose main vector is *Lutzomyia longipalpis* [23]. Table 1 presents all species of *Leishmania* and their respective proven and suspected sandfly vectors and reservoir hosts reported in Neotropical region.

In addition to those listed in Table 1, other species of sandflies have been observed in the Brazilian Amazon region, harboring *Leishmania* spp. such as L. (*Lutzomyia*) *spathotrichia* and L. (*Psathyromyia) dendrophyla* [18].

The detection and identification of the *Leishmania* spp. in phlebotomine species are important to predict the risk of the disease spreading in and around endemic areas, once these species are the main determinants of the clinical outcome in humans. Currently, the use of molecular techniques such as polymerase chain reaction (PCR) has increased the sensitivity and specificity of parasite identification [28]. Based on this technique, L. (*Evandromyia*) *georgii* was reported for the first time to be infected with *Leishmania* spp. in the Brazilian Amazon region [29]. Similarly, L. (*Trichophoromyia*) *ubiquitalis* and L. (*Psychodopygus*) *davisi* were found for the first time to be infected with *Le. lainsoni* in the state of Amazonas, Brazil [30]. These sandflies had already been identified as vectors of *Le. lainsoni* [31] and *Le. brazilienesis* [32], respectively, in the state of Pará (Brazil).

Phlebotomine sandflies are amply distributed in all continents, except in Antarctica. Out of the six genera belonging to the subfamily Phlebotominae, only *Lutzomyia* and *Phlebotomus* harbor the main vectors of human leishmaniasis. The former is restricted to the Neotropical and Neartic regions, where approximately 32 out of more than 500 species described [33] are implicated as vectors, whereas the latter is distributed in all the other regions of the world and comprises important vectors such as *Phlebotomus papatasi* in the Old World, which is the main vector of *Leishmania major* [34,35]. Genus *Lutzomyia* includes the subgenera *Nyssomyia* and *Psychodopygus*, which comprise the most important vectors of CL in the Neotropics, in particular in the Brazilian Amazon region (Table 1; Figures 1 and 2).

| **Parasites** | | **Leishmaniasis in humans** | **Sandfly vectors** | | **Reservoir host** |
|---|---|---|---|---|---|
| **Species** | **Subgenus** | | **Species** | **Subgenus/Group** | |
| *Leishmania chagasi*[Br/A] | *Leishmania* | Visceral and cutaneous* | *Lutzomyia longipalpis*[P]<br>*Lutzomyia cruzi*[P]<br>*Lutzomyia evansi*[P] | *Lutzomyia*<br>*Lutzomyia*<br>Group *Verrucarum* | Canids (*Cerdocyon thou, Speothos venaticus, Canis familiaris*), felines (*Panthera onca, Felis concolor*), marsupials (*Didelphis marsupialis* and *D. albiventris*) |
| *Leishmania enriettii*[Br] | *Leishmania* | Not registered | *Lutzomyia monticola*[S]<br>*Lutzomyia correalimai*[S] | Ungrouped<br>Group *Rupicola* | Rodents (*Cavia porcellus*) |
| *Leishmania mexicana* | *Leishmania* | Cutaneous | *Lutzomyia olmeca olmeca*[P]<br>*Lutzomyia diabolica*[S] | *Nyssomyia*<br>*Lutzomyia* | Rodents (*Ototylomys phyllotis, Nyctomys sumichrasti, Heteromys desmarestianus, Sigmodon hispidus, Neotoma albigula*) |

| Parasites | | Leishmaniasis in humans | Sandfly vectors | | Reservoir host |
|---|---|---|---|---|---|
| **Species** | **Subgenus** | | **Species** | **Subgenus/Group** | |
| *Leishmania pifanoi* | *Leishmania* | Cutaneous | *Lutzomyia flaviscutellata*[S] | *Nyssomyia* | Unknown |
| *Leishmania amazonensis*[Br/A] | *Leishmania* | Cutaneous | *Lutzomyia flaviscutellata*[P]<br>*Lutzomyia o. olmeca*[P]<br>*Lutzomyia reducta*[P] | *Nyssomyia*<br>*Nyssomyia*<br>*Nyssomyia* | Rodents (*Proechimys* spp., *Oryzomys* spp., *Nectomys, Neacomys, Dasyprocta*)<br>Marsupials (*Marmosa, Metachirus, Didelphis, Philander*),<br>fox (*Cerdocyon thous*) |
| *Leishmania aristidesi* | *Leishmania* | Not registered | *Lutzomyia olmeca bicolor*[S] | *Nyssomyia* | Marsupials (*Marmosa robinsoni*), rodents (*Poechmys semispinosus, Dasyprocta punctata*) |
| *Leishmania garnhami* | *Leishmania* | Cutaneous | *Lutzomyia youngi*[S] | Group *Verrucarum* | Marsupials (*Didelphis marsupialis*) |
| *Leishmania venezuelensis* | *Leishmania* | Cutaneous | *Lutzomyia olmeca bicolor*[S]<br>*Lutzomyia rangeliana*[S] | *Nyssomyia*<br>Ungrouped | Domestic cat |
| *Leishmania forattinii*[Br] | *Leishmania* | Not registered | *Lutzomyia ayrozai*[P]<br>*Lutzomyia yuilli*[P] | *Psychodopygus*<br>*Nyssomyia* | Rodents (*Proechimys inheringi*), marsupials (*Didelphis marsupialis*) |
| *Leishmania hertigi* | *Leishmania* | Not registered | Unknown | | Rondent(*Coendou rothschildi*) |
| *Leishmania deanei*[Br/A] | *Leishmania* | Not registered | Unknown | | Rondent (*Coendou p. prehensilis*) |
| *Leishmania braziliensis*[Br/A] | *Viannia* | Cutaneous | *Lutzomyia intermedia*[P]<br>*Lutzomyia whitmani*[P]<br>*Lutzomyia wellcomei*[P]<br>*Lutzomyia davisi*[P]<br>*Lutzomyia complexa*[S] | *Nyssomyia*<br>*Nyssomyia*<br>*Psychodopygus*<br>*Psychodopygus*<br>*Psychodopygus* | Rodents (*Oryzomys concolor, O. capito, O. nigripes, Akodon arviculoides, Proechimys* spp., *Rattus rattus, Rhipidomys leucodactylus, Sigmodon hispidus, Bolomys lasiurus*), marsupials (*Didelphis marsupialis*) |
| *Leishmania peruviana* | *Viannia* | Cutaneous | *Lutzomyia peruensis*[S]<br>*Lutzomyia verrucarum*[S] | *Helcocyrtomyia*<br>Group *Verrucarum* | Rodent (*Phyllotis andinum*), marsupials (*Didelphis marsupialis*) and domestic dog |

http://dx.doi.org/10.5772/60921

| Parasites | | Leishmaniasis in humans | Sandfly vectors | | Reservoir host |
|---|---|---|---|---|---|
| Species | Subgenus | | Species | Subgenus/Group | |
| *Leishmania guyanensis*[Br/A] | *Viannia* | Cutaneous | *Lutzomyia umbratilis*[P]<br>*Lutzomyia anduzei*[P] | *Nyssomyia*<br>*Nyssomyia* | Xenarthrans (*Choloepus didactylus, Tamandua tetradactyla*), rodents and marsupials |
| *Leishmania panamensis* | *Viannia* | Cutaneous | *Lutzomyia trapidoi*[P]<br>*Lutzomyia ylephiletor*[P]<br>*Lutzomyia gomezi*[P]<br>*Lutzomyia* panamensis[P] | *Nyssomyia*<br>*Nyssomyia*<br>*Lutzomyia*<br>*Psychodopygus* | Xenarthrans (*Choloepus hoffmanni, Bradypus infuscatus* and *B. griseus*); racoons (*Bassaricyon gabbi, Nasua nasua, Poto flavus*), primates (*Aotus trivirgatus, Saguinus geoffroyi*), rodents (*Heteromys* spp.) |
| *Leishmania lainsoni*[Br/A] | *Viannia* | Cutaneous | *Lutzomyia ubiquitalis*[P]<br>*Lutzomyia velascoi*[S] | *Trichophoromyia*<br>*Trichophoromyia* | Rodent (*Agouti paca*) |
| *Leishmania naiffi*[Br/A] | *Viannia* | Cutaneous | *Lutzomyia ayrozai*[P]<br>*Lutzomyia panamensis*[P]<br>*Lutzomyia squamiventris*[P] | *Psychodopygus*<br>*Psychodopygus*<br>*Psychodopygus* | Xenarthrans (*Dasypus novemcinctus*) |
| *Leishmania shawi*[Br/A] | *Viannia* | Cutaneous | *Lutzomyia whitmani*[P] | *Nyssomyia* | Primates (*Cebuspaella, Chiropotes satanas*), xenarthrans (*Choloepus didactylus,Bradypus tridactylus*) and racoon (*Nasua nasua*) |
| *Leishmania colombiensis* | *Viannia* | Cutaneous | *Lutzomyia hartmanni*[P]<br>*Lutzomyia gomezi*[P]<br>*Lutzomyia panamensis*[P] | *Helcocyrtomyia*<br>*Lutzomyia*<br>*Psychodopygus* | Xenarthrans(*Choloepus hoffmanni*) |
| *Leishmania equatorensis* | *Viannia* | Not registered | *Lutzomyia hartmanni*[P] | *Helcocyrtomyia* | Xenarthrans (*Choloepus hoffmanni*) and rodent (*Sciurus grantensis*) |
| *Leishmania lindenbergi*[Br/A] | *Viannia* | Cutaneous | *Lutzomyia antunesi*[S] | *Nyssomyia* | Unknown |
| *Leishmania utingensis*[Br/A] | *Viannia* | Not registered | *Lutzomyia tuberculata*[P] | *Viannamyia* | Unknown |

Br/A=Brazil, including Amazon; Br=Brazil, except Amazon; P=proven vector; S=suspect vector. *In Costa Rica, the infection occurs mostly as non-ulcerative skin lesions; Honduras and Nicaragua, the infection is much visceral as skin. Information compiled from Lainson (2010) [23].

**Table 1.** *Leishmania* species with their respective proven and suspect vectors (phlebotomine sandflies) and natural reservoirs (mammals) reported for the Neotropical region.

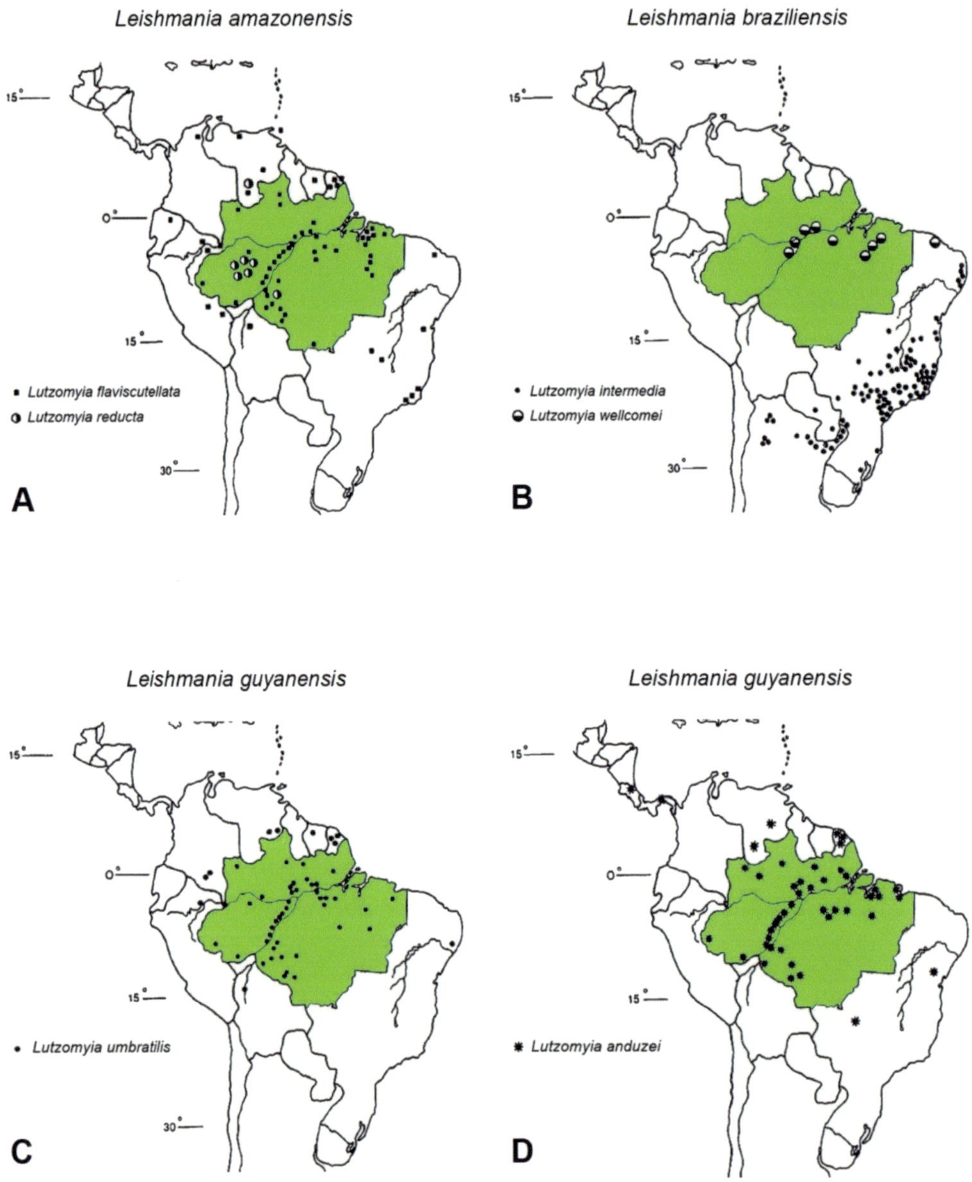


**Figure 1.** Distribution of the sandfly vectors of *Leishmania amazonensis* (A), *Leishmania braziliensis* (B) and *Leishmania guyanensis* (C and D). Highlight in green color corresponding to the Brazilian Amazon region. Map modified from Young and Duncan (1994) [2].

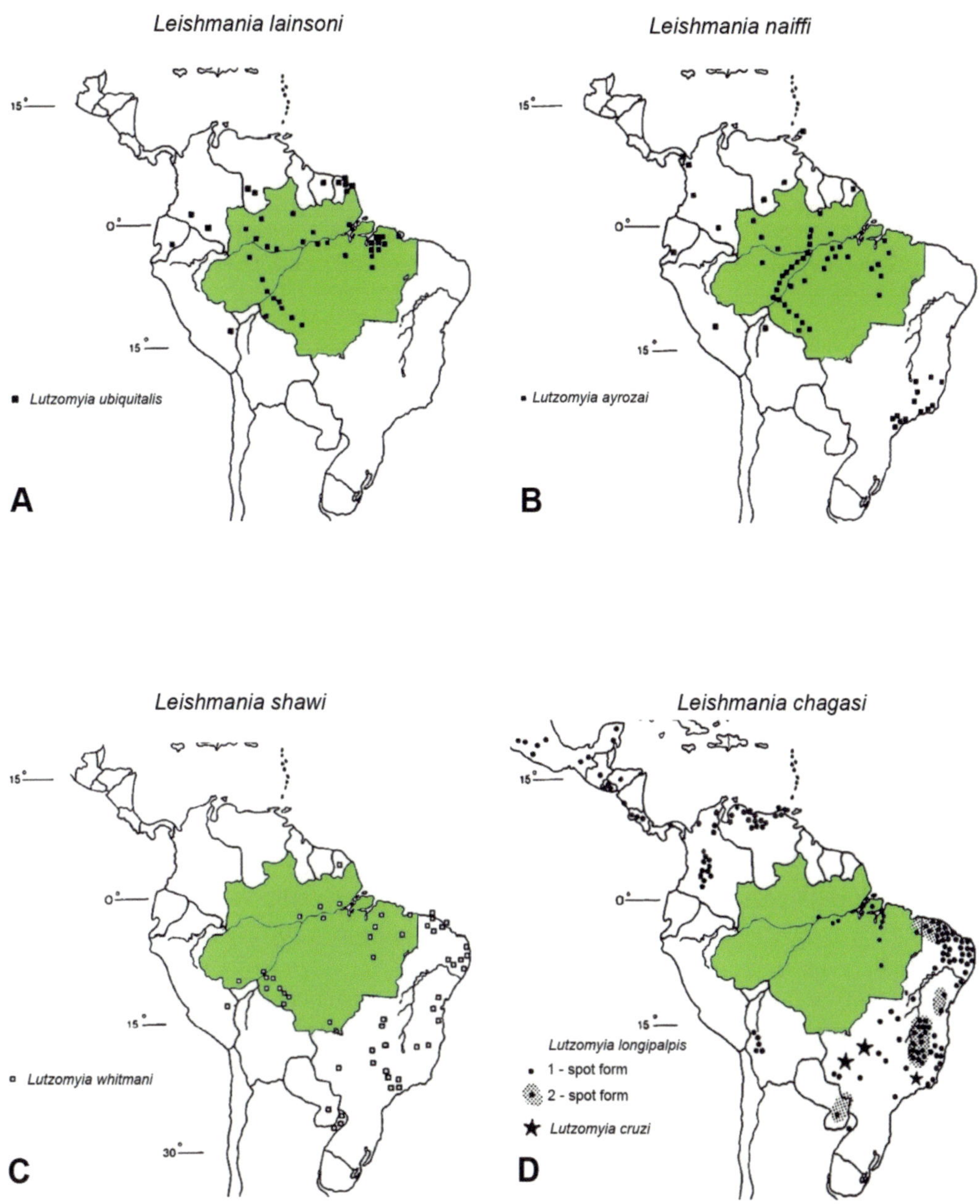


**Figure 2.** Distribution of the sandfly vectors of *Leishmania lainsoni* (A), *Leishmania naiffi* (B), *Leishmania shawi* (C) and *Leishmania chagasi* (D). Highlight in green color corresponding to the Brazilian Amazon region. Map modified from Young and Duncan (1994) [2].

Similar to other insect groups, the Brazilian Amazon hosts a large diversity of sandfly species likely because of the great variety of ecological niches available [36] which are favorable for survival and reproduction. For example, in a single hectare of forest 50 sandfly species were captured [37]. This high level of diversity of insect vectors and also of reservoirs permits the simultaneous circulation of several species of *Leishmania* and is particularly interesting for the dynamic transmission studies of CL in this region [38,39].

In northern South America, in particular in the Brazilian Amazon region, the transmission of CL is associated to *Lutzomyia umbratilis* Ward and Fraiha and *Lutzomyia anduzei* Rozeboom, implicated as principal and secondary vectors of *Le. guyanensis*, respectively. The *Le. guyanensis* cycle is completed in several species of mammals, especially in xenarthrans, the two-toed sloth (*Choloepus didactylus*), considered the main reservoir, and marsupials such as the opossum (*Didelphis marsupialis*) (*Didelphis marsupialis*) [40-43].

## 2. Distribution, biological aspects and population genetics of *Lutzomyia umbratilis*

In the last years, as genetic molecular markers became available, the number of studies on population genetics and evolutionary genetics in sandfly species has significantly increased [44-49], and the results have revealed large intra-population genetic variation, genetically populations structured, genetic lineages and cryptic species complexes. In the case of vector species, the knowledge of the genetic structure of populations and the processes responsible for the differentiation distribution is important for the identification of the disease transmission heterogeneity patterns. Such patterns are often produced by the presence of cryptic species, structured populations and/or genetic lineages, which may show variation in the degrees of anthropophily, susceptibility of females to infection by the pathogen, infection rates and females longevity. The identification of these factors is of paramount importance for developing effective management and vector control strategies.

The diversification patterns (structured populations, lineages, complete speciation) observed in sandfly species have generally been associated to multiple factors, such as climate barriers (or climate events in the past), geographic distances, differences in latitude or altitude, habitat modification, landscape fragmentation caused by anthropogenic actions and others, vegetation type or geographic barriers (rivers, mountains). These factors can reduce the dispersal capacity of sandflies, leading them to become isolated populations and causing loss of genetic diversity and increase of differentiation among the populations, as discussed by Ready et al. [50] with regard to *Lutzomyia whitmani*, by Mukhopadhyay et al. [51] for *Lutzomyia shannoni*, by Uribe-Soto et al. [52] for *L. longipalpis* and by Pech-May et al. [45] for *Lutzomyia cruciata*. Additionally, the low flight capacity of this group of insects which seldom spread over more than 1 km, and the breeding soil type are also factors that may contribute even more to the population isolation and then favor the process of divergence and speciation events.

*Lutzomyiaumbratilis*, the main vector of *Le. guyanensi*, that causes Cutaneous Leishmaniasis (CL), occurs in northern South America, including Bolivia, Brazil, Colombia, French Guyana,

Peru, Suriname and Venezuela [2,53]. In Brazil, *L. umbratilis* has been reported in all states of the northern region, the states of Mato Grosso and Mato Grosso do Sul (Southwest), besides the state of Maranhão and an isolated population in the state of Pernambuco, both in the northeastern region [2, 54,55]. Thus, populations of this species are spread over vast areas, separated by geographic barriers such as the largest rivers, the Amazon and the Negro, in the Brazilian Amazon region. Additionally, sandfly species have very limited dispersal capabilities, usually no more than 1 km [56,57], which favors geographic isolation of the populations. Thus, considering the vast geographic area, with discontinuous distribution, along with the low flight capacity of this insect group, *L. umbratilis* populations could be more susceptible to evolve into differentiated populations, incipient species and, ultimately, reproductively isolated species.

*Lutzomyia umbratilis* has been implicated in the transmission of *Le. guyanensis* in several countries of northern South America, including northern Brazil, and French Guiana and Suriname [58-60]. In the Brazilian Amazon, this species has shown to be highly anthropophilic and has been appointed as the main *Le. guyanensis* vector in the states of Pará [58-60], Amazonas [42,61-63] and Amapá [18] and is probably involved in the transmission in the states of Acre [64] and Rondônia [65]. Moreover, according to the hypothesis of Arias and Freitas [40], the susceptibility of this vector to *Leishmania* seems to vary in the central Brazilian Amazon region. *Lutzomyia umbratilis* populations naturally infected with *Le. guyanensis* have been observed east of the Negro River and north of the Amazonas River; however, there is no report of natural infections by *Leishmania* in this species south of the Amazon River system. Arias and Freitas [40] suggested that the fluvial system formed by the Amazon, Solimões and Negro Rivers may act as a barrier to the *Le. guyanensis* transmission cycle, where *L. umbratilis* populations display distinct degrees of vector competence between the opposite sides of these rivers, suggesting that these populations might represent a species complex or incipient speciation event.

Despite its importance as vector and the probable existence of a cryptic species complex, only few studies have tested the role of the rivers barrier in the genetic subdivision of *L. umbratilis*. A biological study conducted with two *L. umbratilis* populations from Manaus and Manacapuru (left and right banks of the Negro River, respectively) in the Brazilian Amazon region, revealed significant differences in the life cycle, fecundity, fertility, emergence degree and adult longevity between these populations, reflecting intrinsic biological differences [66]. Subsequently, a study that combined morphology, chromosome and isozymes analyses of four *L. umbratilis* populations from this fluvial system showed significant differences in the bristle lengths of 4$^{th}$ instar larvae and in the number and size of the spines of the female genital atrium armature [67]. The latter has been a useful marker for distinguishing closely related species of sandflies [68]. Unfortunately, polytene chromosome analysis was not possible, but the metaphase karyotype was 2n=6. Isozymes did not reveal any differences among the populations [67]. This result may be due to the slow evolution rate, negative selection and the amino acid codon wobble effect. Consequently, isozymes are not informative markers for detecting incipient or recently diverged species. Therefore, the taxonomic status of *L. umbratilis* remains unclear.

*Lutzomyia umbratilis* was described by Ward and Fraiha [69], based on specimens captured in the Jari River region, state of Pará, Brazil. Because of the high morphological similarity between *L. umbratilis* and *L. anduzei*, the former has been wrongly identified as *L. anduzei* in the past. In fact, most of *L. anduzei* specimens found to be naturally infected with *Leishmania* before this date (1977) could actually be *L. umbratilis*. After this date, it has been possible distinguish *L. umbratilis* and *L. anduzei* morphologically, based on the internal and external genitalia of males and females [2,70]. Currently, they can also be identified molecularly by using DNA barcode sequences from *COI* of mitochondrial DNA [70]. The phylogenetic analysis of this dataset found two strongly supported monophyletic clades, although the genetic distances between them, based on the Kimura 2 Parameters (K2P) model, were very small (4.4%), suggesting that these species are very closely related (sister species) [70]. These species have been found infected naturally with *Le. guyanensis* in the Brazilian Amazon, although the studies revealed much higher infection rates in *L. umbratilis* than in *L. anduzei* females, consequently, the former has been recognized as principal vector of this parasite [18,63,71,72].

*L. umbratilis* adults are generally found in the rainforest (primary forest) of the Brazilian Amazon region, with its high humidity and dim light; therefore, the species has been recognized as ombrophilous, as expressed in its name, *L. umbratilis*. This species is further recognized as dendrobatic, because it is associated to tree trunks during the daytime. In the field, its density may vary, depending on the location and of these characteristics, but it seems to be denser in the central Amazon region, tending to reduce its density towards the edges of this region (Alencar, R. B., personal information). *L. umbratilis* adults are captured using aspirators on the bases of tree trunks during daytime and with CDC (Center for Disease Control) miniature light traps at ground level and in the forest canopy at night. These methods have been employed efficiently throughout Brazilian Amazon region [73].

In addition to the isozyme studies mentioned above, the most recent population genetics analyses were performed on the six *L. umbratilis* populations from the two opposite banks of the Amazon and Negro rivers (Table 2; Figure 3) by using a large fragment (1,181 bp) of the *COI* gene (the 3′ end fragment of *COI*) [48] and the Barcode region (663 bp) [70], both from mitochondrial DNA. The aim of these analyses was to assess whether the populations of the opposite banks of these rivers consist of incipient or distinct species. In the study of Scarpassa and Alencar [48], 111 specimens were sequenced and the results revealed 52 haplotypes, reflecting a very large genetic variability for most of the samples examined, except one (Rio Preto da Eva). The genealogical relationships of the haplotypes were accessed using the TCS program [74] at the 95% confidence level. This analysis showed two haplotype groups (lineages), separated by ten mutational steps, but all connected in the network (Figure 4). Similarly, phylogenetic analysis using Bayesian Inference (BI) and inferred under the TIM1+I model, generated two distinct evolutionary lineages (probably clades), with probability support from moderate to slightly high (0.64 and 0.77; Figure 5), suggesting two monophyletic clades. These lineages can be separated by one fixed mutation at position 933 (A ↔ G) of the dataset, and the estimated sequence divergence between them was 1%. Lineage I consisted of four samples from the left bank of the Amazon and Negro rivers, whereas lineage II comprised two samples from the right bank of the Negro river (Figure 3). No haplotypes were shared between samples of the two lineages. Samples from the same clade (within-clades) exhibited low to moderate genetic differentiation ($F_{ST}$ = -0.0390-0.1841), whereas samples from different clades (between clades) exhibited extremely high and significant differentiation ($F_{ST}$ =

0.7100-0.8497; $P < 0.0001$) and fixed differences ($S_f = 1$ to 7) (Table 3). Curiously, the samples from Manacapuru *versus* the samples from the BR-174 Highway, Rio Preto da Eva and Manaus, which are separated by smaller geographic distances (from 59.43 to 96.01 km), displayed more fixed differences ($S_f = 6$ to 7) and no shared polymorphism ($S_s = 0$), whereas, the samples from Manacapuru *versus* the samples from Cachoeira Porteira, which are separated by a larger geographic distance (449.22 km), exhibited less fixed differences ($S_f = 3$) and more shared polymorphisms ($S_s = 2$). Taken together, the evidence of absence of gene flow associated with the high levels of genetic differentiation may be an indicator of genetic discontinuity between these lineages, so they could represent incipient or distinct species. The separation time calculated between these lineages falls in the middle Pleistocene (0.22 Mya), coinciding with the more recent formation of the Amazon and Negro rivers [75], appointed as the most probable evolutionary force. This vicariant event, along with the low dispersal rate of the sandflies, and the amenable environmental conditions for adaptation and also drift are likely to have contributed to the great genetic differentiation between the populations of the opposite banks.

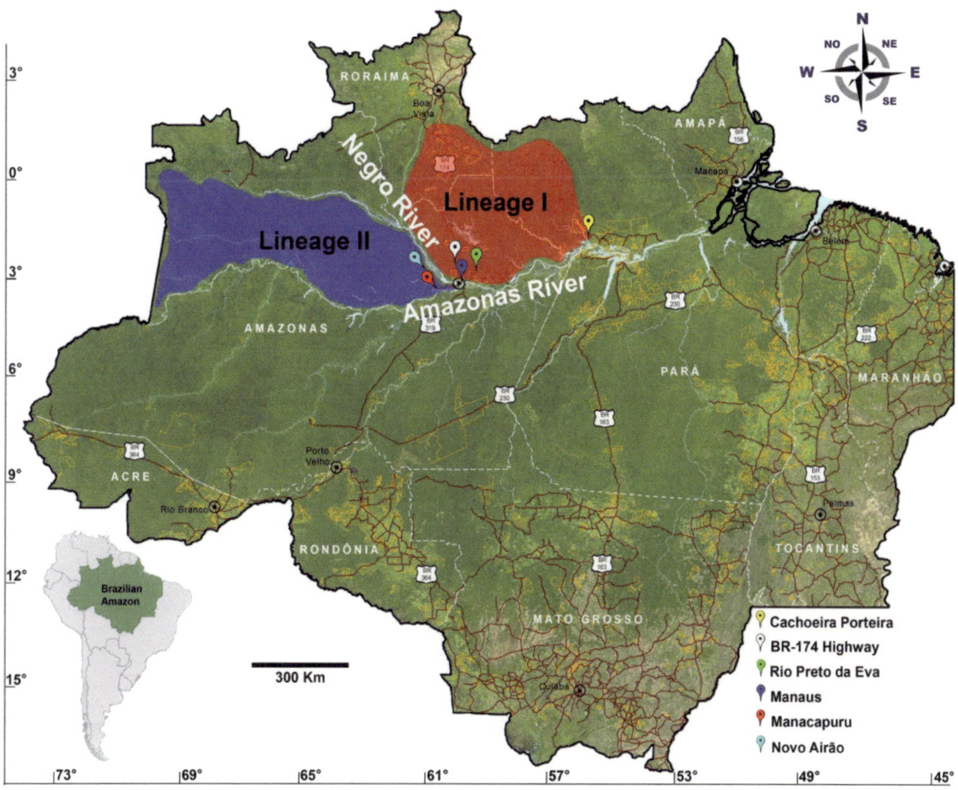


**Figure 3.** Collection sites of *Lutzomyia umbratilis* from the Brazilian Amazon. Geographic distribution inferred of lineage I (in red color); Geographic distribution inferred of lineage II (in blue color). Map modified from Scarpassa and Alencar (2013) [70].

| Species | Localities, State | Co-ordinates | N |
|---|---|---|---|
| | | Latitude; Longitude | |
| *L. umbratilis* | Cachoeira Porteira, Oriximiná, Pará | 1° 28′ S; 56° 22′ W | 18 |
| | BR-174 Highway, Amazonas | 2° 36′ S; 60° 02′ W | 15 |
| | Rio Preto da Eva, Amazonas | 2° 43′ S; 59° 47′ W | 15 |
| | Manaus, Amazonas | 3° 04′ S; 59° 57′ W | 4 |
| | Manacapuru, Amazonas | 3° 14′ S; 60° 31′ W | 24 |
| | Novo Airão, Amazonas | 2° 47′ S; 60° 55′ W | 35 |

N: sample size. **Source:** Scarpassa and Alencar (2012) [48]

**Table 2.** Collection sites and sample sizes of *Lutzomyia umbratilis* from the Brazilian Amazon.

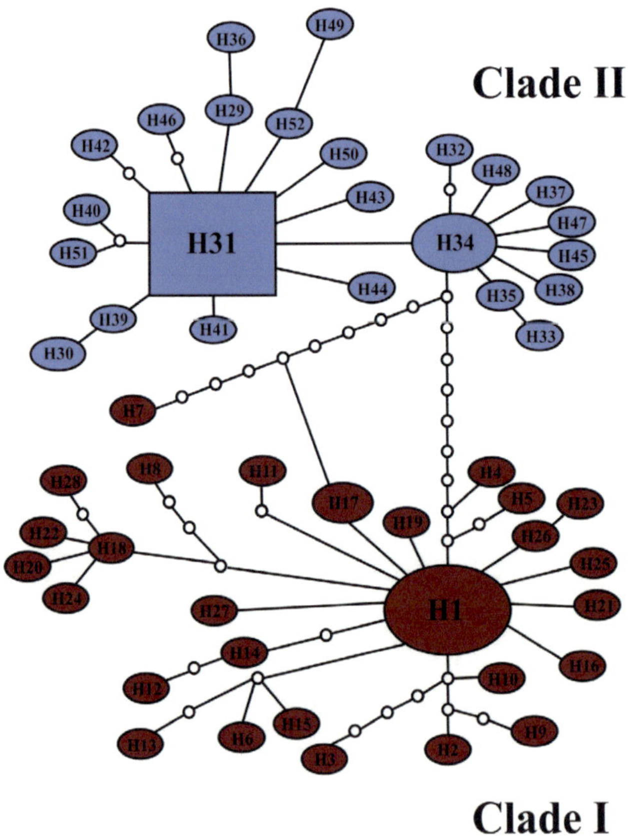


**Figure 4.** Parsimony haplotypes network of the 52 haplotypes observed in *Lutzomyia umbratilis*. H1 to H52, haplotypes. The haplotype circle sizes are proportional to number of individuals observed in each haplotype. Clade I is in red color. Clade II is in blue color. Empty smaller circles represent mutational events. **Source:** Scarpassa and Alencar (2012) [48].

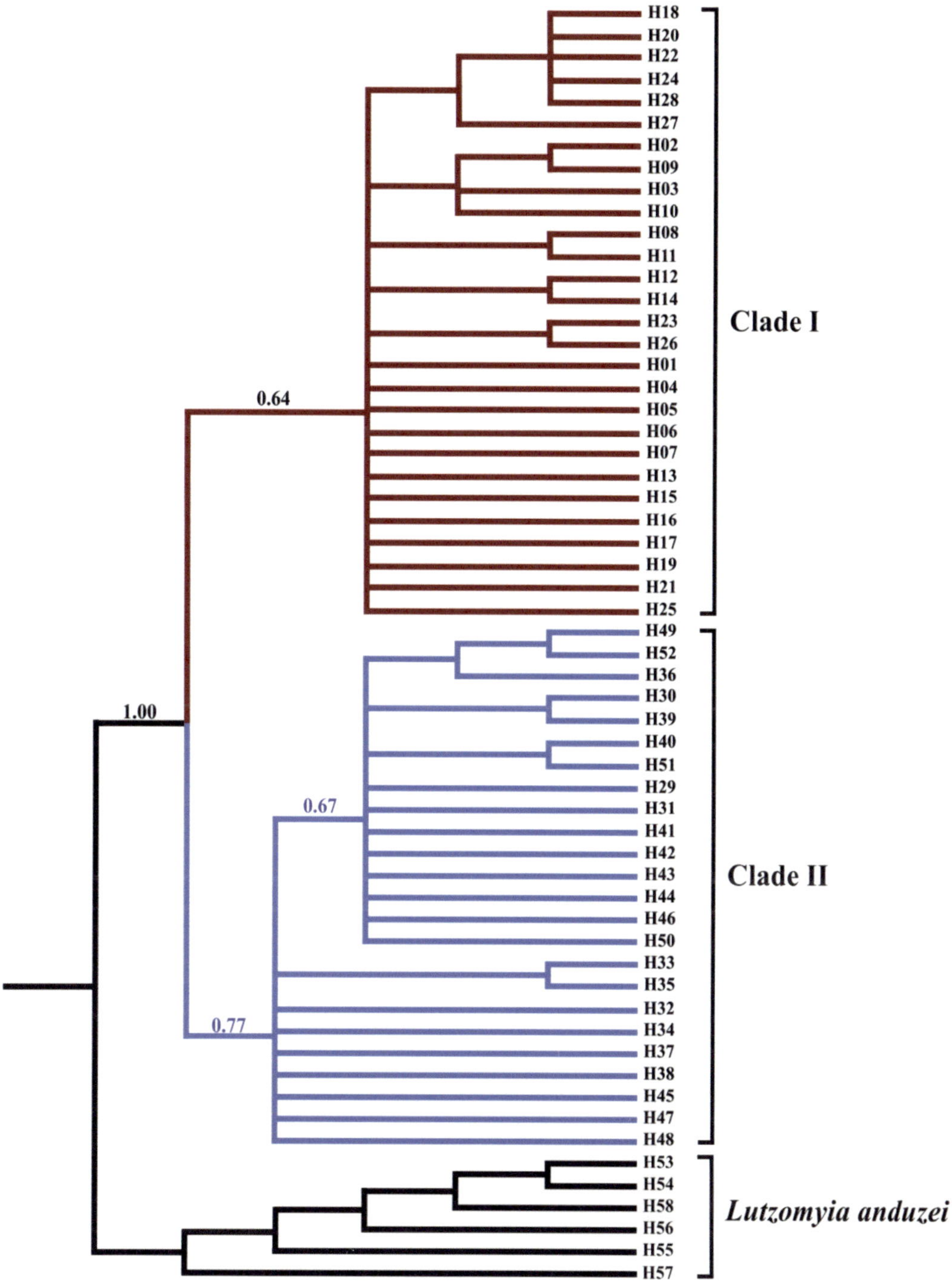


**Figure 5.** Bayesian Inference (BI) topology tree of the 52 haplotypes of *Lutzomyia umbratilis* inferred under the TIM1+I evolutionary model. Numbers above branch represent posterior probabilities obtained in the BI. *Lutzomyia anduzei* was used as outgroup. **Source:** Scarpassa and Alencar (2012) [48].

| Samples | $F_{ST}$ (Km) | K | $D_{xy}$ | $D_a$ | $S_s$ | $S_f$ |
|---|---|---|---|---|---|---|
| Cachoeira Porteira x BR-174 Highway | 0.0522 (368.40) | 3.52 | 0.00297 | 0.00017 | 4 | 0 |
| Cachoeira Porteira x Rio Preto da Eva | 0.0569*** (353.67) | 2.99 | 0.00248 | 0.00017 | 2 | 0 |
| Cachoeira Porteira x Manaus | 0.0230 (394.02) | 3.92 | 0.00332 | 0.00025 | 1 | 0 |
| BR-174 Highway x Rio Preto da Eva | 0.0189 (30.46) | 1.48 | 0.00125 | 0.00002 | 3 | 0 |
| BR-174 Highway x Manaus | -0.0390 (56.29) | 2.20 | 0.00187 | -0.00012 | 3 | 0 |
| Rio Preto da Eva x Manaus | 0.1841 (45.35) | 1.87 | 0.00158 | 0.00008 | 2 | 0 |
| Manacapuru x Novo Airão | 0.0548 (58.74) | 1.81 | 0.00153 | 0.00008 | 4 | 0 |
| Cachoeira Porteira x **Manacapuru** | **0.7100***** (449.22) | 10.19 | **0.00863** | **0.00599** | **2** | **3** |
| BR-174 Highway x **Manacapuru** | **0.8157***** (87.11) | 9.78 | **0.00833** | **0.00673** | **0** | **6** |
| Rio Preto da Eva x **Manacapuru** | **0.8497***** (96.01) | 8.98 | **0.00765** | **0.00653** | **0** | **6** |
| Manaus x **Manacapuru** | **0.8249***** (59.43) | 10.42 | **0.00887** | **0.00699** | **0** | **7** |
| Cachoeira Porteira x **Novo Airão** | **0.7337 ***** (477.49) | 10.55 | **0.00899** | **0.00625** | **6** | **1** |
| BR-174 Highway x **Novo Airão** | **0.8197***** (107.97) | 10.21 | **0.00869** | **0.00705** | **4** | **4** |
| Rio Preto da Eva x **Novo Airão** | **0.8439 ***** (130.14) | 9.43 | **0.00803** | **0.00687** | **1** | **4** |
| Manaus x **Novo Airão** | **0.8269***** (108.76) | 10.84 | **0.00924** | **0.00731** | **2** | **5** |
| **Clade I** x **Clade II** | **0.7776***** | 9.99 | **0.00850** | **0.00660** | **8** | **1** |

$F_{ST}$: pair-wise genetic differentiation; *K:* average number of nucleotide differences between populations; $D_{xy}$: average number of nucleotide substitutions per site between populations; $D_a$: number of net nucleotide substitutions per site between populations; $S_s$: number of shared polymorphisms between pairs of populations; $S_f$: number of fixed differences between pairs of populations. The geographic distance (in km) between localities is represented inside the parentheses. ***$P = 0.00000 \pm 0.0000$, after the Bonferroni correction. **Source:** Scarpassa and Alencar (2012) [48].

**Table 3.** Genetic differentiation among samples and haplotype clade of *Lutzomyia umbratilis*.

Another study was conducted subsequently on these *L. umbratilis* populations, using the Barcode region (663bp) [70]. In the 72 specimens sequenced, 32 haplotypes were observed. In line with the results of the previous study [48], no haplotype was shared between lineages I and II. The genetic distance between the lineages, based on the K2P model, was rather small (0.009 to 0.010); however, they could be identified by one fixed mutation (T ↔ C transition at position 21).

The genetic differentiation observed in these studies supports the biological and morphological differences reported by Justiniano [67] and Justiniano et al. [66]. These results strongly indicate that *L. umbratilis* represents a species complex with recent evolutionary history. Taken together, these findings might explain possible differences in the vector competence of these sandflies, a hypothesis raised by Arias and Freitas [40]. On the other hand, these results do not support the isozyme data, which showed genetic homogeneity among populations. These inconsistencies between markers could be attributed to incomplete lineage sorting, due to recent divergence between *L. umbratilis* lineages (or distinct species) and/or distinct evolution rates of the markers used; for instance, isozymes evolve at a slower rate than mitochondrial DNA and are not informative markers for detecting incipient or recently diverged species.

Little is known about the natural breeding sites of *L. umbratilis* and, consequently, about its biology. This knowledge is important for application in any attempt to create and maintain colonies in laboratory conditions. The maintenance of *L. umbratilis* colonies could be the key to testing the mechanisms of reproductive isolation [66,76,77], as well as the assortative mating features between populations separated by the Negro and Amazon rivers, hypothesized as distinct species. It is particularly important because species that have diverged very recently are expected to share ancestral variation at high proportions, a situation that may confound their phylogenetic reconstruction. In addition, it is likely that in young species, with a recent divergence process, there are fixed differences only in genes involved in the speciation process. The maintenance of *L. umbratilis* colonies in the laboratory would also be important to assess the level of vector competence, based on tests of experimental infection between populations from the opposite river banks.

Another interesting approach could be genomic population studies using multilocus analysis, especially using loci which are involved in the different biologic aspects of *L. umbratilis*. This approach will permit distinguishing the effects of natural selection from those of genetic drift. The importance of this approach resides in the fact that genomic analyses provide more reliable information on historic and demographic events. The effect of a specific locus (outlier locus) helps identifying signs of natural selection in genes involved in the most variable adaptability process, such as those related to vector competence and (or) vector capacity, thus allowing a better understanding of vector status in distinct areas from the Brazilian Amazon.

## 3. Conclusion

The two genetic lineages of *L. umbratilis* found in these studies may represent an advanced speciation process, indicating incipient or distinct species. This suggests that the Amazon and Negro rivers may be acting as effective barriers, as observed in *L. cruciata* [45], preventing gene flow between populations of opposite banks. Such findings have important implications for epidemiology, especially those related to vector competence, which are vital information for surveillance and vector control strategies in northern Brazil. Furthermore, this information may also provide a better knowledge of the evolutionary history of this species complex, as well as *L. umbratilis* represents an interesting example for speciation studies.

Finally, further studies of these populations using other molecular genetic markers, as well as additional sampling along the river banks and within interfluves in the Brazilian Amazon, are clearly needed to allow a more precise estimate of the differentiation, number of clades or distinct species. Studies of this kind are currently under way in our laboratory.

## Acknowledgements

The results of the articles our team cited here were funded by MCTI/INPA, Brazil, and by grants from the Amazonas Research Foundation (FAPEAM-Universal-Amazonas, process number 3111/2012), Brazil, from the INCT-CENBAM/CNPq/FAPEAM/INPA, Brazil, and from the PRO-EQUIPAMENT/CAPES, Brazil.

## Author details

Vera Margarete Scarpassa[1] and Ronildo Baiatone Alencar[2]

*Address all correspondence to: vera@inpa.gov.br

1 Laboratório de Genética de Populações e Evolução de Vetores de Malária e Dengue. Instituto Nacional de Pesquisas da Amazônia (INPA), Manaus, Amazonas, Brazil

2 Universidade do Estado do Amazonas (UEA), Manaus, Amazonas, Brazil

## References

[1] Lane RP. Sandflies. *In* Medical insects and arachnids. Edited by Lane RP, Crosskey RW. London: Chapman and Hall 1993; 78-119.

[2] Young DG, Duncan NA. Guide to the identification and geographic distribution of *Lutzomyia* sandflyies in Mexico, the West Indies, Central and South America (Diptera: Psychodidae). Memoirs of the American Entomological Institute (Gainesville) 1994; 54 1-881.

[3] WORLD HEALTH ORGANIZATION - WHO. Control of the leishmaniasis. Report of a meeting of the WHO Expert Committee on the Control of Leishmaniasis, 22-26 March, Geneva 2010; 5-88.

[4] Reithnger R. Leishmaniases' burden of disease: ways forward for getting from speculation to reality. PLoS Neglected Tropical Diseases 2008; 2 e285. doi:10.1371/ journal.pntd.0000285.

[5] WORLD HEALTH ORGANIZATION - WHO. Leishmaniasis. 2015. Available in: http://www.who.int/tdr/publications/publications/pdf/prl/pr17/leishmaniasis.pdf. Accessed at February 15, 2015.

[6] Gontijo B, Carvalho MLR. Leishmaniose tegumentar americana. Revista Brasileira de Medicina Tropical. 2003; 36(1) 71-80.

[7] Vale ECS, Furtado T. Leishmaniose tegumentar americana: revisão histórica da origem, expansão e etiologia. Anais Brasileiro de Dermatologia 2005; 80(4) 421-428.

[8] Guerra JAO, Ribeiro JAS, Coelho LIARC, Barbosa MGV, Paes MG. Epidemiologia da leishmaniose tegumentar na Comunidade São João, Manaus, Amazonas, Brasil. Caderno de Saúde Pública 2006; 22 2319-2327.

[9] MS/SVS - Ministério da Saúde/Secretaria de Vigilância em Saúde. Manual de Vigilância da Leishmaniose Tegumentar Americana 2010. 2ª ed. – Brasília: Editora do Ministério da Saúde, 180 pp. – (Série A. Normas e Manuais Técnicos).

[10] Marzochi MC. As Leishmanioses no Brasil: as leishmanioses tegumentares. Jornal Brasileiro de Medicina 1992; 63 82-104.

[11] Ministério da Saúde – MS/Fundação Nacional de Saúde – FUNASA. Manual de Controle da Leishmaniose Tegumentar Americana 2000. 5ª ed., Brasília, 62pp.

[12] Basano SA, Camargo LMA. Leishmaniose Tegumentar Americana: histórico, epidemiologia e perspectiva de controle. Revista Brasileira de Epidemiologia 2004; 7(3) 328-337.

[13] Lainson R. The American Leishmaniasis: some observations on their ecology and epidemiology. Transactions of the Royal Society of Tropical Medicine and Hygiene 1983; 77 569-596.

[14] Barrett TV, Senra MS. Leishmaniasis in Manaus, Brazil. Parasitology Today 1989; 5(8) 255-257.

[15] Sá SMA, Sá EV, Diniz AM. Saúde e Qualidade de Vida na Amazônia. *In*: Furtado, L.G. (Org.). *Amazônia, Desenvolvimento, Sociodiversidade e Qualidade de Vida*, UFPA, Belém 1997; 135-145.

[16] Guerra JAO, Talhari S, Paes MG, Garrido M, Talhari JM. Aspectos clínicos e diagnósticos da leishmaniose tegumentar americana em militares simultaneamente expostos à infecção na Amazônia. Revista da Sociedade Brasileira de Medicina Tropical 2003; 36 587-590.

[17] Lainson R, Shaw JJ. Leishmaniasis in Brazil. I. Observations on enzootic rodent leishmaniasis – incrimination of *Lutzomyia flaviscutellata* (Mangabeira) as the vector in the lower Amazonian basin. Transactions of the Royal Society of Tropical Medicine and Hygiene 1968; 62 385-395.

[18] Freitas RA, Naiff RD, Barrett TV. Species Diversity and Flagellate Infections in the Sand Fly Fauna near Porto Grande, State of Amapá, Brazil (Diptera: Psychodidae. Ki-

netosplatida: Trypanosomatidae). Memórias do Instituto Oswaldo Cruz 2002; 97(1) 53-59.

[19] Lainson R, Shaw JJ. Leishmaniasis in Brazil: III. Cutaneous leishmaniasis in an opossum, *Marmo samurina* (Marsupialia, Didelphidae) from the lower Amazon region. Transactions of the Royal Society of Tropical Medicine and Hygiene1969; 63(6) 738-740.

[20] Lainson, R, Shaw JJ. Leishmaniasis in Brazil: V. Studies on the epidemiology of cutaneous leishmaniasis in Mato Grosso State, and observations on two distinct strains of *Leishmania* isolated from man and forest animals. Transactions of the Royal Society of Medicine and Hygiene 1970; 64(5) 654-667.

[21] Naiff RD, Talhari S, Barrett TV. Isolation of *Leishmania guyanensis* of the nasal mucosa. Memórias do Instituto Oswaldo Cruz 1988; 83(4) 529-530.

[22] Center for Food Security and Public Health (CFSPH). Leishmaniasis (cutaneous and visceral). Iowa State of University, College of Veterinary Medicine, Iowa 2009; 1-10.

[23] Lainson, R. Espécies neotropicais de *Leishmania*: uma breve revisão histórica sobre sua descoberta, ecologia e taxonomia. Revista Pan-Amazônica de Saúde 2010; 1 13-32.

[24] Rotureau B. Ecology of the *Leishmania* species in the Guianan eco-region complex. American Journal of Tropical Medicine and Hygiene 2006; 74 81-96.

[25] Silveira FT, Ishikawa EA, De Souza AAA, Lainson R. An outbreak of cutaneous leishmaniasis among soldiers in Belém, Pará State, Brazil, caused by *Leishmania (Viannia) lindenbergi* n. sp. A new leishmaniasis parasite of man in the Amazon region. Parasite 2002; 9 43-50.

[26] Genaro O, Marques MJ, Reis AB, Silva AFF, Michalik MSM, Costa CA, Mayrinc W, Dias M. Leishmaniose Tegumentar Americana. *In*: Neves DP, Melo AL, Genaro O, Linardi PM. Parasitologia Humana 2003; 36-53. ATHENEU, São Paulo-SP.

[27] Rangel EF, Lainson R. Flebotomíneos do Brasil, Fiocruz, Rio de Janeiro 2003; 367 pp.

[28] Cabrera OL, Munstermann LE, Cardenas R, Gutierrez R, Ferro C. Definition of appropriate temperature and storage conditions in the detection of *Leishmania* DNA with PCR in phlebotomine flies. Biomédica (Bogotá) 2002; 22 296-302.

[29] Albuquerque MIC. Fauna de flebotomíneos (Diptera: Psychodidae) e taxa de infecção natural por *Leishmania* spp. (Kinetoplastida: Trypanosomatidae) da Reserva Biológica de Campina – INPA da BR 174, Manaus, Amazonas, Brasil. Masters Thesis 2009; 74 pp.

[30] Pereira Júnior AA. Fauna de flebotomíneos (Diptera: Psychodidae) e taxa de infecção natural por *Leishmania* Ross (Kinetoplastida: Trypanosomatidae) em ambientes de

várzea e de terra firme do município de Tefé, Amazonas, Brasil. Master Thesis 2014; 81 pp.

[31] Silveira FT, Souza AAA, Lainson R, Shaw JJ, Braga RR, Ishikawa EAY. Cutaneous leishmaniasis in the Amazon Region: natural infection of the sandfly *Lutzomyia ubiquitalis* (Psychodidae: Phlebotominidae) by *Leishmania lainsoni* in Pará State, Brazil. Memórias do Instituto Oswaldo Cruz 1991; 86(1) 127-30.

[32] Souza AAA, Silveira FT, Lainson R, Barata IR, Silva MGS, Lima JAN, Pinheiro MSB, Silva FMM, Vasconcelos, LS, Campos, MB, Ishikawa, EAY. Fauna flebotomínica da Serrados Carajás, Estado do Pará, Brasil, e sua possível implicação na transmissão da leishmania tegumentar americana. Revista Pan-Amazônica de Saúde 2010; 1(1) 45-51.

[33] Shimabukuro PHF, Galati, EAB. Checklist dos Phlebotominae (Diptera: Psychodidae) do Estado de São Paulo, Brasil, com comentários sobre sua distribuição greográfica. Biota Neotropical 2011; 11 1-20. http://www. biotaneotropica.org.br/v11n1a/pt/abstract?inventory +bn0361101a2011.

[34] Dantas-Torres F. The role of dogs as reservoirs of *Leishmania* parasites, with emphasis on *Leishmania (Leishmania) infantum* and *Leishmania (Viannia) braziliensis*. Veterinary Parasitology 2007; 149 139-146.

[35] Kakarsulemankhel JK. Leishmaniasis in Pak-Afghan region: a review. International Journal of Agriculture and Biology 2011; 13 611-620.

[36] Aguiar GM, Medeiros WM. Distribuição regional de habitats das espécies de flebotomíneos do Brasil. *In*: Rangel EF, Lainson R (eds). Flebotomíneos do Brasil 2003; 207-256.

[37] Young DG, Arias JR. Flebotomíneos vectores de leishmaniasis en las Americas. Organização Pan-Americana da Saúde. Caderno Técnico 1992; (3).

[38] Grimaldi G Jr, Tesh RB, McMahon-Pratt D. A review of the geographic distribution and epidemiology of leishmaniasis in the New World. American Journal of Tropical Medicine and Hygiene 1989; 41 687-725.

[39] Lainson R, Shaw JJ, Silveira FT, Sousa AAA, Braga RR, Ishikawa EAY. The dermal leishmaniasis of Brazil, with special reference to the eco-epidemiology of the disease in Amazonian. Memórias do Instituto Oswaldo Cruz 1994; 89 435-443.

[40] Arias JR, Freitas RA. Sobre os vetores de leishmaniose cutânea na Amazônia central do Brasil. 2: incidência de flagelados em flebótomos selváticos. Acta Amazônica 1978; 8 387-396.

[41] Arias JR, Freitas RA. On the vectors of cutaneous leishmaniasis in the Central Amazon of Brazil. 4. Sand fly emergence from a "terra firme" forest floor. Acta Amazônica 1982; 12 609-611.

[42] Arias JR, Naiff RD. The principal reservoir host of cutaneous leishmaniasis in the urban area of Manaus, Central Amazon of Brazil. Memórias do Instituto Oswaldo Cruz 1981; 76 279-286.

[43] Arias JR, Miles MA, Naiffi RD, Póvoa MM, Freitas RA, Biancardi CB, Castellón EG. Flagellates infections of Brazilian sandflies (Diptera: Psychodidae): Isolation in vitro and biochemical identification of *Endotrypanum* and *Leishmania*. American Journal of Tropical Medicine and Hygiene 1985; 34 1098-1108.

[44] Zapata S, Mejía L, Le Pont F, León R, Pesson B, Ravel C, Bichaud L, Charrel R, Cruaud C, Trueba G, Depaquit J. A study of a population of *Nyssomyia trapidoi* (Diptera: Psychodidae) caught on the Pacific coast of Equator. Parasites & Vectors 2012; 5 144.

[45] Pech-May A, Marina CF, Vázquez-Domínguez E, Berzunza-Cruz M, Rebollar-Télles EA, Narváez-Zapata JA, Moo-LIanes D, Ibánez-Bernal S, Ramsey JM, Becker I. Genetic structure and divergence in populations of *Lutzomyia cruciata*, a phlebotomine sand fly (Diptera: Psychodidae) vector of *Leishmania mexicana* in southeastern Mexico. Infection, Genetics and Evolution 2013; 16 254-262.

[46] Yamamoto K, Cáceres AG, Gomez EA, Mimori T, Iwata H, Korenaga M, Sakurai T, Katakura K, Hashiguchi Y, Kato H. Genetic diversity of the mitochondrial cytochrome b gene in *Lutzomyia* spp., with special reference to *Lutzomyia peruensis*, a main vector of *Leishmania (Viannia) peruviana* in the Peruvian Andes. Acta Tropica 2013; 126 156-163.

[47] Valderrama A, Tavares MG, Andrade-Filho JD. Phylogeography of the *Lutzomyia gomezi* (Diptera: Phlebotominae) on the Panama Isthmus. Parasites & Vectors 7: 9.

[48] Scarpassa VM, Alencar RB. *Lutzomyia umbratilis*, the main vector of *Leishmaniaguyanensis*, represents a novel species complex? *PLoS ONE* 2012; 7(5) e37341.

[49] Scarpassa VM, Figueiredo AS, Alencar RB. Genetic diversity and population structure in the *Leishmania guyanensis* vector *Lutzomyia anduzei* (Diptera, Psychodidae) from the Brazilian Amazon. Infection, Genetics and Evolution 2015; 31 312-320.

[50] Ready PD, De Souza AA, Rebelo JC, Day J, Silveira FT, Campbell-Lendrum D, Davies CR, Costa JML. Phylogenetic species and domesticity of *Lutzomyia whitmani* at the southeast boundary of Amazonian Brazil. Transaction of the Royal Society Tropical Medicine and Hygiene 1998; 92 159–160.

[51] Mukhopadhyay J, Ghosh K, Ferro C, Munstermann LE. Distribution of phlebotomines and by genotypes (*Lutzomyia shannoni*, Diptera: Psychodidae) across a highly heterogeneous landscape. Journal of Medical Entomology 2001; 38 260–267.

[52] Uribe-Soto SI, Lehmann T, Rowton ED, Vélez IDB, Porter CH. Speciation and population structure in the morphospecies *Lutzomyia longipalpis* (Lutz &Neiva) as derived

from the mitochondrial *ND4* gene. Molecular Phylogenetics and Evolution 2001; 18(1) 84-93.

[53] Azevedo ACR, Lainson R, Souza AA, Fé NF, Feliciangeli DM, Meneses CRV, Rangel EF. Comparative studies of populaitons of *Lutzomyia umbratilis* (Diptera: Psychodidae) in Brazil and Venezuela. Journal of Medical Entomology 2002; 39 587-600.

[54] Forattini, OP. Notas sobre *Phlebotomus* do Território do Amapá, Brasil (Diptera, Psychodidae). Studia Entomologica1960; 11(1-2) 467-480.

[55] Balbino VQ, Marcondes CB, Alexander B, Luna LKS, Lucena MMM, Mendes AC, Andrade PP. First report of *Lutzomyia* (*Nyssomyia*) *umbratilis* Ward & Frahia, 1977 outside of Amazonian region, in Recife, State of Pernambuco, Brazil (Diptera: Psychodidae: Phlebotominae). Memórias do Instituto Oswaldo Cruz 2001; 96 315-317.

[56] Dye C, Davies CR, Lainson R. Communication among phlebotomine sandflies: a field study of domesticated *Lutzomyia longipalpis* populations in Amazonian Brazil. Animal Behaviour 1991; 42 183–192.

[57] Morrison AC, Ferro C, Morales A, Tesh RB, Wilson ML. Dispersal of the sandfly *Lutzomyia long*ipalpis (Diptera: Psychodidae) at an endemic focus of visceral leishmaniasis in Colombia. Journal of Medical Entomology 1993; 30 427–435.

[58] Lainson R, Ward RD, Shaw JJ. Cutaneous Leishmaniasis in north Brazil: *Lutzomyia anduzei* as a major vector. Transaction Royal Society Tropical Medicine and Hygiene 1976; 70(2) 171-172.

[59] Lainson R, Ready PD, Shaw JJ. *Leishmania* in phlebotomid sandflies. VII. On the taxonomic status of *Leishmania peruviana*, causative agent of Peruvian 'uta', as indicated by its development in the sandfly, *Lutzomyia longipalpis*. Proceedings of the Royal Society London Biological Science 1979; 206(1164) 307-318.

[60] Lainson R, Shaw JJ, Póvoa MM. The importance of edentates (sloths and anteaters) as primary reservoirs of *Leishmania braziliensis guyanensis*, causative agent of "pian-bois" in North Brazil. Transaction of the Royal Society Tropical Medicine and Hygiene 1981; 75(4) 611-612.

[61] Arias JR, Freitas RA. On the vectors of cutaneous leishmaniasis in the Central Amazon of Brazil. Acta Amazônica 1977; 7 507-527.

[62] Nery LCR, Lorosa ES, Franco AMR. Feeding preference of the sand flies *Lutzomyia umbratilis* and *L. spathotrichia* (Diptera: Psychodidae: Phlebotominae) in an urban forest patch in the city of Manaus, Amazonas, Brazil. Memórias do Instituto Oswaldo Cruz 2004; 99 571-574.

[63] Pinheiro FG, Luz SLB, Franco AMR. Infecção natural por tripanosomatídeos (Kinetoplastida: Trypanosomatidae) em *Lutzomyia umbratilis* (Diptera: Psychodidae) em áreas de Leishmaniose Tegumentar Americana no Amazonas, Brasil. Acta Amazônica 2008; 38 165-172.

[64] Azevedo ACR, Costa SM, Pinto MCG, Souza JL, Cruz HC, Vidal J, Rangel EF. Studies on the sandfly fauna (Diptera: Psychodidae: Phlebotominae) from transmission areas of American Cutaneous Leishmaniasis in state of Acre, Brazil. Memórias do Instituto Oswaldo Cruz 2008; 103 760-767.

[65] Gil LHS, Araújo MS, Villalobos JM, Camargo LMA, Ozaki LS, Fontes CJF, Ribolla PEM, Katsuragawa TH, Cruz RM, Silva AA, Silva LHP. Species structure of sand fly (Diptera: Psychodidae) fauna in the Brazilian western Amazon. Memórias do Instituto Oswaldo Cruz 2009; 104 955-959.

[66] Justiniano SCB, Chagas AC, Pessoa FAC, Queiroz RG. Comparative biology of two populations of *Lutzomyia umbratilis* (Diptera: Psychodidae) of central Amazonia, Brazil, under laboratory conditions. Brazilian Journal of Biology 2004; 64 227-235.

[67] Justiniano SCB. Biologia comparada de populações de *Lutzomyia umbratilis* (Diptera: Psychodidae) da Amazônia Central Brasileira. Doctoral Thesis. Instituto Nacional de Pesquisas da Amazônia 2004; 151pp.

[68] Valenta DT, Anez N, Tang Y, Killick-Kendrick R. The genital atrium as a good taxonomic character to distinguish between species of phlebotomine sandflies (Diptera: Psychodidae) from Venezuela. Annual of Tropical Medicine and Parasitology 1999; 93 389–399.

[69] Ward RD, Fraiha H. *Lutzomyia umbratilis*, a new species of sandfly from Brazil (Diptera: Psychodidae). Journal of Medical Entomology 1977; 14 313–317.

[70] Scarpassa VM, Alencar RB. Molecular taxonomy of the two *Leishmania* vectors *Lutzomyia umbratilis* and *Lutzomyia anduzei* (Diptera: Psychodidae) from the Brazilian Amazon. Parasites & Vectors 2013; 6 258. http://www.parasitesandvectors.com/content/6/1/258

[71] Arias JR, Freitas RA. On the vectors of cutaneous leishmaniasis in the Central Amazon of Brazil. Acta Amazônica 1977; 7 507-527.

[72] Silva MNT, Castellón EB. Sandflies (Diptera: Psychodidae) naturally infected by *Trypanosoma* (Kinetoplastida: Trypanosomatidae) in urban forest fragments in Manaus city, Amazonas, Brazil. Revista Colombiana de Ciencia Animal 2012; 4(1) 121-129.

[73] Ready PD, Lainson R, Shaw JJ, Ward R. The ecology of *Lutzomyia umbratilis* Ward & Fraiha (Diptera: Psychodidae) the major vector to man of *Leishmania braziliensis guyanensis* in north-eastern Amazonian Brazil. Bulletin of Entomology Resources 1986; 76 21-40.

[74] Clement M, Posada D, Crandall KA. TCS: a computer program to estimate gene genealogies. Molecular Ecology 2000; 9 1657-1660.

[75] Figueiredo J, Hoorn C, Van der Ven P, Soares E. Late Miocene onset of the Amazon River and the Amazon deep-sea fan: Evidence from the Foz do Amazonas Basin. Geology 2009; 37 619–622.

[76] Alencar RB. Emergência de flebotomíneos (Diptera: Psychodidae) em chão de floresta de terra firme na Amazônia Central do Brasil: Uso de um modelo modificado de armadilha de emergência. Acta Amazônica 2008; 37(2) 287-292.

[77] Alencar RB, Queiroz RG, Barrett TV. Breeding sites of phlebotomine sand flies (Diptera: Psychodidae) and efficiency of extraction techniques for immature stages in terra-firme forest in Amazonas State, Brazil. Acta Tropica 2011; 118(3) 204-208.

Chapter 6

# Dirofilariosis and Leishmaniasis in the Northern Region of Serbia

Sara Savic, Branka Vidic, Zivoslav Grgic, Tamas Petrovic, Alekasandar Potkonjak, Aleksandra Cupina, Slavica Vaselek and Dusan Petric

Additional information is available at the end of the chapter

http://dx.doi.org/10.5772/61761

**Abstract**

Research in the field of vector borne diseases and zoonozes became a topic of interest in Serbia, during the last decade. Climate changes in the country (and the region) are evident. Also, significantly is higher frequency of human and animal movement and travel, especially of dogs, within the European countries, but with overseas countries as well. The presence of vectors has already been confirmed in the country and all the surrounding countries. Current research in the domain of infectious diseases in dogs mostly includes diseases which drastically endanger health and population of dogs. Some of those infectious diseases, like dirofilariosis and leishmaniasis, which are found more or less often in dogs, cause clinical symptoms which are not obvious and therefore they represent a danger for public health with dogs acting as reservoirs of the infection.

Vectors necessary for the transmission of dirofilariosis are mosquitoes and for leishmaniasis are sand flies. Vectors of dirofilariosis are mosquitoes. Female mosquitoes which feed on mammals can transfer microfilaria from one infected organism to another non infected one. *Dirofilaria immitis* is a nematode, intravascular parasite that lives in bloodstream of host, usually pulmonary vessels. Prepatent period is at least 6-7 months in definitive hosts. Maturation of organisms in mosquitoes is temperature dependant and over 14oC is needed. Diagnostic methods for dirofilariosis are many, but several serological methods can be used: ELISA modified Knott test, immunoemzyme fast test and then molecular method (PCR), etc.

Leishmaniasis is a vector borne zoonotic disease caused by a pathogen of *Leishmania* species. For the transmission of the disease, sand flies are needed as vectors from

Lutzomyia spp. Female sand flies are bloodsucking organisms which can transfer the pathogen from one host to another during their feeding time. The presence of *Phlebotominae* (commonly known as "sand flies") has been identified in Serbia. The most certain method for diagnostic is demonstration of the parasite from bone marrow, splenic or lymph node aspirates, but there are other less invasive methods, like IFAT (immunofluorescent test) and ELISA (enzyme-linked immunosorbent assay).

Material for the research were samples from dogs and samples of vectors. In total, 292 samples of mosquitoes were collected and identified and 170 of blood samples from dogs were examined for dirofilariosis and leishmaniasis. Methods used in the study were modified Knott test and PCR for dirofilariosis and ELISA test for leismaniasis. For dirofialriosis a total prevalence of the disease in dogs was found to be 15,29%, (with different values from 3-22%) for different groups of dogs (hunting and military dogs, dogs from asylum and pet dogs). Total seroprevalence for all 170 blood samples was 10,59% for leishmaniasis. Overall, there is acually no difference in seroprevalnce for leishmaniosis, between different groups of dogs (hunting and military dogs, dogs from asylum and pet dogs). There is a reasonable doubt that leismaniasis appears as a disease in the Northern part of Serbia, in region of Vojvodina. The presence of vectors has been identified (*Phlebotomus papatasi, Laroussius tobbi*) as well as existing seroprevalence in dogs with and without clinical symptoms. All of this suggests that there is an existence of the reservoirs of infection.

**Keywords:** dirofilariosis, leishmaniasis, diagnostics, dogs

## 1. Introduction

Research in the field of vector-borne diseases and zoonozes became a topic of interest in Serbia during the last decade. Climate changes in the country (and the region) are evident, compared to the weather conditions from 10 or more years ago in terms of higher temperatures during the summer, higher humidity in summer, shorter spring and autumn periods, and shorter period of low temperature during winter. The influence of climate change has already been highlighted [1]. Also, the frequency of human and animal movement and travel, especially of dogs, is significantly higher not only in European countries but also in overseas countries. The importation of dogs is done on a pretty flexible basis with health status analysis only for rabies. The presence of vectors has already been confirmed in the country and all the surrounding countries. Current research in the domain of infectious diseases in dogs mostly includes diseases that drastically endanger health and population of dogs. Some of those infectious diseases, like dirofilariosis and leishmaniasis, which are found more or less often in dogs, cause clinical symptoms that are not so characteristic and expressed. These diseases are zoonozes, and therefore they represent a danger for public health with dogs acting as reservoirs of the infection. For a transmission of vector-borne diseases among dogs and from dogs to humans, vectors are essential because a part of the pathogen's life cycle takes place in vectors.

Dirofilariosis and leishmaniasis were earlier recognized as Mediterranean vector-borne diseases. They both have a zoonotic potential. Vectors necessary for the transmission of dirofilariosis are mosquitoes and for leishmaniasis are sand flies. Today there is evidence of dirofilariosis in different countries around the world and also evidence of presence of vectors for dirofilariosis and leishmaniasis in countries other than Mediterranean [2–5].

Dirofilariosis is a vector-borne zoonosis mostly caused by *Dirofilaria immitis* and *Dirofilaria repens*. Even though dirofilariosis was primary known as a disease found in Mediterranean countries only, it has spread out to the North and West of Europe through the years, so now clinical cases of dirofilariosis can be found in middle Europe, including Serbia [6–12].

The first published research on dirofilariosis in Serbia (ex, like previously known as Yugoslavia) was done during the 1990s, when the first cases were discovered in humans and dogs [13–16]. Since that time, there is a follow-up on dirofilariosis in several regions of Serbia. Diagnostics of dirofilariosis in Serbia has started approximately 10 years ago. Since 2004 until nowadays, veterinary services have started a regular, routine check up in dogs for dirofilariosis. Cases of dirofilariosis (*Dirofilaria immitis* and *Dirofilaria repens*) in Serbia have been found so far both in humans and dogs. Several cases of dirofilariosis in humans have been represented, and few studies have been done [17–22].

The first cases of dirofilariosis in Serbia, in dogs, were discovered as a side finding during dissections [43]. The actual first case of canine dirofilariosis in Serbia was considered to be in a dog imported from USA. A number of studies were done on the outbreaks of dirofilariosis in dogs and seroprevalence in different regions [23–27]. In the northern part of Serbia, Vojvodina province, several studies have been done during the previous period on seroprevalence and diagnostic methods [28–32]. Some research was also done on seroprevalence to dirofilariosis in working and military dogs and in pet dogs [33] (Figure 1).

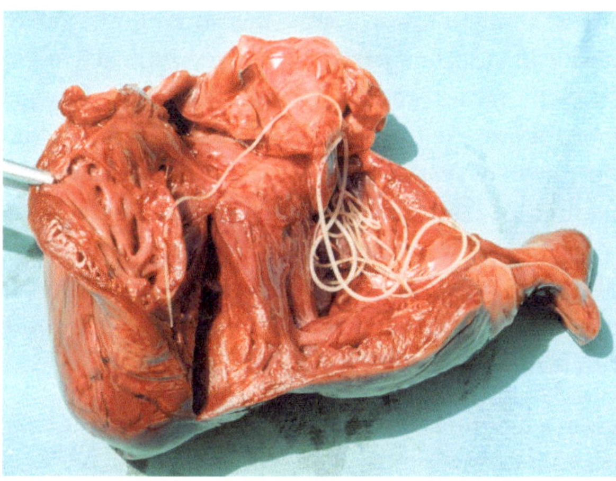

**Figure 1.** *Dirofilaria immitis* found in heart at dissection of a dog.

Vectors of dirofilariosis are mosquitoes. Female mosquitoes that feed on mammals can transfer microfilaria from one infected organism to another noninfected one. Female mosquitoes are vectors that can be found in high numbers in Serbia during the warm period of the year, from May to October. Over 70 mosquito species can be vectors of dirofilariosis out of 3000 mosquito species worldwide. Three of those species can be found in Serbia —*Aedes, Anopheles,* and *Culex* [34].

Dirofilariosis can appear with different severity, from asymptomatic to mild, or it can also progress to fatal. Definitive hosts of the parasite can be domestic dogs and wild candies, such as wolfs, coyotes, and foxes. Reservoirs of dirofilariosis in wildlife are raccoons, wolverines, coyotes, dears, and bears. Dirofilariosis has a zoonotic potential. Humans are not definitive hosts for *Dirofilaria,* but occasionally the disease can occur, most usually under the skin or in the eye.

*Dirofilaria immitis* is a nematode, intravascular parasite that lives in bloodstream of host, usually pulmonary vessels. Prepatent period is at least 6–7 months in definitive hosts. The maturation of organisms in mosquitoes is temperature dependant, and over 14°C is needed. When mosquitoes feed on the blood of an infected dog, they ingest first-stage (L1) larvae (microfilariae), which are produced over many years by the mature heartworm in the dog. Within the mosquito, larvae mature from stage 1 to stage 3. Most of their development takes place in the malphigian tubes of the mosquito. Once developed to the infective (L3) larval stage, they migrate through the body to the head cavities of the mosquito, where they wait to infect another host by leaving the mosquito during the blood meal. The prepatent period between initial infection of the dog and the maturation of the worms into adults living in the heart takes 6 to 7 months in dogs. The (L3) larvae of heartworms deposited by the mosquito into dog's skin grow for a week or two and then molt to the next larval stage (L4) under the skin at the site of the mosquito bite. Then they migrate to the muscles of the chest and abdomen, and 45 to 60 days after infection, they molt to the next larval stage (L5). Between 75 and 120 days after infection, these immature heartworms then enter the bloodstream and are carried through the heart to reside in the pulmonary artery. Over the next 3 to 4 months, they increase in size. Seven months after infection, the adult worms have mated, which has a consequence of the appearance of microfilariae in the blood stream of the host. Microfilariae may circulate in the bloodstream for up to 2 years, waiting for a bloodsucking mosquito. The extrinsic incubation period required to reach the stage when microfilariae become transmittable to another host can vary from 2 to 6 weeks, depending on the temperature. It is possible that there are no evident clinical symptoms in a host for even a year after infection. In humans, *Dirofilaria immitis* never reaches the adult stage, and they can never be found in the heart of humans because humans are accidental hosts [34] (Figure 2).

Dirofilariosis in dogs is most frequently located in the right side of the heart, pulmonal arteries, and rarely in the lungs. Clinical symptoms in dogs are unspecific: lethargy, weakness, fatigue, exercise intolerance, dyspnea, cough, anorexia, weight loss, vomiting, diarrhea, collapse, seizures, and sudden death.

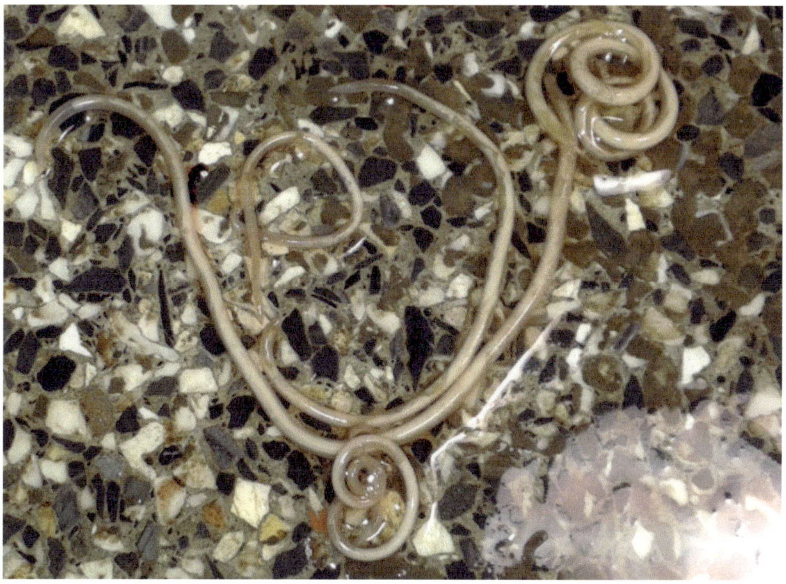

**Figure 2.** *Dirofilaria immitis* taken out from the heart of a dog.

Diagnostic methods for dirofilariosis are many, but several serological methods can be used: ELISA modified Knott test, immunoenzyme fast test, and then molecular method (PCR). Antibodies formed against the antigens of *Dirofilaria* sp. can be detected by ELISA method.

ELISA is a very sensitive and specific test, easy to perform, but it has to be done in a laboratory. There can be a false-positive reaction if there is a cross reaction with another antigen. Also, there can be a false-negative finding, if the analysis is performed too early after the infection and the dog still does not have a level of antibodies high enough (Figure 3).

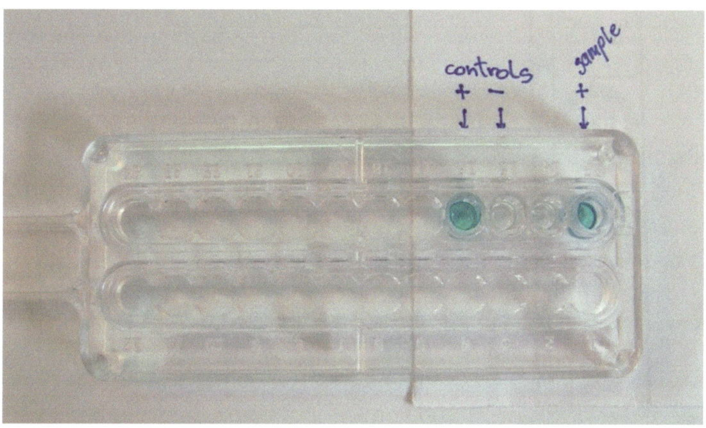


**Figure 3.** ELISA method for diagnostics—positive and negative control and positive and negative samples.

Antibodies formed against *Dirofilria* sp. can also be detected by an immunoenzyme test, usually called "fast" or "snap" tests. It is a user-friendly one- or two-step test that can be performed anywhere. No laboratory conditions are needed for the performance of the test, so it can be done at veterinary practice or even in the field. The results of the tests are ready to be read within 10–15 minutes, and the sensitivity and specificity of fast tests is good compared to the other available tests (Figure 4).

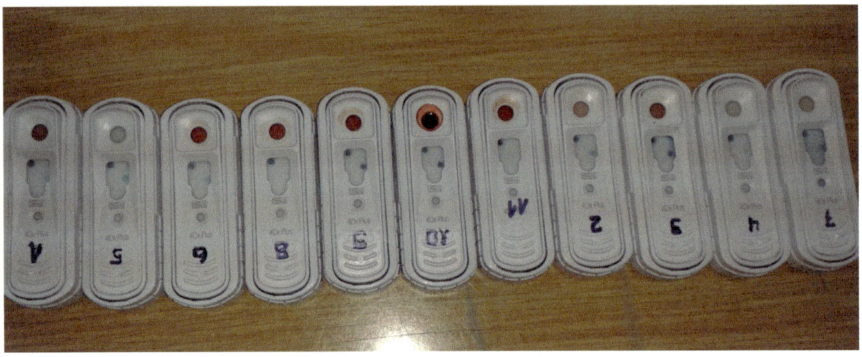

**Figure 4.** Immunoenzyme fast test—positive (two dots) and negative (one dot) findings.

The most "popular" and most used diagnostic test for dirofilariosis among veterinarians is the modified Knott test. With this test, circulating microfilaria from the blood stream can be found, colored, and seen with a microscope. The procedure is not complex but requires some laboratory equipment; time and skills are also needed, with a good knowledge of microfilarial morphology. This method is highly specific and sensitive in dogs, and microfilariae belonging to different species can be determined [35].

PCR is a molecular method with which DNA of *Dirofilaria immitis* is detected. This is a sensitive and accurate method to discriminate microfilariae from other different filarial worms in dogs. It is a good conformation test and a research tool. If dirofilariosis is detected by snap tests, ELISA, or modified Knott test, the presence of the DNA of pathogen can be confirmed by PCR method [36].

Leishmaniasis is a vector-borne zoonotic disease caused by a pathogen of *Leishmania* species. For the transmission of the disease, sand flies are needed as vectors from *Lutzomyia* spp. Female sand flies are bloodsucking organisms that can transfer the pathogen from one host to another during their feeding time. In the overview of human leishmaniasis from 2009, in Europe there are cases described in Greece, Cyprus, France, Italy, Malta, Portugal, Spain, FYROM, and Albania [5]. Later on, there are data published on cases of leishmaniasis in humans in Bulgaria [37], in dogs in Romania [38], and in dogs in Hungary [39].

In Serbia, leishmaniasis is considered, so far, an imported disease, and there is no official data that the disease exists as an autochthonous infection in humans or in animals. There are cases of humans with leishmaniasis in Serbia, but all of them were imported from Montenegro, FYOM (Former Yugoslavia Republic of Macedonia), or Greece during holiday season [40].

http://dx.doi.org/10.5772/61761

There were some notifications about leishmaniasis in dogs during the last several years. Three separate cases of dogs were found with clinical symptoms that could indicate leishmaniasis, and they were found seropositive to leishmaniasis. After therapy, their condition has improved [41, 42].

The presence of *Phlebotominae* (commonly known as "sand flies") has been identified in the southern part of Serbia a long time ago, and these vectors are known in Mediterranean countries as vectors of leishmaniasis. During the late 1950s and early 1960s, studies were done on the presence of *Phlebotominae* in the southern part of Serbia, but after that period, nothing else was published [43]. During a previous period, several dogs were found in the region, as clinical cases suspicious to leishmaniasis (epistaxis, cachexia, pale mucosa, skin problems, blindness, and lethargy), with seropositive findings for this disease [42].

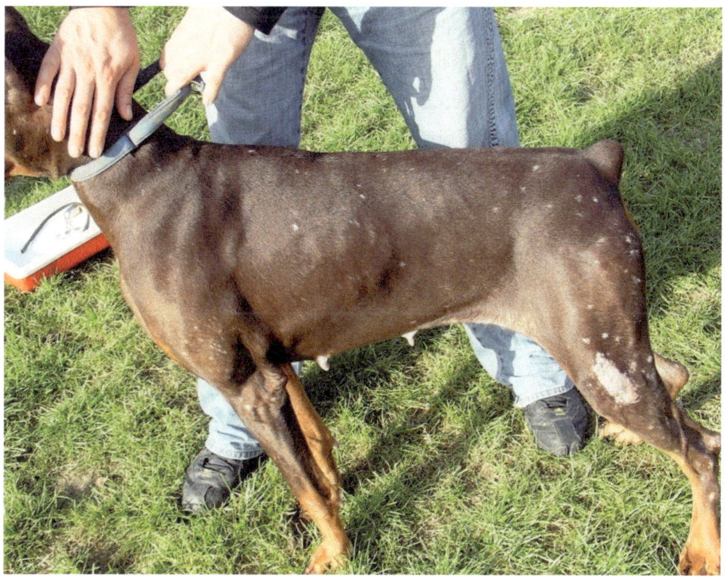

**Figure 5.** Bitch with skin lesions, positive serological finding for leishmaniasis.

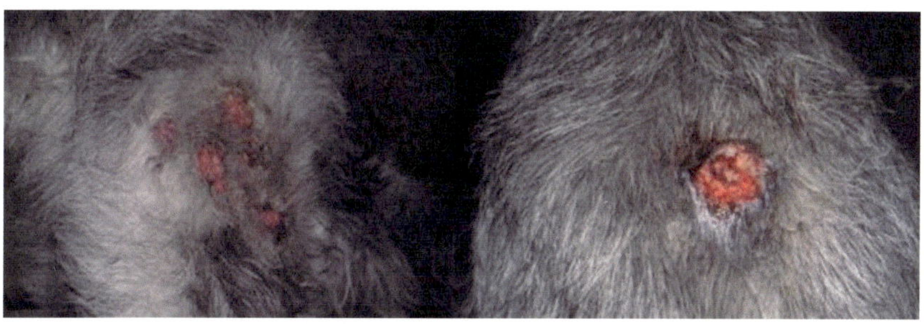

**Figure 6.** Dog with skin lesions, positive serological finding for leishmaniasis.

The first clinical cases of leishmaniasis in humans and dogs in Serbia were infections coming from abroad (Montenegro, Greece, Former Yugoslavia Republic of Macedonia, and Croatia), mostly after summer holidays. Within the last 3 years, positive findings were identified in dogs that have never left their homes in Serbia (Figures 5 and 6) [41, 42].

Domestic and wild canines are the main host species for leishmaniasis, but the domestic dog is the only epidemiologically important reservoir. Causative organisms are protozoa *Leishmania donovani* (in Asia, Middle East, and Africa) and *Leishmania infantum* (in Asia, Middle East, Europe, and South America). The transmission of the disease occurs via sand fly bites, and dogs are the reservoir hosts. Humans are accidental hosts. Transmission of the disease between dogs and humans directly is not possible.

Clinical symptoms of leishmaniasis in dogs are nonspecific. They can be as fever, weakness, lethargy, weight loss, muscle wasting, lymphadenopathy, pallor, anemia, thrombocytopenia, conjunctivitis and eye problems, skin lesions and alopecia, etc.

Diagnostic procedures for leishmaniasis are several. The most certain method is the demonstration of the parasite from bone marrow, splenic, or lymph node aspirates, but there are other less invasive methods too. Serologic tests are most commonly immunofluorescent test (IFAT) and enzyme-linked immunosorbent assay (ELISA) [44].

## 2. Materials and methods

Materials for the research were samples from dogs and samples of vectors. The research was planed as serological examination of dog blood samples for dirofilariosis and leishmaniasis. The vectors (mosquitoes) were collected, identified, and analyzed for the presence of causative agents of dirofilariosis in the northern part of Serbia.

During spring and summer of 2014 (May–September), 292 samples of mosquitoes were collected and identified. Collecting was done with lamps with dry ice. The identification of mosquitoes (for gender and species) was done at Faculty of Agriculture, University of Novi Sad. Vector identification was done with microscopic observation. The analysis of vectors for the presence of causative agent for dirofilariosis was done by a molecular method (PCR). PCR analysis were performed at the Scientific Veterinary Institute of "Novi Sad." The samples were pooled as 20 mosquitoes into one pool. In collected mosquitoes, a molecular method of PCR was performed. DNA extraction was done with commercial kits from Quiagen (QIAmp), during a 2-day protocol. PCR was done according to the prescription of Rishniw et al. [36]. Primers used for PCR analysis were primers 5′–3′, forward: DIDR-F1_for AGTGCGAATTG-CAGACGCATTGAG and reverse: DIDR-R1_rev AGCGGGTAATCACGACTGAGTTGA. Determination was done based on 542 bp for *D. immitis*.

In total, 170 of blood samples from dogs were examined for dirofilariosis and leishmaniasis. Serological analysis for dirofilariosis and leishmaniasis were done from blood samples of dogs obtained by venous punctation. The blood samples were divided into three groups, according to the way of life of the dogs:

- Group of hunting and military dogs (79 samples)—in this group, samples were analyzed from dogs that are actively used for hunting. They had their owners, and they mostly did not receive any preventive treatment against parasites. Not one of these dogs has ever left Serbia.

- Group of dogs from asylum for homeless dogs (64 samples)—in this group were dogs kept in the asylum, but for a long time, and they have all received preventive treatment against parasites annually. Not one of these dogs has ever left Serbia since they were in asylum, but for many of them, the history of their previous life and origin is unknown.

- Group of pet dogs (27 samples)—in this group were dogs that came to veterinary practice for numerous reasons, with nonspecific clinical symptoms, or no clinical symptoms at all. Not one of the owners thought that their dog has dirofilariosis or leishmaniasis. Some of the dogs have received antiparasitic prevention and some did not. Even the ones which did receive preventive treatment did not receive it annually, only during spring and summer. Not one of these dogs has ever left Serbia.

Methods used in the study were the following: modified Knott test and PCR for dirofilariosis and ELISA test for leishmaniasis.

Analysis for dirofilariosis was done with the modified Knott test for the detection of microfilaria in circulation. Analysis for all the samples was done on the same day of sampling or the next day. Samples were taken with anticoagulant. The procedure of the modified Knott test was performed according to the instructions of Genchi et al. [35]. The modified Knott test was done in all the samples—from dogs with clinical symptoms as well as from dogs without any clinical symptoms for dirofilariosis. Positive samples found by the modified Knott test were then selected for molecular analysis to be done by PCR. DNA extraction was done with QIAmp commercial kits for DNA extraction (Quiagen, by the instructions of the producer). After that, a PCR was performed according to the protocol from Rishniw et al. [36]. The same primers were used in the protocol of *Dirofilaria* DNA detection in blood samples as in mosquito samples (primers 5′–3′):

Forward: DIDR-F1_for AGTGCGAATTGCAGACGCATTGAG and

Reverse: DIDR-R1_rev AGCGGGTAATCACGACTGAGTTGA.

Determination was done based on 542 bp for *Dirofilaria immitis*.

For diagnostics of leishmaniasis, same blood samples were used taken from the same dogs. Analysis for leishmaniasis was done by ELISA method (commercial kit by Ingenaza, done by the prescription of the producer). From blood samples, sera samples were obtained by centrifugation. After that, blood sera samples were kept on –20°C until ELISA was performed.

## 3. Results and discussion

### 3.1. Dirofilariosis

Analysis of vectors for dirofilariosis: In total, 292 samples of mosquitoes were collected. After determination, it was found that they belong to *Culex* (*Culex pipiens* and *Culex culex*) and *Aedes* species. The samples were collected as random samples from different locations of the northern part of Serbia. In 292 mosquitoes randomly collected, the presence of DNA of causative agent for dirofilariosis (*Dirofilaria immitis*) was not found. Mosquitoes were collected randomly, and weather conditions during the collection of samples were not favorable. Weather conditions were bad for the lamps and the collection process because there was a lot of wind and often rain during the time of collection. Also, the outside temperature was lower than usual for that the time of the year. The results found after the analysis of mosquito samples indicate that sampling was perhaps not done in the best way. The samples should have been collected at the residence of positive dogs and not from several randomly chosen locations. Also, the weather conditions may have influenced the development of L3 larval stage of microfilariae in the mosquito because the temperature for many days was not too much above 14°C. All of these may have influenced the absence of *Dirofilaria* sp. DNA in mosquito samples.

The results of analysis of blood samples from three groups of dogs (170 samples in total) to dirofilariosis by the modified Knott test are shown in Table 1.

| Group of dogs | Total number of examined dogs | Number of positive dogs | Percentage of positive dogs |
|---|---|---|---|
| Hunting and military dogs | 79 | 18 | 22.78 |
| Dogs from asylum for homeless dogs | 64 | 2 | 3.12 |
| Pet dogs | 27 | 6 | 22 |
| Total | 170 | 26 | 15.29 |

**Table 1.** Results of the analysis of blood samples from three groups of dogs to dirofilariosis

In the group of hunting and military dogs, a seroprevalence for dirofilariosis was found to be 22.78%. In the group of dogs from asylum, a lower seroprevalence for dirofilariosis was found —3.12% and in the group of pet dogs, and seroprevalence for dirofilariosis was found to be 22%. In the case of dirofilariosis, the seroprevalence of the disease in different groups was different. It depended on the received prevention treatment against parasites and the lifestyle of dogs. Seroprevalence was the lowest (3.12%) in dogs living in asylum with regular prevention care. These dogs received preventive treatment monthly during the whole period when mosquitoes can be found (March/April–October). It is important to highlight that even two positive dogs found in asylum were new dogs that came from another place, less than 1 month previously to the sampling. The highest seroprevalence (22.78%) was found in hunting dogs with no prevention treatment in most of the cases. Seroprevalence found in pet dogs was not much different than the one found in hunting dogs. This would refer to the fact that not many pet dogs are under preventive treatment, or even if they are, it is not being repeated enough times. Most of the pet owners are not aware enough of the existence of dirofilariosis as a disease in dogs, and so they believe that it is enough if they give the preventive treatment to their pet dogs once or rarely twice during the whole period of the year when mosquitoes are present (March/April–September). Also, the fact that there are no clinical symptoms in dogs usually for a long time after infection makes the owners believe that their dog is healthy.

During a 2-year period, 170 dog blood samples were analyzed. Most of the dogs did not have any clinical symptoms. Only several dogs had clinical symptoms such as cough, lethargy, tiredness, and heart failure symptoms. The modified Knott test gives us a direct overview into the existence of larvae of *Dirofilaria* (microfilaria) in dogs' circulation. A total average sero-prevalence for the whole three groups of dogs was found to be 15.29%, but the highest seroprevalence was found to be in hunting and military dogs, followed very closely by pet dogs. Hunting and military dogs live in most cases outside in backyards and are in constant contact with vectors. They have a long time of outside activities in the regions where vectors can be found. Also, quite a lot of dogs from this group is not protected constantly with preventive ectoantiparasitic treatment.

The modified Knott test is a fast and reliable diagnostic tool recognized in the world as a method for the detection of microfilaria in circulation of dogs. In veterinary practices, fast tests can be used for routine checkup of patients. However, in the case of positive finding or if there are recognizable clinical symptoms in a dog, a confirmation of diagnosis has to be done with the modified Knott test. With this test, an identification of Dirofilaria can be done with distinction between *Dirofilaria immitis* and *Dirofilaria repens* [35] (Figure 7).

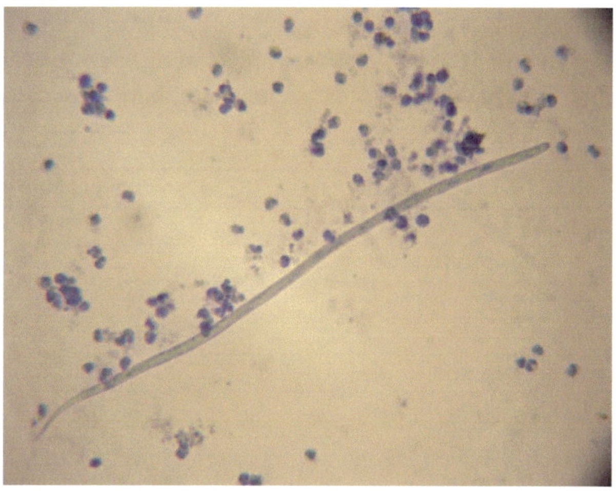

**Figure 7.** Diagnostics of dirofilariosis by the modified Knott test.

After positive samples were found by the modified Knott test, a PCR analysis was done for the conformation of *Dirofilaria immitis*. PCR analysis was done from blood samples of dogs in which microfilariae were found (26 samples). The isolation of *Dirofilaria*'s DNA from 200 μl of blood samples was done with QIAmp set kit (Quiagen). PCR procedure was done as described by Rishniw et al. [36]. PCR is a very sensitive, specific, and accurate method with which determination of *Dirofilaria* species is possible. It is more a research tool than a diagnostic tool because it is a demanding procedure in equipment and skills. From 26 blood samples from dogs in which *Dirofilaria* was found by the modified Knott test, a positive result was found by the PCR method in 24 samples (92.3%) (Figure 8).

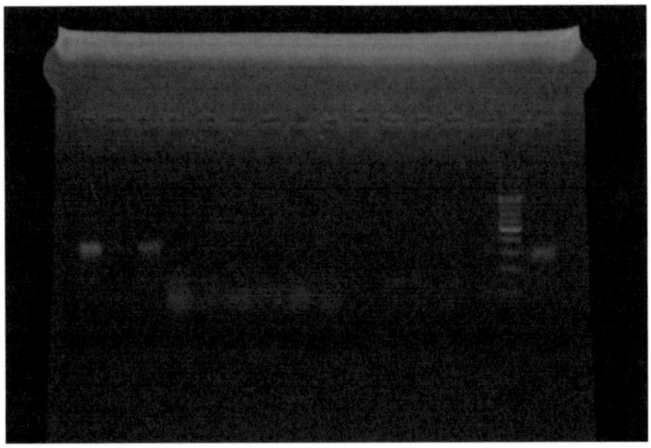

**Figure 8.** PCR reaction for *Dirofilaria immitis* in blood samples of dogs positive to dirofilariosis by the modified Knott test, determination based on 542 bp.

These data can be compared to the data collected during the last several years in the same region by the same authors, shown in Table 2. The first official acknowledgment of dirofilariosis in Serbia was published by Dimitrijevic in 1999 [43]. After that time, several authors have been following the development of this disease in dogs in different regions of Serbia. For the northern part of Serbia, data have been collected for more than 10 years now.

| Year | Percentage of positive dog samples |
|---|---|
| 2003–2004 | 5.9–7 |
| 2006–2007, dogs with no clinical symptoms | 10–11 |
| 2006–2007, dogs with clinical symptoms | 80 |
| 2010 | 14 |
| 2010, only pet dogs | 11 |
| 2011–2013 | 5 human cases |
| 2013–2014 hunting and military dogs, dogs from asylum and pet dogs | 15.29 |

**Table 2.** An overview of data collection during a 10-year period on the seroprevalence of dirofilariosis in dogs in northern Serbia

By comparing the data during the last decade, it can be stated that there is a constant increase of seroprevalence for dirofilariosis in dogs in Serbia over the years. After these findings were published, diagnostic methods for dirofilariosis were introduced into the routine checkup of dogs in veterinary practices—modified Knott test, fast test, and ELISA test. Also, fast tests became available to the practitioners and became the mostly used diagnostic tool in veterinary practices. Preventive treatment is present and offered to the owners, but the awareness of the owners is not quite high enough. Further research on the presence of causative pathogen (*Dirofilaria immitis*) must be done in vectors so that a risk estimation can be made. Definitely, dirofilariosis is present in the northern part of Serbia in the percentage that justifies the fact that this disease should always be considered when looking at a patient in veterinary practice. Also, there are already human cases in the region, so attention should be paid to this disease in the meaning of "One Health" point of view.

Clinical cases of canine dirofilariosis in Serbia are still often found after dissections, and still mostly as a side finding (Figure 9).

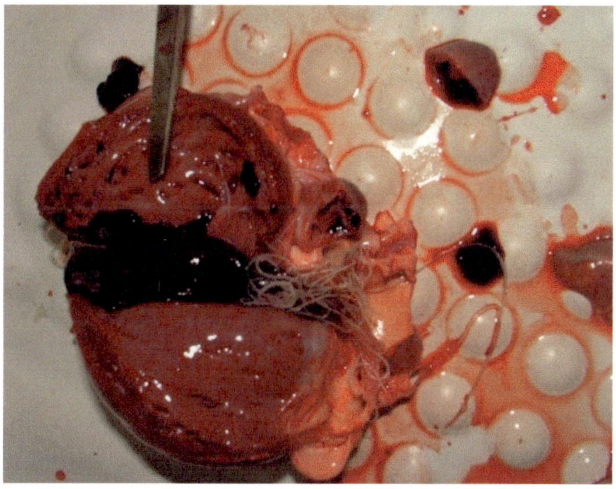

**Figure 9.** Dirofilariosis in one of the military dogs from the survey.

It appears that dirofilariosis is a disease more and more frequent in dogs, so there is more demand for control of health status for dirofilariosis within a routine checkup in dogs. The owners are not enough aware that disease can occur without any clinical symptoms for a certain period of time. During the period of our study, seropositive findings for dirofilariosis were present all the time in dogs, which makes therapy and prevention necessary in the region.

The awareness of the fact that dirofilariosis is a zoonotic disease is higher over the time, and this makes the disease a danger for public health. Cases of human dirofilariosis are also present in the northern part of Serbia but are still neglected within diagnostic procedure. Medical doctors are still not completely aware of the diagnostics of dirofilariosis in humans, and there are still no reliable, noninvasive diagnostic methods on the market [21].

Apart from the modified Knott test done from the blood samples of dogs, an identification of the pathogen has been confirmed by PCR method too. Positive finding were gained by PCR method, at the matching rate of 92.3% with the modified Knott test.

### 3.2. Leishmaniasis

During the same period of study, 170 blood samples were examined for leishmaniasis from dogs that did or did not have clinical symptoms of the disease. After serological testing of the samples, positive findings for leishmaniasis were gained. Blood samples were analyzed for the presence of specific antibodies against *Leishmania* sp. with the ELISA method (Ingezim Leishmania, Ingenasa, 1.5.LSH.K.1). From total number of samples, in 10.59% of samples, the presence of specific antibodies against *Leishmania infantum* was found. It is important to highlight that not one of the examined dogs has ever left their dwelling place. In 18 dogs, positive serological findings for leishmaniasis were obtained. Three of the examined dogs had skin lesions that would not heal and bad skin condition in general.

The findings after the analysis of blood samples from three groups of dogs (170 samples in total) for leishmaniasis with ELISA test are shown in Table 3.

| Group of dogs | Total number of examined dogs | Number of positive dogs | Percentage of positive dogs |
|---|---|---|---|
| Hunting and military dogs | 79 | 8 | 10.12 |
| Dogs from asylum for homeless dogs | 64 | 7 | 10.33 |
| Pet dogs | 27 | 3 | 11.11 |
| Total | 170 | 18 | 10.59 |

**Table 3.** Results of the analysis of blood samples from three groups of dogs for leishmaniasis

In the group of hunting and military dogs, a seroprevalence for leishmaniasis was found to be 10.12%. In the group of dogs from asylum, seroprevalence was found to be 10.33%, and in the group of pet dogs, seroprevalence for leishmaniasis was 11.11%. The total seroprevalence for all 170 blood samples was 10.59% for leishmaniasis. Overall, there is actually no difference in seroprevalence for leishmaniasis between different groups of dogs. There is a similar seroprevalence in all three groups of dogs, unlike the seroprevalence to dirofilariosis. There is a constant presence of causative pathogen among the dog population in the northern part of Serbia. There is a reasonable doubt that leishmaniasis appears as a disease in the northern part of Serbia, in Vojvodina. The presence of vectors has been identified (*Phlebotomus papatasi* and *Laroussius tobbi*) (Vaselek, unpublished data), as well as the existing seroprevalence in dogs with and without clinical symptoms. All of this suggests that there is an existence of the reservoirs of infection. Leishmaniasis in humans has been identified so far only in people who have traveled to Mediterranean countries and not as an autochthonous infection. Due to climate changes, summer temperatures and conditions in the northern part of Serbia are more and more in favor of the life cycle of vectors—sand flies.

In our history, there is evidence of leishmaniasis in humans and in dogs in Serbia, but over 60 years ago. The first autochthonous cases of visceral leishmaniasis were found in the southern part of Serbia (region around city of Nis) back in 1945. During the period of 1946–1949, there were 350 registered cases of human visceral leishmaniasis in Serbia, and some cases were even registered around city of Belgrade [45]. At that same time, about 2% of dogs in the region around city of Nis were found to have asymptomatic leishmaniasis, and dogs were identified as main reservoir of infection [45]. During the period from 1968 to 1969, rare cases of autochthonous visceral leishmaniasis were reported in the southern part of Serbia. At that time, the vectors of leishmaniasis were detected: *P. major*, *P. simici*, and *P. perfiliewi* [46]. In the northern part of Serbia, the disease or vectors have never been identified before. After this period of studies and interest of public into leishmaniasis, no more data were found, and no research has been done until now. No vectors have been identified any more, or they were just not looked for until 50 years later. There is a question on the existence of leishmaniasis in Serbia, but at the moment, there is evidence of the existence of vectors and clinical disease in dogs, with serological conformation of the disease and successful therapy. Today, Serbia is surrounded with several countries that have leishmaniasis for sure (Croatia, Montenegro, and FYROM), countries where vectors are identified so far (Hungary), and countries in which there is also a reasonable doubt that leishmaniasis exists in dogs (Romania). More research has to be done, especially on vectors and reservoirs of the infection, with a precise identification of the pathogen.

## Acknowledgements

This study was supported by the Ministry of Education, Science and Technological Development of the Republic of Serbia (grant TR31084).

## Author details

Sara Savic[1], Branka Vidic[1], Zivoslav Grgic[1], Tamas Petrovic[1], Alekasandar Potkonjak[2], Aleksandra Cupina[3], Slavica Vaselek[3] and Dusan Petric[3]

1 Department of Immunology, Serology and Biochemistry, Scientific Veterinary Institute "Novi Sad," Novi Sad, Serbia

2 Department for veterinary medicine, Agricultural Faculty, University of Novi Sad, Serbia

3 Laboratory for Medical and Veterinary Entomology, Agricultural Faculty, University of Novi Sad, Serbia

## References

[1] Ready PD (2008) Leishmaniasis emergence and climate change. In: S de la Roque, editor. Climate change: the impact on the epidemiology and control of animal diseases. Rev Sci Tech Off Int Epiz. 27(2):399–412.

[2] Jacsó O, Kiss G, Krassóvári D, Kiss HJ, Gyurkovszky M, Fok E. (2014) Epidemiological view about dirofilarioses in dogs of Hungary. Fourth European Dirofilaria and Angiostrongylus Days (FEDAD), 2–4 July, 2014, Budapest, Hungary. Edited by Eva

Fok, Istvan Kucsera, Final Program and Abstracts, Budapest, European Society of Dirofilaria and Angiostrongylus.

[3] Miterpáková M, Iglódyová A, Antolová D, Hurníková Z. (2014) Canine dirofilariosis in Slovakia—the results of 8-year epidemiological research. Fourth European Dirofilaria and Angiostrongylus Days (FEDAD), 2–4 July, 2014, Budapest, Hungary. Edited by Eva Fok, Istvan Kucsera, Final Program and Abstracts, Budapest, European Society of Dirofilaria and Angiostrongylus.

[4] Farkas R1, Tánczos B, Bongiorno G, Maroli M, Dereure J, Ready PD. (2011) First surveys to investigate the presence of canine leishmaniasis and its phlebotomine vectors in Hungary. Vector Borne Zoonotic Dis. 11(7):823–34. doi: 10.1089/vbz.2010.0186. Jan 22.

[5] Ready PD. (2010) Leishmaniasis emergence in Europe. Euro Surveill. 15(10):pii=19505. Available online: http://www.eurosurveillance.org

[6] Draghici S, Jarca A. (2012) Dirofilariasis-case file. European Multicolloquium of Parasitology (EMOP XI). Program and Abstract book, Romania, p. 386.

[7] Hamel D, Silaghi C, Mihalkov A, Maurer U, Pfister K. (2012) Vector-borne infections in imported dogs—a serological and molecular survey. European Multicolloquium of Parasitology (EMOP XI). Program and Abstract book, Romania, p. 300.

[8] Simon F, Gonzles-Miguel J, Morchon R, Mellado I, Del Mar Siles-Luca M. (2012) Proteomic analyses of *Dirofilaria* species. European Multicolloquium of Parasitology (EMOP XI). Program and Abstract book, Romania, p. 234.

[9] Otasevic S, Tasic A, Gabrielli S, Trenkic Bozinovic M, Cancrini G. (2014) Canine and human Dirofilaria infections: what is new in the Balkan Peninsula. Fourth European Dirofilaria and Angiostrongylus Days (FEDAD), 2–4 July, 2014, Budapest, Hungary. Edited by Eva Fok, Istvan Kucsera. Final Program and Abstracts, Budapest, European Society of Dirofilaria and Angiostrongylus.

[10] Diakou A, Kapantaidakis E. (2014) Epidemiology of dirofilariosis in dogs in Greece: previous and last information. Fourth European Dirofilaria and Angiostrongylus Days (FEDAD), 2–4 July, 2014, Budapest, Hungary. Edited by Eva Fok, Istvan Kucsera. Final Program and Abstracts, Budapest, European Society of Dirofilaria and Angiostrongylus.

[11] Margarida Alho A, Gomes L, Pereira da Fonseca I, Meireles J, Madeira de Carvalho L. (2014) Canine dirofilariosis in Lisbon, Portugal, over a 14-year period: prevalence, diagnosis, and routine laboratory approaches. Fourth European Dirofilaria and Angiostrongylus Days (FEDAD), 2–4 July, 2014, Budapest, Hungary. Edited by Eva Fok, Istvan Kucsera. Final Program and Abstracts, Budapest, European Society of Dirofilaria and Angiostrongylus.

[12] Fuehrer H-P, Auer H, Silbermayr K, Duscher GG. (2014) Dirofilaria repens and Dirofilaria immitis in Austria. Fourth European Dirofilaria and Angiostrongylus Days

(FEDAD), 2–4 July, 2014, Budapest, Hungary. Edited by Eva Fok, Istvan Kucsera. Final Program and Abstracts, Budapest, European Society of Dirofilaria and Angiostrongylus.

[13] Kulišić Z, Kranjčić-Zec I, Mitrović S, Radojičić B. (1989) New case of human dirofilariosis in Jugoslavia (serb), 6. Kongres mikrobiologa Jugoslavije Maribor, Proceedings.

[14] Kulišić Z, Milosavljević P. (1994) Modern techniques in diagnostic of dirofilariosis in dogs (serb). Veterinarski Glasnik. 48, 9: 745–9.

[15] Kulišić Z, Mišić Z, Milosavljević P, Popović N. (1995) Dirofilariosis in dogs in Yugoslavia (serb), 8. Symposium of Veterinarians in Serbia, Zlatibor, Proceedings.

[16] Dimitrijević S. (1999) Dirofilarioza ante portas, Clinica Veterinaria 1, Proceedings, p. 58.

[17] Lalošević D. (2004) *Dirofilaria* spp parasite like in mesenterium removed by surgery from mesenterium (serb). Medicinski Pregled, 5–6: 307–8.

[18] Tasić A, Tasić S, Miladinović-Tasić N, Zdravković D, Đorđević. (2007) Dirofilaria repens—potential risk for public health. Acta Medica Medianae; 46(3): 53–6.

[19] Džamić AM, Čolović IV, Arsić-Arsenijević VS, Stepanović S, Boričić I, Džamić Z, Mitrović SM, Rašić DM, Stefanović I, Latković Z, Kranjčić-Zec IF. (2009) Human Dirofilaria repens infection in Serbia. J Helminthol; 83: 129–37.

[20] Tasić S, Stojiljković N, Miladinović-Tasić N, Tasić A, Mihailović D, Đorđević J. (2009) Human subcutaneous dirofilariosis in South Serbia—case report. u: Dirofilaria days (II), Salamanca, Spain, P-12.

[21] Đorđević J, Tasić S, Miladinović-Tasić N, Tasić A. (2010) Diagnosis and clinical value of human dirofilariosis (serb). Acta Facultatis Medicae Naissensis; 27(2): 81–4.

[22] Tasić-Otašević S, Gabrielli S, Tasić A, Miladinović Tasić N, Kostić J, Ignjatović A, Popović Dragonjić L, Milošević Z, Cancrini G. (2014). Seroreactivity to Dirofilaria antigens in people from different areas of Serbia. BMC Infect. Dis; 14: 68.

[23] Tasić A, Katić-Radivojević S, Klun I, Mišić Z, Ilić T, Dimitrijević S. (2003) Prevalence of canine filariasis in some parts of Vojvodina. Veterinary Symposium of Serbia (15), Zlatibor, 09–13. 09., Proceedings.

[24] Tasić A, Tasić S, Miladinović-Tasić N, Zdravković D, Đorđević J. (2007) Prevalence of *Dirofilariae repens* as causative agent of zoonozes in dogs. Acta Facultatis Medicae Naissensis; 24(2): 71–4.

[25] Tasic A, Rossi L, Tasic SA, Miladinovic-Tasic N, Ilic TD, Dimitrijevic SM. (2008) Survey of canine dirofilariasis in Vojvodina, Serbia.

[26] Spasojević-Kosić L, Lalošević V, Lalošević D, Naglić A. (2011) Heart worm disease—a case study. Veterinarski Glasnik; 65(3–4): 257–67.

[27] Spasojević-Kosić L, Lalošević V, Lalošević D, Simin S, Vasić I, Kuruca L. (2012) Prevalence of dirofilariosis in pet dogs in Novi Sad. Saremena Poljoprivreda; 61(3–4): 247–54.

[28] Savić-Jevđenić S, Vidić B, Grgić Ž, Milovanović A. (2004) Fast diagnostic of dirofilariosis in Novi Sad region (serb). Veterinarski Glasnik; 58(5–6): 693–698. ISSN 0350-2457.

[29] Savić-Jevđenić S, Milovanović A, Grgić Ž, Kojić S. (2006) Outspread of dirofilariosis in Novi Sad region-six years later (serb), Proceedings, VIII epizootiological days, Banja Vrdnik, p. 60.

[30] Savić-Jevđenić S, Vidić B, Grgić Ž, Lolić Z. (2007) The appearances of dirofilariosis in Serbia - Vojvodina. First European Dirofilaria Days, Zagreb, Croatia, Proceedings, p. 202.

[31] Savić S, Grgić Z, Vujkov B, Fenjac I, Pajković D, Žekić M. (2009) Determination of canine dirofilariasis by ELISA method and modified Knott's test. Arhiv Veterinarske Medicine; 2(2): 71-77. ISSN 1820-9955.

[32] Savić S, Vidić B, Pajkovič D, Spasojević-Kosić L, Medić S, Potkonjak A, Otašević S. (2014) Overview of dirofilariosis in Serbia during the last ten years 2004–2014 and current status of the disease. Fourth European Dirofilaria and Angiostrongylus Days (FEDAD), 2–4 July, 2014, Budapest, Hungary. Edited by Eva Fok, Istvan Kucsera, Final Program and Abstracts, str. 46, Budapest, European Society of Dirofilaria and Angiostrongylus.

[33] Pajković D, Savić S, Veljković P, Grgić Z. (2010) Study on dirofilariosis in working dogs servicing the Army of Serbia. Arhiv Veterinarske Medicine; 3(2): 53–58.

[34] Newcomb EC, Moorhead A. (2013) Dirofilaria immitis, American Association of Zoo Veterinarians Infectious Disease Committee Manual, 2013 Infectious Disease Manual 2013, 2nd Edition.

[35] Genchi C, Venco L, Genchi M. (2007) Guideline for the laboratory diagnosis of canine and feline *Dirofilaria* infections, *Dirofilaria immitis,* and *D. repens* in dog and cat and human infections. Edited by Genchi C, Rinaldi L, Cringoli Giuseppe. Mappe parasitologiche 8, ISBN 88-89132-14-0, pp. 139–144.

[36] Rishniw M, Barr SC, Simpsom KW, Frongillo MF, Franz M, Dominguez-Alpizar JL. (2006) Discrimination between six species of canine microfilariae by single polymerase chain reaction. Veterinary Parasitology 135, pp. 303–314.

[37] Harizanov R, Rainova I, Tzvetkova N, Kaftandjiev I, Bikov I, Mikov O. (2013) Geographical distribution and epidemiological characteristics of visceral leishmaniasis in Bulgaria, 1988 to 2012, Eurosurveillance, Volume 18, Issue 29, 18 July 2013, Surveillance and outbreak reports.

[38] Mircean V, Dumitrache MO, Mircean M, Bolfa P, Györke A, Mihalca AD. (2014) Autochthonous canine leishmaniasis in Romania: neglected or (re)emerging? Parasit Vectors. 7: 135. http://www.parasitesandvectors.com/content/7/1/135

[39] Tánczos B1, Balogh N, Király L, Biksi I, Szeredi L, Gyurkovsky M, Scalone A, Fiorentino E, Gramiccia M, Farkas R. (2012 July) First record of autochthonous canine leishmaniasis in Hungary. Vector Borne Zoonotic Dis. 12(7): 588–94. doi: 10.1089/vbz.2011.0906. Epub 2012 May 18.

[40] Dakic ZD1, Pelemis MR, Stevanovic GD, Poluga JL, Lavadinovic LS, Milosevic IS, Indjic NK, Ofori-Belic IV, Pavlovic MD. (2009) Epidemiology and diagnostics of visceral leishmaniasis in Serbia. Clin Microbiol Infect. 15(12):1173–6.

[41] Savić-Jevđenić S, Grgić Ž, Vidić B, Vujkov B. (2007) Leishmaniasis in dog—clinical case, IX regional meeting in clinical pathology and therapy in animals Palic, Proceedings, p. 2, Belgrade, Faculty of Veterinary Medicine.

[42] Savić S, Vidić B, Fenjac I, Bekvalac R, Radičević M, Lolić Z. (2010) Leishmaniasis in dogs in Serbia—existence or not? Symposium of Small Animal Practitioners SIVEMAP 2010, Belgrade, Proceedings, pp. 241–243.

[43] Dimitrijević S, Dirofilarioza ante portas. Meeting on Clinical Pathology and Therapy of Animals, Proceedings, Budva, 1999, pp. 58–61.

[44] Fiorello C. (2013) Visceral leishmaniasis. American Association of Zoo Veterinarians Infectious Disease Committee Manual, 2013 Infectious Disease Manual 2013, 2nd Edition.

[45] Simić C. (1957) Protozoe paraziti čoveka i domaćih životinja. Naučna knjiga, Beograd.

[46] Petrović Z. (1980) Epidemiology of kala-azar in Serbia. Belgrade: Institute for Medical Research (Serbian).

# Chapter 7

# Schistosomiasis – Updating Technologies and Diagnostic Approaches in Surveillance Strategies and Clinical Management

Marta Guimarães Cavalcanti and José Mauro Peralta

Additional information is available at the end of the chapter

http://dx.doi.org/10.5772/61310

**Abstract**

*Schistosoma* infection is a poverty-related parasitic infection, being the second most important neglected tropical disease in the world after malaria. Schistosomiasis is caused by five distinct *Schistosoma* species distributed in tropical and subtropical areas. But, imported cases can also be seen in non - endemic areas. Human populations acquire infection after exposure to contaminated water collections. *Schistosoma* infection falls on a large spectrum of clinical manifestations that ranges from absence of signs and symptoms to severe forms of disease. Although morbidity and mortality have been reduced along the years after use of mass drug administration (MDA) in endemic areas, large populations are still at risk of disability-related outcomes on daily basis. Recently, a great deal of debate has been done over two main issues in schistosomiasis management in endemic and non-endemic areas: how to accurately diagnosis *Schistosoma* infections pre and post-therapy in addition to assess morbidity level. Adoption of promising new diagnostic tools and development of new markers of disease progression might change the current scenario by improving schistosomiasis clinical management in both community and institutional settings.

**Keywords:** schistosomiasis, diagnostic tests, markers of therapy response, morbidity, community settings, institutional settings

## 1. Introduction

*Schistosoma* infection is a poverty-related parasitic infection, being the second most important neglected tropical disease in the world after malaria. Schistosomiasis is a blood-fluke-induced infection, which may present with acute and chronic disease forms. Schistosomiasis is caused by five distinct *Schistosoma* species distributed in tropical and subtropical areas. However, imported cases can also been seen in nonendemic areas. Human populations acquire infection after exposure to contaminated fresh water sources like dams, rivers, canals, lakes, and streams. *Schistosoma* infection falls on a large spectrum of clinical manifestations that ranges from absence of signs and symptoms to severe forms of disease. Although morbidity and mortality have been reduced along the years after use of mass drug administration (MDA) in endemic areas, large populations are still at risk of disability-related outcomes on a daily basis. A broad spectrum of clinical manifestations and also asymptomatic infections are observed [1, 2]. Three major species, *Schistosoma haematobium, Schistosoma japonicum,* and *Schistosoma mansoni*, and another two minor species, *Schistosoma mekongi* and *Schistosoma intercalatum*, are recognized as the mainly pathogenic *Schistosoma* species that infect human populations [3, 4]. Parasite transmission occurs after contamination of water collections with *Schistosoma* eggs eliminated by infected individuals, which further develop in the infective form called cercariae in freshwater snails. The release of *Schistosoma* cercariae from snails is followed by skin penetration of the definitive hosts (human and nonhuman species like buffalos in the case of *S. japonicum* or rodents in the case of *S. mansoni* infection). In the latter, *Schistosoma* immature forms evolve to adults that lay eggs, which are spread in the definitive hosts and/or eliminated in the environment through excreta, like urine in the case of *S. haematobium* and stool for the other species. In some areas, nonhuman definitive hosts are also essential to maintain *Schistosoma* life cycle, such as buffalos for *S. japonicum* and rodents for *S. mansoni* [5, 6]. Schistosomiasis world distribution is essentially in tropical and subtropical areas, with more than 90% of infected individuals living in sub-Saharan Africa [7, 8]. However, imported cases of schistosomiasis are also becoming increasingly frequent in nonendemic areas such as Europe. Spotlights were thrown on schistosomiasis in the recent years since elimination is believed to be a reachable goal for some endemic regions on the globe. Education, sanitation policies, and hygiene awareness proved to promote a high impact on infection transmission [9]. Also, field work in different transmission areas shows that chemotherapy plays an evident role in decreasing prevalence, parasite burden, and late morbidity [10].

Recently, a great deal of debate has been done over two main issues in schistosomiasis management in endemic and nonendemic areas: how to accurately diagnosis *Schistosoma* infections before and after therapy in addition to assess morbidity level. The adoption of promising new diagnostic tools and the development of new markers of disease progression might change the current scenario by improving schistosomiasis clinical management in both community and institutional settings.

The diagnosis of active *Schistosoma* infection is based on the demonstration of egg excretion by parasitological methods such as Kato-Katz (K-K), which has a low cost and can be performed in field studies. Direct egg detection achieves 100% specificity and high sensitivities parallel with high parasite burden. However, in individuals with less than 100 eggs per gram (epg), parasitological method loses sensitivity. Non-egg excretors are usually underdiagnosed. Furthermore, the assessment of cure rate is unreliable postchemotherapy use [11, 12]. Moreover, the evaluation of the effectiveness of schistosomiasis control or eradication programs after (mass) chemotherapy is distorted. New approaches have been developed and proposed as complementary or in substitution to K-K. New approaches such as DNA detection assays and rapid tests have evolved in the last years [13]. The accurate assessment of schistosomiasis diagnosis, morbidity determination, and therapy response through new technologies became suitable for use in both institutional as well as community settings. The upgrade of diagnostic technology that encompasses the detection of active infection before chemotherapy and monitoring of treatment response will permit advances in public health policies as well as in individual clinical management [14, 15]. Moreover, the assessment of clinical presentation, the disease stage, and the prognosis have been the object of progresses that go side by side with the development of new image diagnostic apparatus. Also, biochemical, immunological, and molecular markers have been tested for the evaluation of fibrosis, vascular damage, and even cancer [16]. The present review aims to discuss the new surveillance strategies and their impact on schistosomiasis clinical management.

## 2. New diagnostic tools in both community and institutional settings

The laboratory investigation of *Schistosoma* infection consists of different techniques, including parasitological, immunological, and molecular biology methods [17-19]. Frequently, diagnostic approaches are also applied on the monitoring of drug response. In addition, the assessment of morbidity levels can be achieved by using image tests and biochemical markers [20-22]. However, the diagnosis of active *Schistosoma* infection and the monitoring of therapy response as well as the determination of morbidity levels are distinctively assessed at community and institutional settings (Figure 1). Furthermore, in community settings, conventional or investigational tools aim to assess the efficiency of national control programs in the morbidity control and/or elimination of transmission by measuring the prevalence and intensity of infection in intermediary and definitive hosts [23-25]. In contrast, in institutional settings, diagnostic approaches aim to improve clinical management of individual cases.

Traditionally, egg detection by microscopy is the major criteria for active *Schistosoma* infection [24, 26]. Egg excretion can be detected by parasitological methods such as urine filtration and centrifugation methods in the case of *S. haematobium*. Since *S. japonicum*, *S. mansoni*, *S. mekongi*, and *S. intercalatum* eggs are shed in the feces, egg patent infection is detected in fecal samples by parasitological methods such as Kato-Katz test (K-K). The principal characteristics of K-K are as follows: an easy-to-do technique, low cost, reliability, and accurate identification of eggs in the case of *Schistosoma* species. Also, parasitological methods are quantitative. As a result, parasite load can be estimated. Egg counts correlate with the intensity of being <100 eggs per gram (epg), >100-399 epg, and >400 epg designated as light, moderate, and severe infection, respectively, according to WHO guidelines. Furthermore, the assessment of morbidity levels can also be roughly determined. Based on findings in high endemic areas, the elevated number of eggs was associated with severe forms of disease. Both urine filtration and Kato-Katz test have been applied for diagnosis and monitoring therapy response and used in field studies in areas of transmission as well as in institutional settings. Although Kato-Katz are affordable and suitable for low-income areas with individuals presenting with heavy to moderate infections, *Schistosoma* infection diagnosis can be quite tricky to detect in individuals with acute schistosomiasis or light infection living in nonendemic and low-endemic areas when based

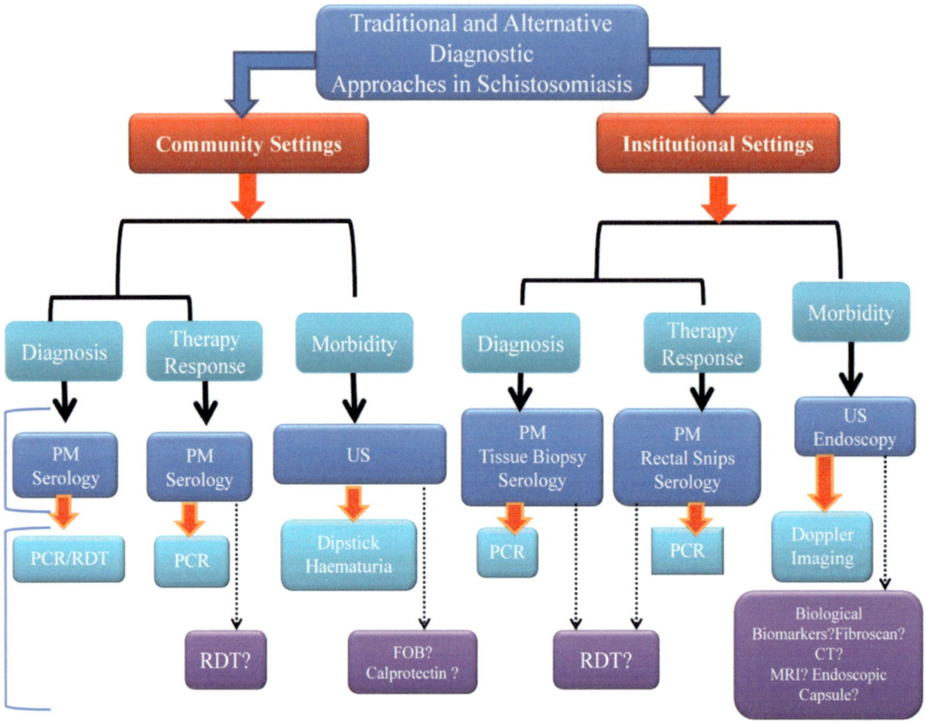


**Figure 1.** Schistosomiasis flowchart for clinical management in community and institutional settings. Conventional and new tools to diagnosis, determination of response to therapy, and morbidity assessment are indicated under community and institutional settings in hierarchic order. Bellow conventional tests, new tools were depicted according to the strength of literature evidence (red boxes). Approaches still under investigation and/or diagnostic platforms that show debatable results are inside the gray boxes. PM: parasitological method; US: ultrasonography; PCR: polymerase chain reaction; RDT: rapid test (POC-CCA /POC-CAA); FOB: fecal occult blood; CT: computed tomography; MRI: magnetic resonance imaging.

solely on microscopy [27]. Lack of egg shedding, one gender-induced infection, and daily variability are some of the causes that directly interfere with the sensitivity of microscopy, thus compromising the detection of *Schistosoma* infection and resulting in the underestimation of "real prevalence" [15, 28]. Moreover, the erratic elimination of *Schistosoma* eggs makes the determination of therapy response uncertain. In addition, some patients may present with severe forms of disease such as neuroschistosomiasis or genital schistosomiasis without any egg excretion detectable [13]. Strategies to overcome the lack of sensitivity of urine filtration and Kato-Katz test include testing replicate samples of urine or stool samples and/or augmenting the number of Kato-Katz slides/sample [29].

Other parasitological methods such as sedimentation, centrifugation, flotation techniques, and miracidium hatching were developed and had improved the diagnosis of light infections by increasing sensitivity [26, 32]. In institutional settings, tissue biopsy such as rectal snips and liver biopsy are largely used to diagnose active infection in non-egg excretors despite its invasiveness [31]. Eventually, surgical specimens reveal previously undiagnosed schistosomiasis. Except for rectal snips, histological examination is not quantitative, lack of information on parasite burden does not preclude clinical assistance.

Albeit the availability of diverse parasitological methods and tissue biopsies as alternatives to the reference test (Kato-Katz), nonparasitological methods were also developed to overcome microscopy false-negative results. This is the case of immunological tests, which have become more useful for showing active infections in recently exposed individuals, such as travelers or chronically infected immigrants residing in nonendemic areas [32]. In areas of transmission, immunodiagnosis is a suitable tool for surveillance in low endemic areas [29]. Several immunodiagnostic tests were developed, but currently the ELISA-based assays using egg antigen, cercarial, or adult worm antigens have been extensively used [33]. In addition, recombinant proteins and peptides have been potential targets [34-36]. Despite its infrequent use in National Programs for Schistosomiasis Control, serology is a potent auxiliary diagnostic approach that permits the diagnosis of non-egg excretors. However, the presence of active infection may be undermined by persistent reactivity despite successful treatment [13, 29]. Although immunoreactivity does not correlate with the intensity of infection, data have demonstrated that isotypic immunoresponse may reflect morbidity levels [37, 38].

Moreover, rapid tests (RDT) for the detection of *Schistosoma* antigens like circulating cathodic (CCA) and anodic (CAA) antigens and DNA detection assays have proven to be an advanced and feasible strategy for diagnosing *Schistosoma* infection despite the absence of their use as routine diagnostic approaches [13, 39]. See detailed comments in Table 1. During active infection, gut-produced *Schistosoma* glycoproteins - POC-CCA and POC-CAA - are detectable in the blood, urine, and stool. At individual level, results revealed that both CAA and CCA ELISA-based assays can be quite sensitive to detect active infection early after exposure in travelers even in the cases of light infections. Also, the tests allow a quantitative assessment of antigen levels, which correlates with the intensity of infection [40]. Point-of-care platforms (POC) have been applied to estimate infection prevalence with high accuracy in field studies in high and moderate endemic areas [41, 42]. Although research groups claim that CCA and CAA might be a suitable substitute for Kato-Katz test, its performance is still debatable in low endemic areas [43, 44]. RDT for hematuria (urogenital schistosomiasis), fecal occult blood (FOB), and calprotectin detection (entero-schistosomiasis) are also point-of-care approaches, which have been shown to have fair association with egg-patent infections with dual use as diagnostic tools and markers of morbidity [25, 45]. Although strong evidences support the usage of hematuria detection by RDTs, larger studies are still necessary to establish the usefulness of FOB and/or calprotectin detection in cases of light infection commonly found in low endemic areas.

## 3. Assessment of morbidity and drug response in community and institutional settings

Sanitation and community health education in addition to chemotherapeutic intervention are measures that effectively contribute to the control and/or elimination of *Schistosoma* infection in several endemic areas and the resolution or attenuation of progressive forms of disease at individual level [10, 46, 47]. However, the determination of the effects of these measures, in particular, drug intervention, still presents as a challenge (Table 1). Tests like microscopy have low sensitivity and underestimate cure rates especially in non-egg excretors. Day-to-day variations in egg excretion contribute to the misdiagnosis of schistosomiasis elimination after treatment [15]. The evaluation of drug response in individuals previously diagnosed by tissue biopsies is also troubled since the procedures might be invasive like brain or spinal cord biopsies in neuroschistosomiasis [48]. In immunoreactive egg and non-egg excretors submitted to PZQ treatment, it was shown that reactivity against several proteins mostly related to parasite musculature or glycolytic metabolism is enhanced after therapy [49]. Immunoreactivity might persist for long periods of time despite effective drug response, although seroconversion may occur in some individuals. Nonetheless, in low-endemic areas, immunodiagnosis has proven to be a valuable tool for schistosomiasis surveillance [50]. Changes in immunoreactivity in controlled areas can be used as an indicator of maintained transmission and/or active infection in community settings [51]. Therefore, the assessment of drug response is a hot topic in the schistosomiasis and development of new tools became an urgent matter (Table 1). Investigations have shown a potential role in drug response assessment with the use of rapid tests and DNA detection assays [14, 52].

| | **Traditional Tools** | | **Investigational Tools** | |
|---|---|---|---|---|
| **Community Settings** | **Tests** | **Characteristics/Observations** | **Tests** | **Characteristics / Observations** |
| **Vector control** | Light Exposure Test (Cercarial shedding detection) | For determination of transmission control, elimination or erradication. Inaccurate. no *species* identification; Test does not detect prepatent infections; no assessment of early post-control measures in snail infection rates. | Antigen Detection | Detection in 2nd week post-infection (pi); secretion by live larvae; group specific. Not commercially available assays. |
| | | | DNA- based assays | Detection in 1st week pi; quantitation of parasite load (real -time PCR; specie-specific identification. Mapping foci of vector snails and monitoring transmission. In house assays. |
| **Non-human Hosts** | Parasitological Methods (Egg detection) | Traditional methods which are simple, cheap and effective for *Schistosoma* detection. | CCA-dipsticks (urine lateral flow test) Serology (IgG/ IgM) | Detection of active infection independent of patent egg-excretion in primate non-humans. Only determination of genus but not species. |

| | Traditional Tools | | Investigational Tools | |
|---|---|---|---|---|
| **Community Settings** | **Tests** | **Characteristics/Observations** | **Tests** | **Characteristics / Observations** |
| | | | | Defines exposure to *Schistosoma*. In chimpanzee populations serology present high sensitivity but reactivity may persist for years after infection has been cleared. Comercial available test. |
| Humans Hosts Sanitation / Education | Questionaries Parasitological Methods (Egg detection) Serology | Questionnaries are applied to identify high - risk populations and permits assessment of *Schistosoma* infection Parasitological tests are quantitative methods. Low price per test. Used for Screening sentinel populations like school children.See more comments below. | DNA- based assays[1] | Identification and mapping of *Schistosoma* endemic areas. DNA based assays are powerful tools for detection of *Schistosoma* active infections. DNA detection show better performance even in light infection (low parasite loads) or despite absence of egg excretion. Mostly tested in "small" studies. |
| **Chemotherapy** | Parasitological Methods (Egg detection) | Microscopy is highly sensitive and specific to detect egg-patent infections. Day-to-day variations on egg excretion is a limitation. Absence of egg excretion post-treatment may not represent response to therapy. Cure rates determined in different *S. mansoni* and *S.haematobium* infections are variable (49.2 to 98.40%) [53, 54]. Understimates reinfection and also incomplete cure. | DNA-based assays[1] | DNA detection has higher sensitivity after use of chemotherapy. Persistent DNA amplification in both egg excretors and non-egg excretors strongly suggest no response to therapy. Presents good performance compared to parasitological methods to determine effect of MDA. Cure rates calculated by different DNA - based assays in distinct populations and by different Schistosoma species may varie from 21.1 - 30.7 to 75.6% [55, 15]. Persistence of DNA amplification until 6 months and post- 6 months after treatment might suggest incomplete infection and reinfection, respectively DNA-based assays for *Schistosoma* infection detection are not currently commercially available. |
| | Serology | Loss of sensitivity of microscopy has been replaced in | Rapid Test | POC-CCA maintains higher sensitivity than parasitological |

| | Traditional Tools | | Investigational Tools | |
|---|---|---|---|---|
| **Community Settings** | **Tests** | **Characteristics/Observations** | **Tests** | **Characteristics / Observations** |
| | | some control programs by serology which may remain reactive for extended periods post effective drug use. In areas submitted to several rounds of chemotherapy, low and/or absence of reactivity might represent control of infection.Long periods of obsevation are necessary to determine *Schistosoma* infection "real status". Reinfection or incomplete cure may not be assessed. | | methods after PZQ use. However, specificity may be compromised by the presence of persistent low reactivity ( trace positive samples) post-chemotherapy.Cure rates may vary from 23.3 - 26.1 to 40.7- 47.8% [42, 54] |
| **Institutional Settings** | | | | |
| **Chemotherapy** | Parasitological Methods (Egg detection) | Assessment of post-therapy response by parasitological methods in clinical wards has similar advantages and limitations as in community settings. In immigrants (long gone from endemic areas) and recently exposed travelers, absence of egg excretion pre-therapy represent an obstacle. Ova detection is inappropriate to determine therapy response in these groups. See above other coments. | DNA-based assays[1] | DNA-based assays are a reliable tool to detect response to therapy in distinct clinical specimens. Absence of DNA amplification correlates with response to therapy in individuals treated in Travel Medicine Clinics [56].In case of therapy failure, maintained DNA amplification correlate with persistence of clinical signs, symptoms and pathological abnormalities associated to therapy failure [57]. Usefulness of DNA-based assays to detect past infection incomplete cure for non re-exposed individuals has to be established with large studies [58]. |
| | Tissue Biopsy | No viable eggs in rectal snips show good correlation with response to therapy. However, tissue biopsy (rectal snips, liver biopsies) are invasive procedures. And, lack of ova | | |

| | Traditional Tools | | Investigational Tools | |
|---|---|---|---|---|
| **Community Settings** | **Tests** | **Characteristics/Observations** | **Tests** | **Characteristics / Observations** |
| | | detection may not represent absence of active infection [59]. | | |
| | Serology | Immunoreactivity persistence for years after effective therapy is the major limitation. Negative seroconversion representes response to therapy and it is observed in some individuals [56]. But, assessment of therapy failure is mostly difficult [59]. | | |
| **Transplant** | Tissue Biopsy | Donnor and organ-recipients from endemic areas with / without transaminase alterations can be screened by tissue biopsy [60]. But, negative tissue samples do not rule out active infection. | DNA- based assays[1] | Further studies are necessary. |

[1]**DNA based assay** - conventional PCR, real-time PCR and LAMP (Loop-mediated isothermal amplification)

**Table 1.** Effectiveness of interventions in surveillance programs and monitoring therapy response in clinical management: use of traditional and investigational tools.

RDTs for antigen detection have been largely used for population studies to evaluate post-therapy response and efficacy [42, 43]. In areas of moderate and high endemicity, therapy response represented by decrease or disappearance of antigen detection may represent cure. However, in light infections, rapid test accuracy is reduced with maintained antigen detection in individuals without infection. The use of antigen detection assays is a debatable matter to measure posttherapy response. In contrast, DNA assays seem to be a suitable marker of drug response. Cure is determined by the absence of DNA amplification postchemotherapy use, while persistent DNA amplification correlates with nonresponse to therapy [15].

Schistosomiasis presents as a large spectrum of manifestations and disease severity during acute and chronic phases. Usually, imaging tests and/or biological markers are required to confirm diagnosis, to assess morbidity, and to stage disease progression [21, 22]. Image tests such as ultrasonography became revolutionary to assess urogenital *S. haematobium* infection and *S. mansoni* liver disease [61]. In both community and institutional settings, conventional ultrasound (US) examination is a well-standardized test to assess bladder and liver fibrosis, which is the hallmark of disease progression in urinary and intestinal schistosomiasis, respectively [62-65]. US predicts disease prevalence rates and is a reliable noninvasive indicator of morbidity levels which aloud disease staging [64, 66]. However, morbidity measurement in a multivariate clinical manifestation infection like schistosomiasis is no easy task. Targeting one compartment to measure schistosomiasis morbidity might not be enough since some clinical presentations can affect a single compartment like in neuroschistosomiasis and others. In intestinal *Schistosoma* infection, independent hepatosplenic forms are the most common clinical presentation after asymptomatic *S. mansoni* infection. However, in contrast to hepatic schistosomiasis, the study of disease progression by using image and/or biochemical markers is still poorly developed [21]. Promising new approaches such as capsule endoscopy have been introduced, but large-scale studies are still necessary to evaluate the usefulness of the method [67]. In hepatosplenic forms, vascular gastropathy and colopathy can be indicators of portal hypertension severity [68]. The assessment of vascular alterations in superior gastrointestinal tract are used to determine schistosomiasis levels of morbidity through the use of upper digestive endoscopy in association with conventional ultrasonography and Doppler imaging [66]. In institutional settings, transient elastography, magnetic resonance, and computerized tomography might give supplementary information regarding fibrosis progression and vascular status, although standardization is necessary especially for disease staging [22, 69]

## 4. Conclusion

In community settings, concerns have been increasing on the effectiveness of schistosomiasis control interventions like MDA over the years. The low accuracy of the reference test to detect active *Schistosoma* infection and the improper estimates of cure rates jeopardize the truthful analysis of drug intervention, which compromises the effectiveness of surveillance systems. In clinical settings, underdiagnosed schistosomiasis and inadequate morbidity assessment also increase the burden on public and private health systems. In order to change this scenario, new diagnostic tools, markers of treatment response, and morbidity assessment have been developed over the years showing promising results. Nonetheless, efforts still have to be made to find a single cheap and easy-to-do approach that is suitable and reliable for diagnosis, treatment evaluation, and disease staging in community and institutional settings.

## Author details

Marta Guimarães Cavalcanti[1,2] and José Mauro Peralta[2*]

*Address all correspondence to: peralta@micro.ufrj.br

1 Serviço de Doenças Infecciosas e Parasitárias, Hospital Universitário Clementino Fraga Filho, Universidade Federal do Rio de Janeiro, Rio de Janeiro, Brazil

2 Departmento de Imunologia, Instituto de Microbiologia Paulo de Góes, Universidade Federal do Rio de Janeiro, Rio de Janeiro, Brazil

## References

[1] Lambertucci JR. Acute schistosomiasis mansoni: revisited and reconsidered. Mem Inst Oswaldo Cruz. 2010; 105(4):422-435.

[2] Barsoum RS, Esmat G, El-Baz. Human schistosomiasis: clinical perspective: review. J Adv Res. 2013; 4(5):433-444.

[3] McManus DP, Gray DJ, Li Y, Feng Z, Williams GM, Stewart D, Rey-Ladino J, Ross AG. Schistosomiasis in the People's Republic of China: the era of the Three Gorges. Clin Microbiol Rev. 2010; 23(2):442-466.

[4] Walker AJ. Insights into the functional biology of schistosomes. Parasit Vectors. 2011; 4:203.

[5] Ribeiro AC, Maldonado Júnior A, D'Andrea PS, Vieira GO, Rey L. Susceptibility of *Nectomys rattus* (Pelzen, 1883) to experimental infection with *Schistosoma mansoni* (Sambon, 1907): a potential reservoir in Brazil. Mem Inst Oswaldo Cruz. 1998; 93 Suppl 1:295-299.

[6] McGarvey ST, Zhou XN, Willingham AL 3rd, Feng Z, Olveda R. The epidemiology and host-parasite relationships of *Schistosoma japonicum* in definitive hosts. Parasitol Today. 1999; 15(6):214-215.

[7] Hotez PJ, Kamath A. Neglected tropical diseases in sub-Saharan Africa: review of their prevalence, distribution, and disease burden. PLoS Negl Trop Dis. 2009; 3(8):e412.

[8] WHO: Schistosomiasis. http://www.who.int/mediacentre/factsheets/fs115/en/

[9] Esrey SA, Potash JB, Roberts L, Shiff C. Esrey SA, Potash JB, Roberts L, Shiff C. Effects of improved water supply and sanitation on ascariasis, diarrhoea, dracunculiasis, hookworm infection, schistosomiasis, and trachoma. Bull World Health Organ. 1991; 69(5):609-621.

[10] Touré S, Zhang Y, Bosqué-Oliva E, Ky C, Ouedraogo A, Koukounari A, Gabrielli AF, Bertrand S, Webster JP, Fenwick A. Two-year impact of single praziquantel treatment on infection in the national control programme on schistosomiasis in Burkina Faso. Bull World Health Organ. 2008; 86(10):780-787.

[11] Rabello A, Pontes LA, Dias-Neto E. Recent advances in the diagnosis of *Schistosoma* infection: the detection of parasite DNA. Mem Inst Oswaldo Cruz. 2002; 97 Suppl 1:171-172.

[12] Enk MJ, Oliveira e Silva G, Rodrigues NB. Diagnostic accuracy and applicability of a PCR system for the detection of *Schistosoma mansoni* DNA in human urine samples from an endemic area. PLoS One. 2012; 7(6):e38947.

[13] Cavalcanti MG, Silva LF, Peralta RH, Barreto MG, Peralta JM. Schistosomiasis in areas of low endemicity: a new era in diagnosis. Trends Parasitol. 2013; 29(2):75-82.

[14] Downs JA, Kabangila R, Verweij JJ, Jaka H, Peck RN, Kalluvya SE, Changalucha JM, Johnson WD, van Lieshout L, Fitzgerald DW. Detectable urogenital schistosome DNA and cervical abnormalities 6 months after single-dose praziquantel in women with *Schistosoma haematobium* infection. Trop Med Int Health. 2013; 18(9):1090-1096.

[15] Vinkeles Melchers NV, van Dam GJ, Shaproski D, Kahama AI, Brienen EA, Vennervald BJ, van Lieshout L. Diagnostic performance of *Schistosoma* real-time PCR in urine samples from Kenyan children infected with *Schistosoma haematobium*: day-to-day variation and follow-up after praziquantel treatment. PLoS Negl Trop Dis. 2014; 8(4):e2807.

[16] Sousa-Figueiredo JC, Basáñez MG, Khamis IS, Garba A, Rollinson D, Stothard JR. Measuring morbidity associated with urinary schistosomiasis: assessing levels of excreted urine albumin and urinary tract pathologies. PLoS Negl Trop Dis. 2009; 3(10):e526

[17] Hoy AM, Lundie RJ, Ivens A, Quintana JF, Nausch N. Forster T, Jones F, Kabatereine NB, Dunne DW, Mutapi F, Macdonald AS, Buck AH. Parasite-derived MicroRNAs in host serum as novel biomarkers of helminth infection. PLoS Negl Trop Dis. 2014; 8(2):e2701.

[18] Carneiro TR, Peralta RH, Pinheiro MC, Oliveira SM, Peralta JM, Bezerra FS. A conventional polymerase chain reaction-based method for the diagnosis of human schistosomiasis in stool samples from individuals in a low-endemicity area. Mem Inst Oswaldo Cruz. 2013; 108(8):1037-1044.

[19] Gordon CA, Acosta LP, Gray DJ, Olveda RM, Jarilla B, Gobert GN, Ross AG, McManus DP. High prevalence of *Schistosoma japonicum* infection in carabao from Samar Province, the Philippines: implications for transmission and control. PLoS Negl Trop Dis. 2012; 6(9): e1778.

[20] Voieta I, de Queiroz LC, Andrade LM, Silva LC, Fontes VF, Barbosa A Jr, Resende V, Petroianu A, Andrade Z, Antunes CM, Lambertucci JR. Imaging techniques and histology in the evaluation of liver fibrosis in hepatosplenic schistosomiasis mansoni in Brazil: a comparative study. Mem Inst Oswaldo Cruz. 2010; 105(4):414-421.

[21] Domingues AL, Medeiros TB, Lopes EP. Ultrasound versus biological markers in the evaluation of periportal fibrosis in human *Schistosoma mansoni*. Mem Inst Oswaldo Cruz. 2011:106(7):802-807.

[22] Lambertucci JR. Revisiting the concept of hepatosplenic schistosomiasis and its challenges using traditional and new tools. Rev Soc Bras Med Trop. 2014; 47(2):130-136.

[23] Mutapi, Improving diagnosis of urogenital schistosome infection. Expert Rev Anti Infect Ther. 2011; 9(10):863-865.

[24] Colley DG, Bustinduy AL, Secor WE, King CH. Human schistosomiasis. Lancet. 2014; 383(9936):2253-2264.

[25] Stothard JR, Stanton MC, Bustinduy AL, Sousa-Figueiredo JC, Van Dam GJ, Betson M, Waterhouse D, Ward S, Allan F, Hassan AA, Al-Helal MA, Memish ZA, Rollinson D. Diagnostics for schistosomiasis in Africa and Arabia: a review of present options in control and future needs for elimination. Parasitology. 2014; 141(14):1947-1961.

[26] Gray DJ, Ross AG, Li YS, McManus DP (2011). Diagnosis and management of schistosomiasis. BMJ. 2011; 342:d2651.

[27] Coltart CE, Chew A, Storrar N, Armstrong M, Suff N, Morris L, Chiodini PL, Whitty CJ. Schistosomiasis presenting in travellers: a 15 year observational study at the Hospital for Tropical Diseases, London. Trans R Soc Trop Med Hyg. 2015; 109(3):214-220.

[28] Degarege A, Legesse M, Medhin Gm Teklehaymanot T, Erko B. Day-to-day fluctuation of point-of-care circulating cathodic antigen test scores and faecal egg counts in children infected with *Schistosoma mansoni* in Ethiopia. BMC Infect Dis. 2014; 14:210.

[29] Gonçalves MM, Barreto MG, Peralta RH, Gargioni C, Gonçalves T, Igreja RP, Soares MS, Peralta JM. Immunoassays as an auxiliary tool for the serodiagnosis of *Schistosoma mansoni* infection in individuals with low intensity of egg elimination. Acta Trop. 2006; 100(1-2):24-30.

[30] Coelho PM, Jurberg AD, Oliveira AA, Katz N. Use of a saline gradient for the diagnosis of schistosomiasis. Mem Inst Oswaldo Cruz. 2009; 104:720-723.

[31] Olveda DU, Olveda RM, Lam AK, Chau TN, Li Y, Gisparil AD 2nd, Ross AG. Utility of diagnostic imaging in the diagnosis and management of schistosomiasis. Clin Microbiol. 2014; 3(2):142.

[32] WHO (2013). http://www.who.int/mediacentre/factsheets/fs115/en/

[33] Chand MA, Chiodini PL, Doenhoff MJ. Development of a new assay for the diagnosis of schistosomiasis, using cercarial antigens. Trans R Soc Trop Med Hyg. 2010; 104:255-258.

[34] Zhou XH, Wu JY, Huang XQ, Kunnon SP, Zhu XQ, Chen XG. Identification and characterization of *Schistosoma japonicum* Sjp40, a potential antigen candidate for the early diagnosis of schistosomiasis. Diagn Microbiol Infect Dis. 2010; 67:337-345.

[35] de Oliveira EJ, Kanamura HY, Takei K, Hirata RD, Valli LC, Nguyen NY, de Carvalho Rodrigues I, de Jesus AR, Hirata MH. Synthetic peptides as an antigenic base in an ELISA for laboratory diagnosis of schistosomiasis mansoni. Trans R Soc Trop Med Hyg. 2008; 102:360-366.

[36] Ludolf F, Patrocínio PR, Corrêa-Oliveira R, Gazzinelli A, Falcone FH, Teixeira-Ferreira A, Perales J, Oliveira GC, Silva-Pereira RA. Serological screening of the *Schistosoma mansoni* adult worm proteome. PLoS Negl Trop Dis. 2014; 8(3):e2745.

[37] Ramírez RM, Ceballos E, Alarcón de Noya B, Noya O, Bianco N. The immunopathology of human schistosomiasis: III. Immunoglobulin isotype profiles and response to praziquantel. Mem Inst Oswaldo Cruz. 1996; 91(5):593-599.

[38] Negrão-Corrêa D, Fittipaldi JF, Lambertucci JR, Teixeira MM, Antunes CM, Carneiro M. Association of *Schistosoma mansoni*-specific IgG and IgE antibody production and clinical schistosomiasis status in a rural area of Minas Gerais, Brazil. PLoS One. 2014; 9(2):e88042.

[39] Nausch N, Dawson EM, Midzi N, Mduluza T, Mutapi F, Doenhoff MJ. Field evaluation of a new antibody-based diagnostic for *Schistosoma haematobium* and *S. mansoni* at the point-of-care in northeast Zimbabwe. BMC Infect Dis. 2014; 14:165.

[40] van Lieshout L, Polderman AM, Deelder AM. Immunodiagnosis of schistosomiasis by determination of the circulating antigens CAA and CCA, in particular in individuals with recent or light infections. Acta Trop. 2000; 77(1):69-80.

[41] Tchuem Tchuenté LA, Kueté Fouodo CJ, Kamwa Ngassam RI, Sumo L, Dongmo Noumedem C, Kenfack CM, Gipwe NF, Nana ED, Stothard JR, Rollinson D. Evaluation of circulating cathodic antigen (CCA) urine-tests for diagnosis of *Schistosoma mansoni* infection in Cameroon. PLoS Negl Trop Dis. 2012; 6(7):e1758.

[42] Coulibaly JT, N'Gbesso YK, Knopp S, N'Guessan NA, Silué KD, van Dam GJ, N'Goran EK, Utzinger J. Accuracy of urine circulating cathodic antigen test for the diagnosis of *Schistosoma mansoni* in preschool-aged children before and after treatment. PLoS Negl Trop Dis. 2013; 7(3):e2109.

[43] Sousa-Figueiredo JC, Betson M, Kabatereine NB, Stothard JR. The urine circulating cathodic antigen (CCA) dipstick: a valid substitute for microscopy for mapping and point-of-care diagnosis of intestinal schistosomiasis. PLoS Negl Trop Dis. 2013; 7(1):e2008.

[44] van Dam GJ, Xu J, Bergquist R, de Dood CJ, Utzinger J, Qin ZQ, Guan W, Feng T, Yu XL, Zhou J, Zheng M, Zhou XN, Corstjens PL. An ultra-sensitive assay targeting the circulating anodic antigen for the diagnosis of *Schistosoma japonicum* in a low-endemic area, People's Republic of China. Acta Trop. 2015; 141(Pt B):190-197.

[45] King CH, Bertsch D. Meta-analysis of urine heme dipstick diagnosis of *Schistosoma haematobium* infection, including low-prevalence and previously-treated populations. PLoS Negl Trop Dis. 2013; 7(9):e2431.

[46] Martins-Leite P, Gazzinelli G, Alves-Oliveira LF, Gazzinelli A, Malaquias LC, Correa-Oliveira R, Teixeira-Carvalho A, Silveira AM. Effect of chemotherapy with praziquantel on the production of cytokines and morbidity associated with schistosomiasis mansoni. Antimicrob Agents Chemother. 2008;52(8):2780-2786.

[47] Silva PC, Leal TV, Domingues AL. Treatment and education reduce the severity of schistosomiasis periportal fibrosis. Rev Soc Bras Med Trop. 2013; 46(4):472-477.

[48] Lambertucci JR, Souza-Pereira SR, Carvalho TA. Simultaneous occurrence of brain tumor and myeloradiculopathy in schistosomiasis mansoni: case report. Rev Soc Bras Med Trop. 2009; 42(3):338-341.

[49] Mutapi F, Burchmore R, Mduluza T, Foucher A, Harcus Y, Nicoll G, Midzi N, Turner CM, Maizels RM. Praziquantel treatment of individuals exposed to *Schistosoma haematobium* enhances serological recognition of defined parasite antigens. J Infect Dis. 2005;192(6):1108-1118.

[50] Ramírez RM, Ceballos E, Alarcón de Noya B, Noya O, Bianco N. The immunopathology of human Schistosomiasis-III. Immunoglobulin isotype profiles and response to praziquantel. Mem Inst Oswaldo Cruz. 1996; 91(5):593-599.

[51] Wami WM, Nausch N, Bauer K, Midzi N, Gwisai R, Simmonds P, Mduluza T, Woolhouse M, Mutapi F. Comparing parasitological vs serological determination of *Schistosoma haematobium* infection prevalence in preschool and primary school-aged children: implications for control programmes. Parasitology. 2014; 141(14):1962-1970.

[52] Gomes LI, Enk MJ, Rabello A. Diagnosing schistosomiasis: where are we? Rev Soc Bras Med Trop. 2014; 47(1):3-11.

[53] Garba A, Lamine MS, Barkiré N, Djibo A, Sofo B, Gouvras AN, Labbo R, Sebangou H, Webster JP, Fenwick A, Utzinger J. Efficacy and safety of two closely spaced doses of praziquantel against *Schistosoma haematobium* and *S. mansoni* and re-infection patterns in school-aged children in Niger. Acta Trop. 2013; 128(2):334-344.

[54] Lamberton PH, Kabatereine NB, Oguttu DW, Fenwick A, Webster JP. Lamberton PH, Kabatereine NB, Oguttu DW, Fenwick A, Webster JP. Sensitivity and specificity of multiple Kato-Katz thick smears and a circulating cathodic antigen test for *Schistosoma mansoni* diagnosis pre- and post-repeated-praziquantel treatment. PLoS Negl Trop Dis. 2014; 8(9):e3139.

[55] Pontes LA, Oliveira MC, Katz N, Dias-Neto E, Rabello A. Comparison of a polymerase chain reaction and the Kato-Katz technique for diagnosing infection with *Schistosoma mansoni*. Am J Trop Med Hyg. 2003; 68(6):652-656.

[56] Wichmann D, Poppert S, Von Thien H, Clerinx J, Dieckmann S, Jensenius M, Parola P, Richter J, Schunk M, Stich A, Zanger P, Burchard GD, Tannich E. Prospective European-wide multicentre study on a blood based real-time PCR for the diagnosis of acute schistosomiasis. BMC Infect Dis. 2013; 13:55.

[57] Kato-Hayashi N, Yasuda M, Yuasa J, Isaka S, Haruki K, Ohmae H, Osada Y, Kanazawa T, Chigusa Y. Use of cell-free circulating schistosome DNA in serum, urine, semen, and saliva to monitor a case of refractory imported schistosomiasis hematobia. J Clin Microbiol. 2013 51(10):3435-3438.

[58] Wichmann D, Panning M, Quack T, Kramme S, Burchard GD, Grevelding C, Drosten C. Diagnosing schistosomiasis by detection of cell-free parasite DNA in human plasma. PLoS Negl Trop Dis. 2009; 3(4):e422.

[59] Helleberg M, Thybo S. High rate of failure in treatment of imported schistosomiasis. J Travel Med. 2010; 17(2):94-99.

[60] Mahmoud KM, Sobh MA, El-Agroudy AE, Mostafa FE, Baz ME, Shokeir AA, Ghoneim MA. Impact of schistosomiasis on patient and graft outcome after renal transplantation:10 years' follow-up. Nephrol Dial Transplant. 2001;16(11):2214-2221.

[61] Koukounari A, Sacko M, Keita AD, Gabrielli AF, Landouré A, Dembelé R, Clements AC, Whawell S, Donnelly CA, Fenwick A, Traoré M, Webster JP. Assessment of ultrasound morbidity indicators of schistosomiasis in the context of large-scale programs illustrated with experiences from Malian children. Am J Trop Med Hyg. 2006; 75(6):1042-1052.

[62] Akpata R, Neumayr A, Holtfreter MC, Krantz I, Singh DD, Mota R, Walter S, Hatz C, Richter J. The WHO ultrasonography protocol for assessing morbidity due to *Schistosoma haematobium*. Acceptance and evolution over 14 years. Systematic review. Parasitol Res. 25 February 2015 (published on line).

[63] el Scheich T, Holtfreter MC, Ekamp H, Singh DD, Mota R, Hatz C, Richter J. The WHO ultrasonography protocol for assessing hepatic morbidity due to *Schistosoma mansoni*. Acceptance and evolution over 12 years. Parasitol Res. 2014;113(11): 3915-3925.

[64] Abebe N, Erko B, Medhin G, Berhe N. Clinico-epidemiological study of *Schistosomiasis mansoni* in Waja-Timuga, District of Alamata, northern Ethiopia. Parasit Vectors. 2014;7:158.

[65] Wu YM, Xu N, Hu JY, Xu XF, Wu WX, Gao SX, Zhu WJ, Wu WL, Shen XZ, Wang JY, Wu SD. A simple noninvasive index to predict significant liver fibrosis in patients with advanced schistosomiasis japonica. Parasitol Int. 2013;62(3):283-288.

[66] Pinto-Silva RA, Queiroz LC, Azeredo LM, Silva LC, Lambertucci JR. Ultrasound in schistosomiasis mansoni. Mem Inst Oswaldo Cruz. 2010; 105(4):479-484.

[67] Betson M, Sousa-Figueiredo JC, Rowell C, Kabatereine NB, Stothard JR. Intestinal schistosomiasis in mothers and young children in Uganda: investigation of field-applicable markers of bowel morbidity. Am J Trop Med Hyg. 2010;83(5):1048-1055.

[68] Ganc RL, Malheiros CA, Nakakubo S, Szutan LA, Ganc AJ. Small-bowel lesions caused by portal hypertension of schistosomal origin: a capsule endoscopy pilot study. Small-bowel lesions caused by portal hypertension of schistosomal origin: a capsule endoscopy pilot study. Gastrointest Endosc. 2010; 71(4):861-866.

http://dx.doi.org/10.5772/61310

[69] Esmat G, Elsharkawy A, El Akel W, Fouad A, Helal K, Mohamed MK, Attia D, Khattab H, Doss W, Labib S. Fibroscan of chronic HCV patients coinfected with schistosomiasis. Arab J Gastroenterol. 2013;14(3):109-112.

Chapter 8

# Praziquantel and Arachidonic Acid Combination — An Innovative Approach to the Treatment of Schistosomiasis

Hatem Tallima, Kevin Hadley and Rashika El Ridi

Additional information is available at the end of the chapter

http://dx.doi.org/10.5772/61185

## Abstract

Schistosomiasis is a debilitating disease caused by trematode worms of the genus *Schistosoma*. Three members *Schistosoma mansoni*, *Schistosoma haematobium*, and *Schistosoma japonicum* are responsible for the great majority of human infections. Schistosomiasis is widespread in sub-Saharan Africa, several countries of the Middle East, South America, and South-East Asia. Vaccination against the infection would be the most reliable way to combat the infection and decrease or interrupt its transmission, but a commercial vaccine is still unavailable. Praziquantel (PZQ) is the only drug considered for schistosomiasis treatment as it is effective against the major human schistosomes, commercially available, cost-affordable, and elicits limited side-effects. Several reports documented the highly significant PZQ efficacy in treatment of light infections in areas of low *S. mansoni* and *S. haematobium* endemicity and PZQ use. Chemotherapy with PZQ alone of patients residing in regions of high schistosome endemicity and afflicted with light, moderate, or heavy infection is not efficacious. Accordingly, we propose implementation of cost-affordable arachidonic acid (ARA), a polyunsaturated omega-6 fatty acid and efficacious in vitro and in vivo schistosomicide, for oral therapy of children with *Schistosoma mansoni* and *Schistosoma haematobium* light infection, as adjunct to PZQ for cure of children with moderate and heavy infections, and for counteracting schistosome resistance to PZQ that arises in endemic areas exposed to repeated and intense PZQ mass treatment campaigns.

**Keywords:** Praziquantel, Arachidonic acid, Schistosomiasis, Chemotherapy, Combination chemotherapy

## 1. Introduction

Schistosomiasis is a debilitating disease caused by dioecious (having separate sex) trematode worms of the genus Schistosoma. Three members, *Schistosoma mansoni, Schistosoma haematobium,* and *Schistosoma japonicum,* are responsible for the great majority of human infections. Schistosomiasis is also called snail fever as the schistosomes' life cycle comprises asexual reproduction in an appropriate, fresh water snail. Actually, it is the presence of the specific snail vector that determines the prevalence of the disease, as infection is exclusively caused by the larvae (termed cercariae) shed by infected snails. The cercariae of *S. mansoni, S. haematobium,* and *S. japonicum* swim in fresh water and soon die if they fail to land on the skin of humans or other suitable mammalian hosts. The cercariae then penetrate the epidermis, linger there for one (*S. japonicum*) to three (*S. mansoni, S. haematobium*) days or more until extensive biochemical changes end by setting a protective, outer double-lipid bilayer armor. The larvae, now termed schistosomula, exit to the dermis and then make their way into dermal venous capillaries, en route to the lung and then liver. There the parasites start to feed and rapidly grow and mature, and the male carrying the female into its ventral gynecophoric groove or "schist" migrate to permanent residence in the inferior mesenteric (*S. mansoni, S. japonicum*) or the peri-vesical (*S. haematobium*) venous plexus. Until then, the worms are nearly innocuous causing very limited harm, especially in endemic regions. With the onset of female parasite egg deposition, harm starts and progresses into overt diseases [1-5].

To continue the life cycle, the ova must egress the mammalian host vasculature to the exterior to locate the intermediate snail host where asexual reproduction takes place. The parasite dwelling is nearest to the outlets of the lower colon and rectum via feces and the urinary bladder with urine. Eggs release proteolytic and other hydrolytic enzymes to transit the blood capillaries, and thereafter the large intestine (or urinary bladder) wall into the lumen. Besides releasing host matrix digestive enzymes, *S. mansoni* and *S. haematobium* additionally depend on the sharp, lateral and terminal spine, respectively. The massive daily egg migration, trapping, and calcification lead to edema, congestion, ulcers, lesions, petechial hemorrhage, necrosis, hyperplastic and hypertrophic changes, fibrosis, and excessive nodules and polyps formation in the intestine, symptoms collectively known as intestinal schistosomiasis [1, 2]. Continuous egg transit via the wall of the lower urinary tract to the lumen causes even more damage to the urinary tract and bladder, the severe symptoms of urinary schistosomiasis [3]. Beside the egg-induced overt mechanical injury and lesions, the presence of parasite molecules within the extracellular matrix signals danger and expectedly contributes to intense and prolonged generation of inflammatory mediators [4].

The "plat de resistance" is still away, as the most severe injury does not result from the eggs that escape to the exterior but from the eggs that fail to do so. Eggs trapped in the wall of the intestine or urinary tract drift and eventually accumulate in tissues of other organs, namely the liver, where they remain viable for approximately three weeks, and release soluble egg antigens (SEA) via their microscopic pores. The host responds to these insults through vigorous immunologic reactions. These intense immunological reactions are injurious to the host, not the egg that remains unscathed, until its viability becomes exhausted. Lymphocytes, eosinophils, basophils, and macrophages accumulate around the egg in attempt to prevent its contents from seeping and disseminating, thus forming large granulomas. The granulomas gradually begin to encompass the entire organ, progressing to fibrosis with excessive accumulation of collagen and extracellular matrix proteins, obstructive vascular lesions, vascular hypertension, neo angiogenesis, splenomegaly, esophageal varices, and signs of hepatocellular (*S. mansoni*) or kidney (*S. haematobium*) failure [1-3, 5].

The transiting eggs-induced mechanical injury and the immunological reactions to the entrapped eggs manifest into colitis, diarrhea, blood in stool or urine, abdominal discomfort and pain, urodynamic abnormalities, fatigue, lower exercise and work tolerance, impaired cognitive capacities, and retarded development. Chronic infection leads to organ dysfunction, intense vascular complications, and additionally, predisposes to other even more severe viral and bacterial infections, cancer development, and ultimately death [1-3, 5].

Detection of eggs in stool specimens is the gold standard for diagnosis of the infection. In chronic infections, i.e., in adults residing in endemic areas, continuous egg deposition and migration via the wall of the lower intestine and the urinary bladder and tracts generate fibrosis in the submucosa and hypertrophy in the muscularis mucosa, and consequently, a barrier is raised to the usual route of ova transit from the surrounding veins to the lumen of the gut or urinary bladder [2, 3]. Expectedly, the gold standard method of egg detection is entirely unreliable in chronic infections. Diagnostic methods based on serological detection of antibodies to the parasite antigens do not lack sensitivity, but lack specificity and additionally may not be used to monitor the outcome of therapy or to differentiate between present and past infection. Diagnostic methods based on antigen detection in serum, urine or stool, and saliva lack both sensitivity and specificity and together with the methods based on molecular biology advances are cumbersome, costly, and none has been adapted for routine screening in endemic regions, all situated in the developing world [5 and references therein, 6]. Epidemiological surveys are costly and require thorough scientific and political involvement, both often failing in developing countries. Based on the above, it may be foreseen that the figures on the prevalence of schistosomiasis, namely 252 million infected, are a gross underestimate. Yet, it is certain that the figures of 800 million persons, namely children, residing in rural areas are at risk of the infection, and yearly deaths as high as 200,000 are correct [6-9]. Schistosomiasis is widespread in sub-Saharan Africa, several countries of the Middle East, South America, and South-East Asia [6-10]. Vaccination against the infection would be the most reliable way to combat the infection and decrease or interrupt its transmission, but a commercial vaccine is still an unmet clinical need. Praziquantel is the only drug considered for schistosomiasis treatment as it is effective against the major human schistosomes, commercially available, cost-affordable, and elicits limited side-effects [reviewed in 5, 11, 12].

## 2. Chemotherapy

### 2.1. Praziquantel

#### *2.1.1. Structure and schistosomicidal effects in vitro and in experimental animals*

Praziquantel (PZQ), $C_{19}H_{24}N_2O_2$ (2-cyclohexylcarbonyl-4-oxo-1,2,3,6,7,11*b*-hexahydro-4*H*-pyrazino[2,1-a]iso-quinolin-4-one) (Figure 1) is a hydrophobic molecule of molecular weight

312.4 g/mole, for all this lengthy formula, smaller than the molecular weight of cholesterol 386.6 g/mole), which schistosomes cannot synthesize de novo and rely on absorption from the host via the tegument [13].

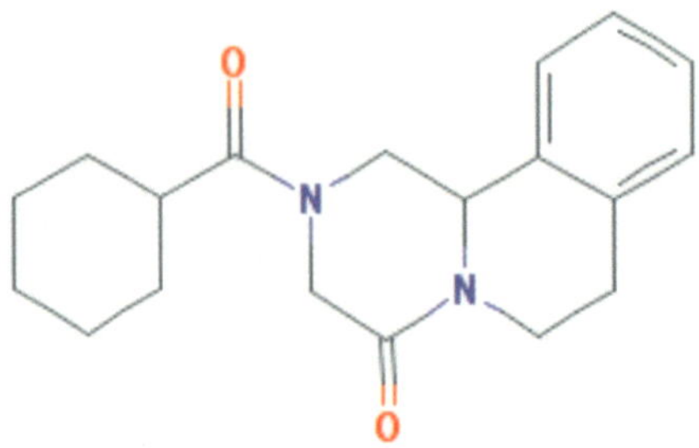


**Figure 1.** Structure of praziquantel.

Because of its small molecular weight and hydrophobic nature, PZQ may access and interact with the schistosome outer lipid bilayer, expectedly causing disruption, degeneration, and disintegration. Adult *S. mansoni* were exposed in vitro to 1, 10, or 100 μg/ml PZQ for 5, 15, 30, or 60 minutes, and examined by light and electron microscopy. Severe body contraction and complete cessation of movement were associated with the appearance of numerous small areas of vacuolization and vesicle formation distributed all over the parasite surface, their number increasing with PZQ concentration and exposure time and eliciting disruption of the apical tegumental layer [14, 15].

Mice orally treated with 500 mg/kg PZQ seven weeks following infection with *S. mansoni* showed dislodgment of the worms from the veins of the intestine to the portal circulation, and pronounced vacuolization of the tegument as early as one hour after treatment, indicating that in vitro and in vivo likewise, PZQ suddenly and abruptly affects the worm physiology. Soon after, neutrophils and eosinophils attached to the bleb-like vacuoles and succeeded in infiltrating the interior of the worms leading to progressive internal lysis and eventually total disintegration [15]. Yet, several reports indicated that 21- and 28-day worms are less sensitive to PZQ action in vivo [16, 17].

Lung-stage schistosomula were recovered one hour after treatment of 6-day *S. mansoni*-infected mice with 0 or 200 mg/kg PZQ, and examined by indirect membrane immunofluorescence using chronic infection serum. Larvae recovered from untreated mice were entirely negative, a finding we repeatedly confirmed decades later [11, 12 and references therein]. Larvae harvested from PZQ-treated hosts revealed exposure of hitherto hidden surface membrane molecules, likely consequent to interaction of PZQ with the lung-stage schistosomula apical lipid bilayer [18]. Proven PZQ-mediated exposure of larval and adult *S. mansoni* surface membrane antigens to hitherto barred antibody access suggested that PZQ in vivo action is due to the synergy between its direct effect on the worm and host-immune effectors, principally antibody-dependent cell- and complement-mediated cytotoxicity and granulocytes cytolytic action [19-22].

Praziquantel was shown to be equally effective against *S. haematobium* and *S. japonicum* in vitro and in vivo, inducing spastic paralysis, tegumental vacuolation and disruption, and surface membrane exposure to host antibodies and other immune effectors [23-25].

### 2.1.2. Mechanism of action

The pyrazino-isoquinoline ring system of PZQ represents a completely novel structure in anti-helminthic chemotherapy, and additionally, its schistosomicidal mode of action is not intuitively clear [26]. The most immediate PZQ effect, at least in vitro, is dramatic parasite contraction and spastic paralysis, followed by outer membrane vacuolation, blebbing, and disruption. Thus, one hypothesis to explain PZQ mode of action is that the drug inserts itself in the membrane, destabilizes the double lipid bilayer [27-29], and subsequently interacts with muscle filaments. Due to its size and hydrophobic nature, PZQ likely intercalates within the phospholipid molecules of the worm apical lipid leaflets, undergoes hop diffusion in the plasma membrane, and permeates to access tegumental actin, myosin, and/or tropomyosin [27-30]. Adult worms' surface spines are crystalline structures consisting of filaments of actin that interact directly with the apical and basal membranes [31, 32]. Actin is present in the surface membrane tubercles and in the tegument [33]. More importantly, actin molecules are known to form a mesh or fence underneath surface plasma membranes [30, 34, 35]. Putative interaction of PZQ with actin in spines, tubercles, and tegument would affect its polymerization status, leading to surface membrane disruption. Pre-incubation of parasites in the presence 30 mM magnesium before exposure to PZQ prevented contraction and tegumental disintegration in all worms [36]. This finding, coupled with the recent report showing magnesium-dependent modulation of myosin and actin functions, [37] may be construed to indicate that PZQ directly interacts with the parasite myosin and actin.

We have taken advantage of the Claisen Condensation Reaction to irreversibly bind the otherwise inert PZQ to cellulose acetate membrane and thus use affinity chromatography to isolate the parasite surface membrane molecule(s) that most selectively bind to PZQ. Amino acid microsequencing and immunogenicity studies indicated that PZQ preferably binds to schistosome actin at the exclusion of other adult worm surface membrane antigens. We have proposed that PZQ accesses actin of schistosomes and induces its polymerization, with subsequent parasite contraction and tegument disruption [38, 39]. Cytochalasin B disrupts actin polymerization by capping the fast-growing end of actin filaments. Pre-treatment of adult *S. mansoni* with cytochalasin B did not entirely prevent worm contraction and immobility, yet rendered the parasites refractory to killing by even exceedingly high PZQ concentrations. The results may easily be construed to indicate that PZQ-mediated actin polymerization is the major mechanism of PZQ killing [40]. Ramaswamy and colleagues expressed the cDNA library of *S. mansoni* on the surface of T7 bacteriophages and screened the displayed proteins with labeled PZQ. The results indicated PZQ binds to the N-terminal end of myosin light chain and to actin, and further revealed that *S. mansoni* myosin light chain is phosphorylated in vivo upon binding to PZQ [41].

The second major PZQ effect is abnormal calcium influx in the worm, leading to hypothesizing that voltage-gated calcium channel(s) on the surface of the worm is the elusive target of PZQ action [42-46]. However, Cioli and colleagues failed to detect the correlation between PZQ-induced intra-worm calcium influx and parasite death [47]. In support, incubation of *S. mansoni* worms in the presence of seven different calcium channel blockers gave insignificant protection against PZQ lethal action except for nicardipine and nifedipine, which nevertheless did not prevent the spastic paralysis observed in worms observed in schistosomes exposed to PZQ, and allowed 50% of the worms to be killed by 3 μM PZQ. In contrast, all worm survived exposure to 36 μM PZQ following pre-treatment with the actin depolymerizing agent, cytochalasin B [40].

*2.1.3. Safety and efficacy*

Extensive use of PZQ for treatment and control of schistosomiasis requires a comprehensive understanding of efficacy and safety:

a. **Of various doses for different Schistosoma species.** PZQ is active against all schistosome species that infect humans. A multicenter, randomized, controlled trial of the efficacy and safety of single-dose PZQ at 40 mg/kg versus 60 mg/kg for treating intestinal schistosomiasis in the Philippines (*S. japonicum*), Mauritania, Tanzania, and Brazil (*S. mansoni*) enrolled 856 patients, aged 10-19 years and with ≥ 100 eggs per gram of feces (epg). A total of 666 (78%) reported adverse reactions, mostly abdominal pain, at 4 hours after administration with no highly significant differences between doses. Both doses were highly effective, as in Day 21 cure rates were 91.7% (86.6%-98% at individual sites) with 40 mg/kg and 92.8% (88%-97%) with 60 mg/kg, suggesting there is no significant efficacy advantage of the 60 versus standard 40 mg/kg for therapy of intestinal schistosomiasis. Of note, there were no differences in efficacy outcomes with variations in transmission and infection intensities across the sites [48]. A meta-analysis of comparative and non-comparative clinical trials on PZQ clinical efficacy and tolerability for intestinal and urinary schistosomiasis, involved 19,500 patients, largely children, in 24 countries and 82 sites. Again, approximately 60% of the subjects receiving 40 mg/kg PZQ reported adverse reactions, namely abdominal pain. The WHO-recommended dose of PZQ 40 mg/kg achieved within 8 weeks cure rates of 94.7% (92.2-98.0) for *S. japonicum*, 77.1% (68.4-85.1) for *S. haematobium*, 76.7% (71.9-81.2) for *S. mansoni*, and 63.5% (48.2-77.0) for mixed *S. haematobium/S. mansoni* infections; the data revealed efficacy in some sites was significantly lower than expected [49].

b. **For low, moderate, and heavy infections.** In a study performed in 2009-2010, PZQ-mediated cure rates in 588 school-age children of *S. mansoni* endemic El Rouse village in Kafr El Sheikh at 4 weeks after a single PZQ dose of 40 mg/kg were 83%, 76%, and 54% for light (<100 epg), moderate (100-400 epg), and heavy (>400 epg) infection, respectively, indicating that pre-treatment intensity of infection has a great influence on PZQ efficacy [50]. Decrease of cure rates with increasing pre-treatment egg counts was also observed among 611 *S. mansoni*-infected schoolchildren from three schools in northeast Ethiopia. Side-effects and symptoms, especially abdominal cramps, vomiting, diarrhea, and dizziness were reported by 91% of the children and were more pronounced in those with high pre-treatment egg excretion [51]. Among 253 *S. mansoni*-infected children in western

Côte d'Ivoire treated with 60 mg/kg PZQ, there was a significant (P<0.01) association between cure rate and intensity of infection prior to treatment with highest cure rates observed in light infections [reviewed in 52]. Highest cure rates against *S. haematobium* infection among 675 primary schoolchildren in Zimbabwe were observed in those with light baseline infection; yet, a wide range of observed mild and transient side effects were not associated with egg intensity [53]. The remarkably low cure rates obtained from people with heavy *S. mansoni* or *S. haematobium* infections led King et al. [54] to advocate the repeat of PZQ treatment 2-8 weeks after the first dose. We have recently performed a study involving 260 *S. mansoni*-infected schoolchildren in Kafr El Sheikh, Egypt. Cure rates 6 weeks after a single dose of 40 mg/kg PZQ were 60%, 42%, and 20% for light, moderate, and heavy infections, respectively [55], fully supporting the observation that PZQ efficacy greatly decreases with the increase of baseline infection levels.

c. **In areas of low endemicity/limited PZQ treatment versus areas of high endemicity and massive, repeated PZQ administration**. In our recent study involving 66 school-age children in low *S. mansoni* endemicity villages of Menoufiya, Egypt, PZQ cure rates at 4 weeks following treatment with a single dose of 40 mg/kg PZQ, were 87% and 83% for light and moderate infections, respectively, significantly higher than cure rates achieved in the high *S. mansoni* endemicity villages of Kafr El Sheikh [55, 56]. Our findings fully support the observations of King et al. [54] who reported that for subjects with *S. mansoni* or *S. haematobium* infection, cure rates were higher in communities having lower initial prevalence. Indeed, in Cameroon regions with low prevalence of schistosomiasis, and in Senbete Town, northeast of Ethiopia, treatment of schoolchildren with a single dose of 40 mg/kg body weight resulted into cure rates of 80-95%, with the majority of children reporting drug-related symptoms and malaise as late as 24 hours after treatment [57, 58]. Conversely, a single oral dose at 40 mg/kg body weight induced only approximately 60% reduction in prevalence and epg in <10-14 year-old schoolchildren In Wondo Genet, southern Ethiopia, region with school age children prevalence rate of 75%, i.e., high-risk communities. Approximately 83% of *S. mansoni*-infected children complained of headache, nausea, abdominal pain, bloody stool, vomiting, and fever at 24 hour post-treatment. These symptoms were associated with age ($P<0.001$) and pre-treatment intensity of infection ($P<0.05$) [59].

A study was performed along the high endemicity shores of Lake Victoria after 12.5 years of massive and repeated PZQ use involving 178 *S. mansoni*-infected men. The overall cure rate after a single PZQ dose was 66% ranging from 36% to 82%. Of note, treatments administered in 2006 were significantly more likely to result in cure failures than treatments administered in 2004, the year in which PZQ efficacy was highest [60]. Similar observation was also reported for *S. mansoni*-infected schoolchildren in Kafr El Sheikh, Egypt. Thus, in a study performed in 2009-2010, PZQ-mediated cure rates in school-age children of *S. mansoni* high endemicity El Rouse village in Kafr El Sheikh were 83%, 76%, and 54% for light, moderate, and heavy infection, respectively, 4 weeks after a single PZQ dose of 40 mg/kg [50]. These cure rates were distinctly higher than those obtained in in the same areas at 6 weeks after PZQ therapy, suggesting reduction in PZQ efficacy 3 years later, following intense and repeated PZQ administration [55].

### *2.1.4. Evidence for worm resistance to PZQ*

Twenty years after its introduction, PZQ remains the drug of choice despite treatment failures and emergence of resistance being reported.

First indications on worm resistance to PZQ appeared in the Senegal River Basin, whereby 117 out of 130 selected subjects (87%) were infected with *S. mansoni* with overall geometric mean epg of 478. The overall cure rate 4 weeks after treatment with single standard PZQ dose was only 42%. However, cure rate after a second round of treatment rose to 76%, suggesting the low cure rate observed after one treatment was probably the result of a combination of high infection intensity and the maturation of pre-existing pre-patent *S. mansoni* infections [61]. Exceedingly low cure rates but similar conclusions were reached by Gryseels et al. [62], advocating there is no convincing evidence for emergence of PZQ-resistant *S. mansoni* in Senegal, and that the exceptionally low cure rates can be attributed to high initial worm loads and intense transmission in this area. However, low PZQ cures were again reported in children living in villages in Senegal River Basin with intense *S. mansoni* and *S. haematobium* transmission. Additionally, high prevalence and high infection intensity of *S. mansoni* and *S. haematobium* were still evident despite multiple rounds of chemotherapy, leading to the recommendation of new treatment regimens to control schistosomiasis in the school-age population [63].

Evidence for some degree of *S. mansoni* resistance to PZQ has been obtained using parasites taken from treated, but uncured human patients in Egypt and Senegal and in a laboratory isolate of *S. mansoni* subjected to successive passages under drug pressure, raising the need for alternative drugs to treat PZQ-resistant schistosomiasis [64-66]. Yet, there was no increase in drug failure, despite 10 years of therapeutic pressure in some Nile Delta villages where there had been resistant infections and worms with decreased response to PZQ [67]. In contrast to this optimistic note, a British traveler returning from East Africa failed to be cured despite several rounds of standard PZQ doses and no opportunity for re-infection [68]. In addition, there are several schistosomiasis cases caused by *S. haematobium* infections in which repeated standard treatment failed to clear the infection [69]. Isolates of *S. mansoni* obtained from patients from Kisumu, Kenya continuously exposed to infection as a consequence of their occupations as car washers or sand harvesters showed reduced PZQ susceptibility that was associated with previous PZQ treatment of the patient [70]. Recently, miracidia were hatched from eggs obtained from seven Kenyan car washers and used to infect snails. Shed cercariae were used to establish in mice a laboratory *S. mansoni* strain with significantly reduced PZQ sensitivity that was achieved within only 5 generations by administering increasing PZQ doses to the infected mice; the parasites were eventually able to withstand a normally lethal dose [71].

### *2.1.5. Proposed mechanism(s) for PZQ resistance*

Resistance to a drug is defined as "genetically transmitted loss of sensitivity in a parasite population that was previously sensitive to the drug". Schistosomicidal action of oxamniquine (OXA) and hycanthone is dependent on activation by sulfotransferase enzymatic esterification and this ultimately results in the production of an electrophilic moiety capable of alkylating DNA [72, 73]. Resistance of *S. mansoni* to OXA was attributed to loss-of-function mutations in a gene on chromosome 6 that was found to be encoding the enzyme, sulfotransferase [74]. Unlike OXA and hycanthone, there is no evidence PZQ interacts with schistosome DNA, inducing mutation(s) responsible for the drug inefficacy. It was then proposed that massive use of the drug would select for parasites harboring "genes" that confer resistance to the drug [75]. The presence of gene(s) that confer resistance to PZQ is not excluded, especially that a proportion of adult worms consistently survive treatment, and the drug is ineffective against immature worms. Yet, PZQ-resistant and susceptible worms did not show differences at 15 microsatellite genotypic markers [76].

Voltage-gated calcium channels that have been implicated in PZQ action did not show differences in the encoding cDNA sequence or expression levels among PZQ-susceptible and PZQ-resistant isolates [42-46, 77]. Adenosine triphosphate binding cassette (ABC) multi-drug transporters, especially the P glycoprotein, which shows selectivity for hydrophobic molecules, are predominantly localized in schistosome excretory system. Evidence for association between schistosome multi-drug transporters and PZQ resistance has been recently presented [78-81 and references therein].

On the other hand, Botros et al. [82] reported that laboratory-maintained *S. mansoni* isolates obtained from Egyptian patients resistant to PZQ cure failed to display PZQ-induced tegumental damage, implying changes in tegument characteristics in PZQ-unresponsive worms. Changes in parasite tegument properties in PZQ-resistant *S. mansoni* isolates were associated with decreased stability, reproductive fitness, and immunogenicity [65]. We recently proposed that the decrease in PZQ efficacy may be explained if repeated and intensive PZQ use selects for the worms with tighter outer lipid bilayer shield consequent to higher percentage of cholesterol and sphingomyelin (SM) and/or less active tegument-associated neutral sphingomyelinase (nSMase) [83]. The result would be worm progeny, able to prevent or decrease access of even molecules of 312 Da such as PZQ [55]. Schistosomes showing PZQ insusceptibility were documented to incur serious biological costs [65, 78], a strong support to our assumption.

## 2.2. Arachidonic acid

### 2.2.1. *Structure, biological sources, and functions*

Arachidonic acid (ARA) is a polyunsaturated fatty acid, i.e., the 20 carbon-chain contains more (#4) than one double bond, the first starting at position 6 from the last = omega carbon (methyl terminus opposite the COOH end). The formula is $C_{20}H_{32}O_2$, 20:4(ω-6). All double bonds are in a *cis* position (hydrogen atoms are on the same side of the double bonds) and, hence, ARA is also termed all-*cis*-5,8,11,14-eicosatetraenoic acid (Figure 2). ARA has an average mass of 304.467 Da and adopts a dominant hairpin conformation [84].

ARA is present throughout the body and comprises the greatest % weight of total fatty acids among long chain poly-unsaturated fatty acids (LC-PUFAs). It is present as a structural component in animal and human cell membrane phospholipids, especially phosphatidylethanolamine, phosphatidylcholine, and phophatidylinositol. It is particularly abundant in skeletal muscles, the brain, and liver. ARA nutrition appears to serve various important roles throughout the human (and mammalian) life-cycle. Throughout pregnancy, ARA, along with

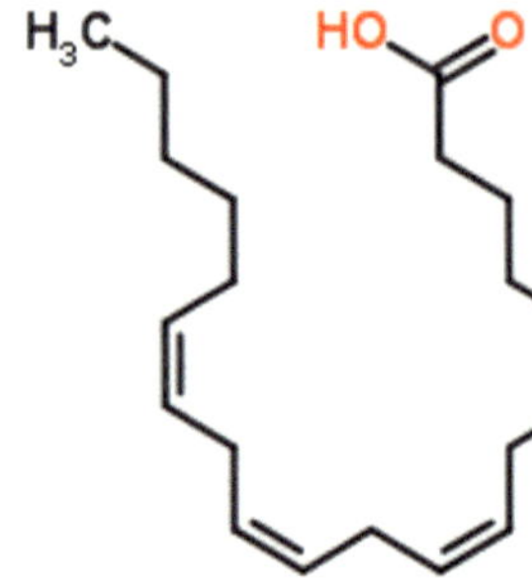


**Figure 2.** Structure of arachidonic acid.

other fats and nutrients, originates from the maternal diet and is supplied via the placenta to support the development of the growing fetus.

Between the third trimester of pregnancy and second year of neonatal life, the human brain undergoes a remarkable increase in the rate of growth. During this period, mass and volume increase more than 10-fold, and achieve >40% of the average-sized adult brain. These changes in size are mirrored by the accumulation of ARA in the brain [85, 86]. A major hallmark of mammalian birth is the sudden transition, following partuition, from the placenta as the source of prenatal nutrition, onto mother's milk as the main source from which to acquire nutrients. On average, ARA comprises 0.47±0.13% of total fatty acids in human milk [87]. The concentration of ARA in human milk varies between individuals and populations due, at least in part, to the presence of polymorphisms in the genes involved in the endogenous synthesis of LC-PUFAs [88].

The amount of LC-PUFA intake by infants has been estimated based upon the assumptions that the fat content in human milk is 3.8 g/dL, and that average daily intake is 780 mL/day [89]. Using these values, average daily intake of ARA can be estimated to be approximately 140 mg. In addition, it is possible to compare the estimated average intake levels by infants to those of post-weaned individuals, due to the availability in the U.S. of annually collected data from dietary surveys [90].

The results from such a comparison reveal an interesting trend related to the levels of ARA consumed as individuals advance from pre- to post-weaning stages of human development. The average amount of dietary intake by toddler and preschool-age children (2-5 years) is approximately 80 mg. A modest increase in the absolute level of intake of approximately 20% occurs by school-age (6-11 years). Intake then decreases by adolescence (12-19 years), and once again approximates the average levels obtained through nursing. These differences in the amount of ARA consumed in the diet may initially seem to be marginal, until they are considered on a per weight basis. A change of approximately 20-fold in body mass occurs as humans develop from infancy to adulthood (i.e., ~3 kg to ~60 kg). Therefore, on a per weight basis, the amount of preformed ARA consumed daily by mid-adolescence is ≤ 5% relative to the estimated amount per kg of intake for infants.

Although ARA is synthesized endogenously by the desaturation and elongation of linoleic acid (18:2n-6), results from experimental efforts consistently point to a need for ARA availability through dietary sources in order to elevate ARA in plasma and other tissues. In addition, associations between experimentally-defined endpoints and changes in the status of ARA reported in numerous investigations support the notion of a minimum required threshold in the concentrations of esterified and/or unesterified ARA in tissues or circulating pools [91].

The importance of preformed dietary ARA in supporting healthy immune functions has been demonstrated by investigations comparing the effects of supplementation using refined, microbial-derived ARA as triglycerides (TG) or unsupplemented formula and human milk on immune ability in pre-term and term infants. In an investigation involving infants born before 37 weeks of gestation, infants were provided with a control formula, or that same formula supplemented with 0.49% (wt/wt) of ARA, in addition to DHA [92-94]. After a period of 4 weeks, immunologic parameters were assessed from both groups and the results compared to those obtained from human milk-fed infants. The status of ARA in phospholipids was equivalent in the human milk-fed and LC-PUFA+formula-fed infants, and in both cases, significantly greater compared to infants fed with the control formula. In addition, effects on lymphocyte populations, cytokine production, and antibody maturation in formula-fed infants supplemented with LCPUFAs were consistent with those observed for human milk-fed infants.

More recently, healthy full-term, formula-fed infants supplemented with ≤ 190 mg/day ARA for a period of at least 8 weeks, showed fewer incidence of symptoms commonly associated with infections of the upper respiratory tract, in addition to fewer incidents of diarrhea. Importantly, the combined results from these investigations provide a clear example of the utility of preformed LC-PUFA in the diet to support the ability of infants to respond to immune challenges. In each case, the availability of preformed LC-PUFAs in the diet was associated with a preferred response to immune challenges, in contrast to results obtained from the use of formulations that contained adequate (i.e., 16% wt/wt) 18:2n-6 [95].

Animal models have also been used to explore possible roles and functions of LC-PUFAs, including ARA, in immune-related activities. In piglets fed with formula enriched with supraphysiological levels of ARA resulted in maximal enrichment of intestinal mucosal within 8 days of initiating treatment. In addition, enrichment showed a dose-dependent response of intestinal mucosal phospholipid ARA concentration to dietary ARA in formula [96].

These results along with data from the human studies indicate that dietary intake of microbial-derived ARA supports enrichment of ARA phospholipids in tissues. In addition, intake of sufficient levels of dietary ARA may support mucosal immunity against pathogenic agents, during periods of rapid growth and development in humans and other mammals. Overall, these and other results may not be surprising considering the large number of metabolic pathways and signaling cascades in which ARA is involved.

Arachidonic acid is essentially incorporated into cell phospholipids; in humans, approximately 10% of phopholipids in liver and plasma contain ARA [97-100]. N-arachidonoyl-phosphatidylethanol- amine leads via multiple pathways to anandamide, an endogenous cannabinoid neurotransmitter [101]. Arachidonic acid is liberated from phospholipids by the action of phospholipase A2, and then produces eicosanoids, prostaglandins, leukotrienes, and other essential bioactive products via the action of three types of oxygenases, cyclooxygenase (COX), lipoxygenase (LOX), and cytochrome P450. There is evidence that exogenous, plasma unesterified ARA may effectively compete with endogenous ARA for these enzymes, predominantly located on the nuclear and endoplasmic reticulum membrane. Some resultant eicosanoids are pro-inflammatory and vasoconstrictive, such as prostaglandin $E_2$, thromboxane $A_2$, and leukotriene $B_4$, and some are anti-inflammatory and anti-aggregatory such as prostacyclin and lipoxin $A_4$ [97-100]. Indeed, shortly after inflammation is initiated, neutrophils that enter the tissue promote the switch of arachidonic acid-derived prostaglandins and leukotrienes to lipoxins, which induce resolution of the inflammation via termination of neutrophil recruitment and release of reparatory cytokines, such as transforming growth factor-beta [102].

### *2.2.2. Dietary intake in humans*

In humans ARA is acquired directly from the diet or is derived by desaturation-elongation of linoleic acid (10-20 g daily) in the liver and in extra-hepatic tissues. ARA preference for acylation and transacylation reactions favors its partition in tissue phospholipids rather than adipose tissue and plasma triglycerides. Absorption of ingested ARA occurs in the endothelium of the intestinal lumen of the small intestine. Absorbed ARA is transported to various tissues and cells throughout the body by lipoproteins and acylated into *sn*-2 position of unesterified lysophospholipids, where it may remain until released by the enzymatic activation of phospholipase A2.

There is considerable evidence of the importance of ARA nutrition during early childhood development. ARA levels in circulation correlate positively with length to weight ratio and head circumference in neonates [91, 103]. In addition, the rate of ARA accretion by the brain increases exponentially during the brain growth-spurt, during the last trimester of pregnancy and into the first year of neonatal growth [85, 86]. Tissue lipid data indicate that a 70 kg human contains 50-100 g ARA distributed between cell cytosolic and membrane compartments. It was estimated that on average, Australian diet provides ARA intake of 130 mg/day for males and 96 mg/day for females. Survey data for the intake of dietary ARA indicates a range of 80 to 190 mg/day. Intake of ARA provided by a typical Japanese diet was calculated to be 300 mg/day, respectively [104 and references therein]. To my knowledge, there is no information on the amounts of ARA diets in poor rural areas provide to children and pregnant women, but values are expectedly far less than those reported above. That is of concern as ARA is known to be essential for proper development of the brain and muscles in the fetus and in infants [91, 93, 105].

### *2.2.3. Safety/adverse effects*

We recently conducted clinical trials on the safety of ARA intake in 20 and 90 Egyptian school-age children of Menoufiya and Kafr El Sheikh Governorate, respectively. Arachidonic acid oral capsules, containing 396 mg ARA (ARASCO®) per capsule, were provided by DSM (DSM Nutritional Products, Columbia, MD). Children were given10 mg/kg/day (approximately 400 mg daily) for 15 days over 3 weeks, i.e., 5 days per week. Not a single child reported the slighted malaise or adverse reaction during, and 6 weeks after, treatment. A panel of analyses indicated that biochemical profiles were either unchanged or ameliorated following ARA therapy in all children [55, 56]. These results fully confirm the reports on safety of ARA in athletes supplemented with 1,000 mg for 50 days [106]. Regarding immunological analyses, intake of approximately 400 mg ARA/day for 15 days led to significant ($P$<0.0001) decrease of *S. mansoni*-infected Egyptian schoolchildren plasma levels of interleukin (IL)-10 and interferon-gamma (IFN-$\gamma$), thus rendering the plasma cytokine profile of the treated children nearer to normal [55, 56]. Our findings are consistent with the observational studies showing that higher ARA intake was associated with lower levels of inflammatory markers and sequelae [107, 108].

The most serious adverse reaction reported for ARA was causing platelet aggregation in adults given 6 g ARA/day for 2 to 3 weeks [109]. However, approximately 0.5 g ARA daily intake for 15 days over 3 weeks did not alter platelet counts or blood coagulation parameters in *S. mansoni*-infected schoolchildren [55, 56], and healthy adults given 1.7 g ARA daily for 50 consecutive days [106]. In a double-blind, placebo-controlled study, supplementation of Japanese healthy adults with 838 mg/day ARA for 2 weeks led to no changes in platelet aggregation [104].

### *2.2.4. Schistosomicidal effects in vitro and in experimental animals*

The first indication on ARA schistosomicidal action was evident as we exposed ex vivo lung-stage larvae of *S. mansoni* and *S. haematobium* to 0-500 μM ARA. Incubation in the presence of 10-20 μM ARA for 30 minutes induced exposure of otherwise hidden parasite surface membrane antigens to specific antibody binding. Higher ARA concentration or exposure time led to irreversible death of the larvae and destruction of their surface membrane. The mono-unsaturated omega-9 fatty acid, oleic acid (the major, 78.6%, fatty acid in olive oil) alone or in conjunction with linoleic acid (as in corn oil), were able to expose the larval surface membrane antigens to antibody binding but did not induce attrition or membrane disruption. The study suggested that ARA is a schistosomicide for young larvae, with *S. haematobium* being more sensitive than *S. mansoni* [110]. Experiments with inhibitors and activators of neutral sphingomyelinase (nSMase) further indicated that ARA schistosomicidal effect is due, at least in part, to its ability to activate the parasite tegument-associated, magnesium-dependent nSMase [83].

Developing and adult *S. mansoni* and *S. haematobium* worms were also susceptible to in vitro schistosomicidal action whereby 2.5 and 5 mM ARA elicited irreversible killing of ex vivo 4-, 5-, and 6-week-old *S. mansoni* and 9-, 10-, and 12-week-old *S. haematobium* worms, within 3-4 hours, depending on the parasite age, even when worms were maintained in up to 50% fetal calf serum. Juvenile (3-week-old) *S. mansoni* were more sensitive to ARA as 100% irreversible attrition was noted 1 hour after exposure to 2.5 and 5 mM concentration of ARA. Of note, ARA-mediated worm attrition was prevented by concurrent incubation with nSMase inhibitors such as $CaCl_2$ or GW4869, providing another evidence for the mechanism of ARA schistosomicidal action. Scanning and transmission electron microscopy revealed that ARA-mediated adult worm killing was associated with spine destruction, membrane blebbing, and disorganization of the apical membrane structure [111]. Expectedly, otherwise sequestered adult worm surface membrane antigens were accessible to specific antibody binding as judged by indirect membrane immunofluorescence. Additionally, addition of serum antibodies and peripheral blood mononuclear cells from patently infected hosts significantly enhanced ARA-mediated adult *S. mansoni* and *S. haematobium* attrition in vitro, suggesting that immune effectors strongly enhance ARA-mediated schistosomicidal effect [112].

Schistosomicidal activity of ARA was evident in vivo as a single oral dose of 500 and 1000 mg/kg pure ARA administered to mice 7 and 35 days after *S. mansoni* infection, respectively elicited significant ($P<0.01$) reduction of approximately 40% in worm burden, documenting the ARA susceptibility of larval and adult worms. *Schistosoma haematobium* appeared even more sensitive as a single oral dose of 1000 mg/kg ARA administered 70 days after infection induced highly significant ($P=0.003$) reduction of 57.5% in worm burden evaluated 20 days later. Oral administration of mice with 300 mg/kg ARA incorporated in infant formula for 15 successive days led to even more highly significant ($P<0.0005$) reduction of approximately 60% and 80% *S. mansoni* and *S. haematobium* worm burden, respectively [111]. These results were extended and entirely confirmed in hamster hosts where a series of 4 experiments for *S. mansoni* and *S. haematobium* indicated that ARA oral administration after patency led to highly significant ($P<0.02$-$<0.001$) reduction in worm burden accompanied with significant ($P<0.05$) decrease in worm egg load [112]. No adverse reactions were noted in any treated mouse or hamster. Additionally, no significant differences were noted among schistosome-infected and ARA-treated hamsters regarding serum total triglycerides and cholesterol levels, fatty acids relative percentages, erythrocytes and platelet count, and prothrombin and partial thromboplastin time, all evaluated in blood samples obtained 2 hours after ARA administration [112].

### *2.2.5. Mechanism of schistosomicidal action*

We have previously shown that sphingomyelin (SM) in the schistosome apical lipid bilayer is the major responsible for the sieving properties of the outer membrane, which readily allows entry of nutrient molecules of <600 Da such as water, sugars, fatty acids, and cholesterol, while it prevents access of larger molecules, namely host antibodies (>150,000 Da), via interacting with surrounding water molecules to form a tight hydrogen barrier [83]. We have been able to use quasi-elastic neutron scattering to formally demonstrate the existence of the hydrogen barrier around schistosomes, and shown it is stronger in lung-stage larvae than adult worms and *S. mansoni* than *S. haematobium*. We have also shown that the hydrogen barrier collapses following nSMase activation and SM hydrolysis [113, 114].

We have predicted, and provided evidence for, the existence of schistosome tegument-associated magnesium-dependent nSMase as early as 2006 [83]. The existence of the enzyme was formally demonstrated in 2009 following the analysis of *S. mansoni* complete genome [115]. The enzyme nucleotide and amino acid (aa) sequences were later fine-tuned [116]. We succeeded in cloning and sequencing 836 bp near the 5′ end of *S. haematobium* nSMase-encoding mRNA. The predicted amino acid sequences corresponded to aa18- aa277 in the *S. mansoni* counterpart with 96% identities and 98% positives, and contained the conserved domains characterizing the exonuclease-endonuclease-phosphatase (EEP) superfamily [12,

117]. The complete *S. haematobium* genome and the complete sequence of the nSMase were published by Young et al. in 2012 [118].

We have been able to demonstrate the presence of nSMase in the tegument of adult *S. mansoni* and *S. haematobium* using enzymatic, immunologic, and immune-histochemical assays, and further shown that ARA was particularly potent in stimulating nSMase enzymatic activity, entirely supporting our previous findings using larvae and adult worms [12, 83, 110-114, 117, and references therein].

#### 2.2.6. *Efficacy in school-age children*

In Menoufiya villages of low *S. mansoni* prevalence, efficacy of ARA in treatment of school-age children with <100 epg was highly comparable to that of PZQ + Placebo (Pbo) with percent cure of 78% (11/14) and 85% (12/14), respectively, and similar levels of reduction in geometric mean egg counts (GMEC) in uncured patients. However, the efficacy of ARA in treatment of schoolchildren with 100-400 epg was significantly ($P<0.0001$) lower than for PZQ regarding cure rate (44% and 83%, respectively) and reduction in GMEC in uncured children, suggesting that ARA is indicated for treatment of light *S. mansoni* infection in children. In Kafr El Sheikh villages of high *S. mansoni* endemicity and where intensive mass PZQ treatment campaigns were implemented for 10 consecutive years, the efficacy of ARA in the treatment of school children with light infection (<100 epg) was highly comparable to that of PZQ + Pbo with percent cure of 50% and 60%, respectively. Efficacy of ARA and PZQ was again comparable in school-age children with heavy infection (800-1000 epg) leading to 21% and 20% cure rate, and 64% and 81% reduction in GMEC in uncured children, respectively. The results indicated that either PZQ or ARA are moderately efficacious for treatment of light *S. mansoni* infection in regions of elevated schistosomiasis prevalence, and neither should be used alone for treatment of children with heavy infections, especially those residing in regions of intense endemicity [55, 56].

It is important to assess the efficacy of ARA for treatment of *S. haematobium*. We expect high cure rates as larval and adult *S. haematobium* worms are shown in in vitro, and in vivo experiments in mice and hamsters to be more susceptible to ARA than *S. mansoni* [12, 83, 110-114-117].

### 2.3. PZQ and arachidonic acid combination for treatment of human schistosomiasis

#### 2.3.1. *Evidence for safety and efficacy in children*

Intake of PZQ + ARA was as safe as for PZQ or ARA alone regarding metabolic panels or immunological parameters of *S. mansoni*-infected schoolchildren. Regarding efficacy, ARA and PZQ synergized for a spectacular cure of all lightly- and moderately-infected children residing in the low endemicity villages of Menoufiya, Egypt. In the high endemicity areas of Kafr El Sheikh, combining ARA and PZQ resulted into higher cure rates than mono-therapies for light, moderate, and heavy infection. For light infection, mono-therapy cure rate of 50-60% was increased to 83% with the ARA + PZQ regimen. For the children with heavy infection,

PZQ and ARA mono-therapy induced 20% cure rates, while cure rate of 78% was achieved with the drug combination [55, 56].

Combination of PZQ-oxamniquine (OXA) was assayed in randomized, non-blinded, dose-ranging trials in treatment of Malawi and Zimbabwe schoolchildren with low, moderate, and heavy infection. Cure rates were not available for Malawi children, while it reached 89% with the higher dose (20 and 10 mg/kg for PZQ and OXA, respectively) for children in Zimbabwe. No direct comparisons were reported for PZQ and OXA mono-therapy, and accordingly, synergistic effect was not documented [119-121]. Additionally, opposite to PZQ and ARA, OXA is effective against *S. mansoni* but not *S. haematobium* [121].

PZQ and artemether or artesunate in combination resulted in a protection rate of about 80%, slightly higher than PZQ mono-therapy for treatment of schistosomiasis haematobium and japonicum in two field trials [122, 123]. In a field trial in high *S. mansoni* endemicity Senegalese villages, 1- to 60-year-old (median=18 years) patients with moderate *S. mansoni* infection were treated with PZQ, artesunate, or both drugs in combination (35-39 individuals per study arm). Cure rates were 44% for PZQ, 23% for artesunate, and 69% for the drugs combined. Combination of PZQ and artesunate appeared clearly synergistic, but the efficacy was obviously lower than for PZQ + ARA [123, 124]. This study revealed that efficacy of artemisinin derivative alone against *S. mansoni* is not evident and, furthermore, was not observed in *S. haematobium* infections [122]. Most importantly, artemether, and artemisin derivatives are used for malaria therapy; artemisinin resistance in *Plasmodium falciparum* is now prevalent across mainland Southeast Asia, and poses a threat to the control and elimination of malaria [125].

### *2.3.2. Molecular basis for efficacy*

There were no reduction in efficacy of artemether and artesunate in killing PZQ-resistant and PZQ-susceptible *S. japonicum* worms in mice treated 7 and 8 or 35 and 36 days post-infection [126]. Opposite findings were observed regarding ARA, as its efficacy was as low as that of PZQ in treating schoolchildren with heavy *S. mansoni* infection, residing in areas where massive PZQ campaigns were applied for 10 consecutive years [55]. This finding implies that *S. mansoni* worms were resistant to mono-therapy with either PZQ or ARA. That has led us to propose that resistance to PZQ and ARA is attributed to continuous PZQ use, eliciting selection for worms with tight upper lipid bilayer, consequent to excessive SM synthesis and content or lower nSMase activity. Progeny of these worms would prevent access of even the 312 Da PZQ molecules, and would be less susceptible to ARA-mediated nSMase activation. Exposure of such worms to PZQ would not lead to their demise, yet likely facilitate ARA-mediated nSMase activation, SM hydrolysis and worm attrition. Exposure of these worms to ARA would lead to nSMase activation that is not lethal, yet sufficient to now allow entry of PZQ to perform its schistosomicidal action. Our proposition was supported by the considerable increase in cure rates in all children treated with PZQ + ARA versus the drugs' mono-therapy. The increase in cure rates was most highly significant ($P<0.0001$) for children with heavy infections were cure rates with either PZQ or ARA alone were 20% and attained 78% with the drugs combined.

We shall test this hypothesis via evaluation of the cholesterol/SM content and nSMase activity in worms derived from cercariae obtained from communities of low prevalence/low PZQ use and high endemicity/intense PZQ administration. For documenting hypothesized mechanism for ARA counteraction of worm resistance to PZQ, larvae and worms that are progeny of entirely PZQ susceptible and strongly resistant breeds will be incubated with micromolar concentrations of ARA and then evaluated for responsiveness to PZQ, cholesterol/SM content, and nSMase activity.

## 3. Conclusions and recommendations

We may conclude that PZQ or ARA treatment shows considerable efficacy uniquely in the treatment of light infections in areas of low *S. mansoni* endemicity and PZQ use. Even then, efficacy never reaches 100%, except when PZQ and ARA are combined. Chemotherapy with PZQ alone for patients residing in regions of high *S. mansoni* endemicity and afflicted with light, moderate, or heavy infection is not efficacious. Hence, it is recommended to implement optimal treatment regimens with PZQ in conjunction with ARA.

## Acknowledgements

Experiments related to ARA efficacy and safety in mice and hamsters were supported by the Science and Technology Development Fund, Egypt, grants Nos. 144 and 2073 to R. El Ridi. For clinical trials in Menoufiya and Kafr El Sheikh, funding was provided by DSM North America, Columbia, Maryland.

## Author details

Hatem Tallima[1], Kevin Hadley[2] and Rashika El Ridi[1*]

*Address all correspondence to: rashikaelridi@hotmail.com

1 Zoology Department, Faculty of Science, Cairo University, Cairo, Egypt

2 Human Evidence Department, DSM North America, Columbia, Maryland, USA

## References

[1] Barsoum RS, Esmat G, El-Baz T. Human schistosomiasis: Clinical perspective: Review. Journal of Advanced Research. 2013;4(5):433-444.

[2] El Baz T, Esmat G. Hepatic and intestinal schistosomiasis: Review. Journal of Advanced Research. 2013;4(5):445-452.

[3] Barsoum RS. Urinary schistosomiasis: Review. Journal of Advanced Research. 2013;4(5):453-459.

[4] Bhardwaj R, Skelly PJ. Purinergic signaling and immune modulation at the schistosome surface? Trends in Parasitology. 2009;25(6):256-260.

[5] Othman A, El Ridi R. Schistosomiasis. In: Bruschi F. (ed.) Helminth Infections and Their Impact on Global Public Health. The Netherlands:Springer; 2014. p49-92.

[6] Chitsulo L, Loverde P, Engels D. Schistosomiasis. Nature Reviews Microbiology. 2004;2(1):12-13.

[7] WHO Technical Report Series 912: Prevention and control of schistosomiasis and soil-transmitted helminthiasis. Who Geneva, 2002 http://whqlibdoc.who.int/trs/WHO_TRS_912.pdf.

[8] King CH. Parasites and poverty: The case of schistosomiasis. Acta Tropica. 2010;113(2):95-104.

[9] Hotez PJ, Alvarado M, Basáñez MG, Bolliger I, Bourne R, Boussinesq M, et al. The global burden of disease study 2010: Interpretation and implications for the neglected tropical diseases. PLoS Neglected Tropical Diseases. 2014;8(7):e2865.

[10] World Schistosomiasis Risk Chart. 2012 Edition. International Association for Medical Assistance to Travellers. www.IAMAT.Org.

[11] El Ridi RAF, Tallima HA-M. Novel therapeutic and prevention approaches for schistosomiasis: Review. Journal of Advanced Research. 2013;4(5):467-478.

[12] El Ridi R, Tallima H. Solving the riddle of the lung-stage schistosomula paved the way to a novel remedy and an efficacious vaccine for schistosomiasis. In: El Ridi R. (ed.) Parasitic Diseases - Schistosomiasis. Croatia: Intech Open; 2013. p179-202. www.intechopen.com/books/parasitic-diseases-schistosomiasis.

[13] Meyer F, Meyer H, Bueding E. Lipid metabolism in the parasitic and free-living flatworms, *Schistosoma mansoni* and *Dugesia dorotocephala*. Biochimica Biophysica Acta. 1970;210(2):257-266.

[14] Becker B, Mehlhorn H, Andrews P, Thomas H, Eckert J. Light and electron microscopic studies on the effect of praziquantel on *Schistosoma mansoni*, *Dicrocoelium dendriticum*, and *Fasciola hepatica* (Trematoda) in vitro. Zeitschrift fur Pflanzenernahrung und Bodenkunde. 1980;63(2):113-128.

[15] Mehlhorn H, Becker B, Andrews P, Thomas H, Frenkel JK. In vivo and in vitro experiments on the effects of praziquantel on *Schistosoma mansoni*. A light and electron microscopic study. Arzneimittel-Forschung. 1981;31(3a):544-554.

[16] Sabah AA, Fletcher C, Webbe G, Doenhoff MJ. *Schistosoma mansoni*: Chemotherapy of infections of different ages. Experimental Parasitology. 1986;61(3):294-303.

[17] Shaw MK. *Schistosoma mansoni*: Stage-dependent damage after in vivo treatment with praziquantel. Parasitology. 1990;100(Pt 1):65-72.

[18] Flisser A, McLaren DJ. Effect of praziquantel treatment on lung-stage larvae of *Schistosoma mansoni* in vivo. Parasitology. 1989;98(Pt 2):203-211.

[19] Brindley PJ, Sher A. The chemotherapeutic effect of praziquantel against *Schistosoma mansoni* is dependent on host antibody response. Journal of Immunology. 1987;139(1):215-220.

[20] Brindley PJ, Sher A. Immunological involvement in the efficacy of praziquantel. Experimental Parasitolology. 1990;71(2):245-248.

[21] Doenhoff MJ, Modha J, Lambertucci JR, McLaren DJ. The immune dependence of chemotherapy. Parasitology Today. 1991;7(1):16-18.

[22] Fallon PG, Cooper RO, Probert AJ, Doenhoff MJ. Fallon PG, Fookes RE, Wharton GA. Temporal differences in praziquantel- and oxamniquine-induced tegumental damage to adult *Schistosoma mansoni*: implications for drug-antibody synergy. Parasitology. 1996;112(Pt 1):47-58.

[23] Webbe G, James C. A comparison of the susceptibility to praziquantel of *Schistosoma haematobium, S. japonicum, S. mansoni, S. intercalatum* and *S. mattheei* in hamsters. Zeitschrift fur Pflanzenernahrung und Bodenkunde. 1977;52(2):169-177.

[24] James C, Webbe G, Nelson GS. The susceptibility to praziquantel of *Schistosoma haematobium* in the baboon (*Papio anubis*) and of *S. japonicum* in the vervet monkey (*Cercopithecus aethiops*). Zeitschrift fur Pflanzenernahrung und Bodenkunde. 1977;52(2): 179-194.

[25] Andrews P. A summary of the efficacy of praziquantel against schistosomes in animal experiments and notes on its mode of action. Arzneimittel-Forschung. 1981;31(3a):538-541.

[26] Köhler P. The biochemical basis of anthelmintic action and resistance. International Journal for Parasitology. 2001;31(4): 336-345. Review.

[27] Harder A, Goossens J, Andrews P. Influence of praziquantel and Ca2+ on the bilayer-isotropic-hexagonal transition of model membranes. Molecular and Biochemical Parasitology. 1988;29(1):55-59.

[28] Schepers H, Brasseur R, Goormaghtigh E, Duquenoy P, Ruysschaert JM. Mode of insertion of praziquantel and derivatives into lipid membranes. Biochemical Pharmacolology. 1988;37(8):1615-16 23.

[29] Lima SF, Vieira LQ, Harder A, Kusel JR. Altered behaviour of carbohydrate-bound molecules and lipids in areas of the tegument of adult *Schistosoma mansoni* worms damaged by praziquantel. Parasitology. 1994;100(Pt 4):469-477.

[30] Kusumi A, Nakada C, Ritchie K, Murase K, Suzuki K, Murakoshi H, Kasai RS, Kondo J, Fujiwara T. Paradigm shift of the plasma membrane concept from the two-dimensional continuum fluid to the partitioned fluid: high-speed single-molecule tracking of membrane molecules. Annual Review of Biophysics and Biomolecular Structure. 2005;34:351-378. Review.

[31] Cohen C, Reinhardt B, Castellani L, Norton P, Stirewalt M. Schistosome surface spines are "crystals" of actin. The journal of Cell biology. 1982;95(3):987-988.

[32] Zhou Y, Podesta RB. Surface spines of human blood flukes (*Schistosoma mansoni*) contain bundles of actin filaments having identical polarity. European Journal of Cell Biology. 1989Feb;48(1):150-153.

[33] Abbas MK, Cain GD. Actin and intermediate-sized filaments of the spines and cytoskeleton of *Schistosoma mansoni*. Parasitological Research. 1987;73(1):66-74.

[34] Viola A, Gupta N. Tether and trap: regulation of membrane-raft dynamics by actin-binding proteins. Nature Reviews Immunology. 2007;7(11):889-896. Review.

[35] Morone N. Freeze-etch electron tomography for the plasma membrane interface. Methods in Molecular Biology. 2010;657:275-86.

[36] Bricker CS, Depenbusch JW, Bennett JL, Thompson DP. The relationship between tegumental disruption and muscle contraction in *Schistosoma mansoni* exposed to various compounds. Zeitschrift fur Pflanzenernahrung und Bodenkunde. 1983;69(1): 61-71.

[37] Trivedi DV, Muretta JM, Swenson AM, Thomas DD, Yengo CM. Magnesium impacts myosin V motor activity by altering key conformational changes in the mechanochemical cycle. Biochemistry. 2013;52(27):4710-4722.

[38] Tallima H, El Ridi R. Praziquantel binds *Schistosoma mansoni* adult worm actin. International Journal of Antimicrobial Agents. 2007;29(5):570-575.

[39] Tallima H, El Ridi R. Re: Is actin the praziquantel receptor? International Journal of Antimicrobial Agents. 2007;30(6):566-567.

[40] Pica-Mattoccia L, Valle C, Basso A, Troiani AR, Vigorosi F, Liberti P, Festucci A, Cioli D. Cytochalasin D abolishes the schistosomicidal activity of praziquantel. Experimental Parasitology. 2007;115(4):344-351.

[41] Gnanasekar M, Salunkhe AM, Mallia AK, He YX, Kalyanasundaram R. Praziquantel affects the regulatory myosin light chain of *Schistosoma mansoni*. Antimicrobial Agents and Chemotherapy 2009;53(3):1054-1060.

[42] Kohn AB, Anderson PA, Roberts-Misterly JM, Greenberg RM. Schistosome calcium channel beta subunits. Unusual modulatory effects and potential role in the action of

the antischistosomal drug praziquantel. Journal of Biological Chemistry. 2001;276(40):36873-36876.

[43] Kohn AB, Lea J, Roberts-Misterly JM, Anderson PA, Greenberg RM. Structure of three high voltage-activated calcium channel alpha1 subunits from *Schistosoma mansoni*. Parasitology. 2001;123(Pt 5):489-497.

[44] Kohn AB, Roberts-Misterly JM, Anderson PA, Khan N, Greenberg RM. Specific sites in the Beta Interaction Domain of a schistosome Ca2+ channel beta subunit are key to its role in sensitivity to the anti-schistosomal drug praziquantel. Parasitology. 2003;127(Pt 4):349-356.

[45] Kohn AB, Roberts-Misterly JM, Anderson PA, Greenberg RM. Creation by mutagenesis of a mammalian Ca(2+) channel beta subunit that confers praziquantel sensitivity to a mammalian Ca(2+) channel. International Journal for Parasitology. 2003;33(12):1303-1308.

[46] Salvador-Recatalà V, Greenberg RM. Calcium channels of schistosomes: unresolved questions and unexpected answers. Wiley Interdisciplinary Review of Membrane Transport and Signaling. 2012;1(1):85-93.

[47] Pica-Mattoccia L, Orsini T, Basso A, Festucci A, Liberti P, Guidi A, Marcatto-Maggi AL, Nobre-Santana S, Troiani AR, Cioli D, Valle C. *Schistosoma mansoni*: lack of correlation between praziquantel-induced intra-worm calcium influx and parasite death. Experimental Parasitology. 2008;119(3):332-335.

[48] Olliaro PL, Vaillant MT, Belizario VJ, Lwambo NJ, Ouldabdallahi M, Pieri OS, Amarillo ML, Kaatano GM, Diaw M, Domingues AC, Favre TC, Lapujade O, Alves F, Chitsulo L. A multicentre randomized controlled trial of the efficacy and safety of single-dose praziquantel at 40 mg/kg vs. 60 mg/kg for treating intestinal schistosomiasis in the Philippines, Mauritania, Tanzania and Brazil. PLoS Neglected Tropical Diseases. 2011;5(6):e1165.

[49] Zwang J, Olliaro PL. Clinical efficacy and tolerability of praziquantel for intestinal and urinary schistosomiasis-a meta-analysis of comparative and non-comparative clinical trials. PLoS Neglected Tropical Diseases. 2014;8(11):e3286.

[50] Barakat R, El Morshedy H. Efficacy of two praziquantel treatments among primary school children in an area of high *Schistosoma mansoni* endemicity, Nile Delta, Egypt. Parasitology. 2011;138(4):440-446.

[51] Berhe N, Gundersen SG, Abebe F, Birrie H, Medhin G, Gemetchu T. Praziquantel side effects and efficacy related to *Schistosoma mansoni* egg loads and morbidity in primary school children in north-east Ethiopia. Acta Tropica. 1999;72(1):53-63.

[52] Utzinger J, N'Goran EK, N'Dri A, Lengeler C, Tanner M. Efficacy of praziquantel against *Schistosoma mansoni* with particular consideration for intensity of infection. Tropical Medicine and International Health. 2000;5(11):771-778.

[53] Midzi N, Sangweme D, Zinyowera S, Mapingure MP, Brouwer KC, Kumar N, Mutapi F, Woelk G, Mduluza T. Efficacy and side effects of praziquantel treatment against *Schistosoma haematobium* infection among primary school children in Zimbabwe. Transactions of the Royal Society of Tropical Medicine and Hygiene. 2008;102(8): 759-766.

[54] King CH, Olbrych SK, Soon M, Singer ME, Carter J, Colley DG. Utility of repeated praziquantel dosing in the treatment of schistosomiasis in high-risk communities in Africa: A systematic review. PLoS Neglected Tropical Diseases. 2011;5(9):e1321.

[55] Barakat R, Abou El-Ela N, Sharaf S, El Sagheer O, Selim S, Tallima H, Bruins MJ, Hadley KB, El Ridi R. Efficacy and safety of arachidonic acid for treatment of school-age children in *Schistosoma mansoni* high endemicity regions. American Journal of Tropical Medicine and Hygiene. 2015;92(4):797-894.

[56] Selim S, El Sagheer O, El Amir A, Barakat R, Hadley K, Bruins MJ, El Ridi R. Efficacy and safety of arachidonic acid for treatment of *Schistosoma mansoni*-infected children in Menoufiya, Egypt. American Journal of Tropical Medicine and Hygiene. 2014;91(5):973-981.

[57] Tchuem Tchuenté LA, Momo SC, Stothard JR, Rollinson D. Efficacy of praziquantel and reinfection patterns in single and mixed infection foci for intestinal and urogenital schistosomiasis in Cameroon. Acta Tropica. 2013;128(2):275-283.

[58] Reta B, Erko B. Efficacy and side effects of praziquantel in the treatment for *Schistosoma mansoni* infection in school children in Senbete Town, northeastern Ethiopia. Tropical Medicine and International Health. 2013;18(11):1338-1343.

[59] Erko B, Degarege A, Tadesse K, Mathiwos A, Legesse M, 2012. Efficacy and side effects of praziquantel in the treatment of *Schistosomiasis mansoni* in schoolchildren in Shesha Kekele Elementary School, Wondo Genet, Southern Ethiopia. Asian Pacific Journal of Tropical Biomedicine. 2012;2(3):235-239.

[60] Black CL, Steinauer ML, Mwinzi PN, Evan Secor W, Karanja DM, Colley DG. Impact of intense, longitudinal retreatment with praziquantel on cure rates of schistosomiasis mansoni in a cohort of occupationally exposed adults in western Kenya. Tropical Medicine and International Health. 2009;14:450-457.

[61] Picquet M, Vercruysse J, Shaw DJ, Diop M, Ly A. Efficacy of praziquantel against *Schistosoma mansoni* in northern Senegal. Transactions of the Royal Society of Tropical Medicine and Hygiene. 1998;92(1):90-93.

[62] Gryseels B, Mbaye A, De Vlas SJ, Stelma FF, Guissé F, Van Lieshout L, Faye D, Diop M, Ly A, Tchuem-Tchuenté LA, Engels D, Polman K. Are poor responses to praziquantel for the treatment of *Schistosoma mansoni* infections in Senegal due to resistance? An overview of the evidence. Tropical Medicine and International Health. 2001;6(11):864-873.

[63] Webster BL, Diaw OT, Seye MM, Faye DS, Stothard JR, Sousa-Figueiredo JC, Rollinson D, 2013. Praziquantel treatment of school children from single and mixed infection foci of intestinal and urogenital schistosomiasis along the Senegal River Basin: monitoring treatment success and re-infection patterns. Acta Tropica. 2013;128(2): 292-302.

[64] Ismail M, Botros S, Metwally A, William S, Farghally A, Tao LF, Day TA, Bennett JL. Resistance to praziquantel: Direct evidence from *Schistosoma mansoni* isolated from Egyptian villagers. American Journal of Tropical Medicine and Hygiene. 1999;60(6): 932-935.

[65] [65]William S, Sabra A, Ramzy F, Mousa M, Demerdash Z, Bennett JL, Day TA, Botros S. Stability and reproductive fitness of *Schistosoma mansoni* isolates with decreased sensitivity to praziquantel. International Journal for Parasitology. 2001;31(10):1093-1100.

[66] Doenhoff MJ, Kusel JR, Coles GC, Cioli D. Resistance of *Schistosoma mansoni* to praziquantel: Is there a problem? Transactions of the Royal Society of Tropical Medicine and Hygiene. 2002;96(5):465-469.

[67] Botros S, Sayed H, Amer N, El-Ghannam M, Bennett JL, Day TA. Current status of sensitivity to praziquantel in a focus of potential drug resistance in Egypt. International Journal for Parasitolology. 2005;35(7):787-791.

[68] Lawn SD1, Lucas SB, Chiodini PL. Case report: *Schistosoma mansoni* infection: failure of standard treatment with praziquantel in a returned traveller. Transactions of the Royal Society of Tropical Medicine and Hygiene. 2003;97(1):100-101.

[69] Wang W, Wang L, Liang YS. Susceptibility or resistance of praziquantel in human schistosomiasis: A review. Parasitological Research. 2012;111(5):1871-1877.

[70] Melman SD, Steinauer ML, Cunningham C, Kubatko LS, Mwangi IN, Wynn NB, Mutuku MW, Karanja DM, Colley DG, Black CL, Secor WE, Mkoji GM, Loker ES. Reduced susceptibility to praziquantel among naturally occurring Kenyan isolates of *Schistosoma mansoni*. PLoS Neglected Tropical Diseases. 2009;3(8):e504.

[71] Mwangi IN, Sanchez MC, Mkoji GM, Agola LE, Runo SM, Cupit PM, Cunningham C. Praziquantel sensitivity of Kenyan *Schistosoma mansoni* isolates and the generation of a laboratory strain with reduced susceptibility to the drug. International Journal for Parasitology: Drugs and Drug Resistance. 2014;4(3):296-300.

[72] Cioli D, Pica-Mattoccia L, Archer S. Drug resistance in schistosomes. Parasitology Today. 1993;9(5):162-166.

[73] Pica-Mattoccia L, Dias LC, Moroni R, Cioli D. *Schistosoma mansoni*: Genetic complementation analysis shows that two independent hycanthone/oxamniquine-resistant strains are mutated in the same gene. Experimental Parasitology. 1993;77(4):445-449.

[74] Valentim CL, Cioli D, Chevalier FD, Cao X, Taylor AB, Holloway SP, Pica-Mattoccia L, Guidi A, Basso A, Tsai IJ, Berriman M, Carvalho-Queiroz C, Almeida M, Aguilar

H, Frantz DE, Hart PJ, LoVerde PT, Anderson TJ. Genetic and molecular basis of drug resistance and species-specific drug action in schistosome parasites. Science. 2013;342(6164):1385-1389.

[75] Fallon PG, Tao LF, Ismail MM, Bennett JL. Schistosome resistance to praziquantel: Fact or artifact? Parasitology Today. 1996;12(8):316-320.

[76] Blanton RE1, Blank WA, Costa JM, Carmo TM, Reis EA, Silva LK, Barbosa LM, Test MR, Reis MG. *Schistosoma mansoni* population structure and persistence after praziquantel treatment in two villages of Bahia, Brazil. International Journal for Parasitology. 2011;41(10):1093-1099.

[77] Valle C, Troiani AR, Festucci A, Pica-Mattoccia L, Liberti P, Wolstenholme A, Francklow K, Doenhoff MJ, Cioli D. Sequence and level of endogenous expression of calcium channel beta subunits in *Schistosoma mansoni* displaying different susceptibilities to praziquantel. Molecular and Biochemical Parasitology. 2003 31;130(2):111-115.

[78] [78]Greenberg RM. New approaches for understanding mechanisms of drug resistance in schistosomes. Parasitology. 2013;140(12):1534-1546.

[79] Kasinathan RS, Sharma LK, Cunningham C, Webb TR, Greenberg RM. Inhibition or knockdown of ABC transporters enhances susceptibility of adult and juvenile schistosomes to Praziquantel. PLoS Neglected Tropical Diseases. 2014;8(10):e3265

[80] Greenberg RM. Schistosome ABC multidrug transporters: From pharmacology to physiology. International Journal for Parasitology: Drugs and Drug Resistance. 2014;4(3):301-309.

[81] Greenberg RM. Ion channels and drug transporters as targets for anthelmintics. Current Clinical Microbiology Reports. 2014;1(3-4):51-60.

[82] William S, Botros S, Ismail M, Farghally A, Day TA, Bennett JL. Praziquantel-induced tegumental damage in vitro is diminished in schistosomes derived from praziquantel-resistant infections. Parasitology. 2001;122(Pt 1):63-66.

[83] El Ridi R, Tallima H. Equilibrium in lung schistosomula sphingomyelin breakdown and biosynthesis allows very small molecules, but not antibody, to access proteins at the host-parasite interface. Journal of Parasitology. 2006;92(4):730-737.

[84] Rich MR. Conformational analysis of arachidonic and related fatty acids using molecular dynamics simulations. Biochimica Biophysica Acta. 1993;1178(1):87-96.

[85] Martinez M. (1992). Tissue levels of polyunsaturated fatty acids during early human development. The Journal of Pediatrics. 1992;120(4):S129-S138.

[86] Carlson SE, Werkman SH, Peeples JM, Wilson WM 3rd. Growth and development of premature infants in relation to omega 3 and omega 6 fatty acid status. World Review of Nutrition and Dietetics 1994;75:63-69.

[87] Brenna JT, Varamini B, Jensen RG, Diersen-Schade DA, Boettcher JA, Arterburn LM. Docosahexaenoic and arachidonic acid concentrations in human breast milk worldwide. The American Journal of Clinical Nutrition. 2007;85(6):1457-1464.

[88] Scholtz SA, Kerling EH, Shaddy DJ, Li S, Thodosoff JM, Colombo J, Carlson SE (2014). Docosahexaenoic acid (DHA) supplementation in pregnancy differentially modulates arachidonic acid and DHA status across FADS genotypes in pregnancy. Prostaglandins, Leukotrienes and Essential Fatty Acids (PLEFA). 2014; pii: S0952-3278(14)00186-0. doi: 10.1016/j.plefa.2014.10.008, in press.

[89] Innis SM. Fatty acids and early human development. Early human development. 2007;83(12):761-766.

[90] U.S. Department of Agriculture, Agricultural Research Service, Beltsville Human Nutrition Research Center, Food Surveys Research Group (Beltsville, MD) and U.S. Department of Health and Human Services, Centers for Disease Control and Prevention, National Center for Health Statistics (Hyattsville, MD). *What We Eat in America, NHANES 2009-2010 Data: Dietary Interview - Total Nutrients Intakes -- First Day (DR1TOT_C).* (2009, September). Available from: http://www.ars.usda.gov/SP2UserFiles/Place/80400530/pdf/0910/Table_1_NIN_GEN_09.pdf [accessed 1/22/15].

[91] Carlson SE, Werkman SH, Peeples JM, Cooke R J, Tolley EA. Arachidonic acid status correlates with first year growth in preterm infants. Proceedings of the National Academy of Sciences USA. 1993;90(3):1073-1077.

[92] Field CJ, Thomson CA, Van Aerde JE, Parrott A, Lien E, Clandinin MT. Lower proportion of CD45R0+ cells and deficient interleukin-10 production by formula-fed infants, compared with human-fed, is corrected with supplementation of long-chain polyunsaturated fatty acids. Journal of Pediatric Gastroenterology and Nutrition. 2000;31(3):291-299.

[93] Birch EE, Garfield S, Hoffman DR, Uauy R, Birch DG. A randomized controlled trial of early dietary supply of long-chain polyunsaturated fatty acids and mental development in term infants. Developmental Medicine and Child Neurology. 2000;42(3): 174-181.

[94] Lapillonne A, Pastor N, Zhuang W, Scalabrin DM. Infants fed formula with added long chain polyunsaturated fatty acids have reduced incidence of respiratory illnesses and diarrhea during the first year of life. BMC Pediatrics. 2014:14(1):168.

[95] Field CJ, Van Aerde JE, Robinson LE, Thomas Clandinin M. Effect of providing a formula supplemented with long-chain polyunsaturated fatty acids on immunity in full-term neonates. British Journal of Nutrition. 2008;99(1):91-99.

[96] Hess HA, Corl BA, Lin X, Jacobi SK, Harrell RJ, Blikslager AT, Odle J. Enrichment of intestinal mucosal phospholipids with arachidonic and eicosapentaenoic acids fed to suckling piglets is dose and time dependent. The Journal of Nutrition. 2008;138(11): 2164-2171.

[97] Thomas JM, Hullin F, Chap H, Douste-Blazy L. Phosphatidylcholine is the major phospholipid providing arachidonic acid for prostacyclin synthesis in thrombin-stimulated human endothelial cells. Thrombosis Research. 1984;34(2):117-123.

[98] Zhou L, Vessby B, Nilsson A. Quantitative role of plasma free fatty acids in the supply of arachidonic acid to extrahepatic tissues in rats. Journal of Nutrition. 2002;132(9):2626-2631.

[99] Brash AR. Arachidonic acid as a bioactive molecule. The Journal of Clinical Investigation. 2001;107(11):1339-1345.

[100] Zhou L, Nilsson A. Sources of eicosanoid precursor fatty acid pools in tissues. Journal of Lipid Research. 2001;42(10):1521-42. Review.

[101] Wang J, Ueda N. Biology of endocannabinoid synthesis system. Prostaglandins and Other Lipid Mediators. 2009;89(3-4):112-129.

[102] Serhan CN, Savill J. Resolution of inflammation: The beginning programs the end. Nature Immunology. 2005;6(12):1191-1197.

[103] Leaf AA, Leighfield MJ, Costeloe KL, Crawford MA. Long chain polyunsaturated fatty acids and fetal growth. Early Human Development. 1992;30(3):183-191.

[104] Kusumoto A, Ishikura Y, Kawashima H, Kiso Y, Takai S, Miyazaki M. Effects of arachidonate-enriched triacylglycerol supplementation on serum fatty acids and platelet aggregation in healthy male subjects with a fish diet. British Journal of Nutrition. 2007;98(3):626-635.

[105] Kohn G, Sawatzki G, van Biervliet JP, Rosseneu M. Diet and the essential fatty acid status of term infants. Acta Paediatrica Supplement. 1994;402:69-74.

[106] Roberts MD, Iosia M, Kerksick CM, Taylor LW, Campbell B, Wilborn CD, Harvey T, Cooke M, Rasmussen C, Greenwood M, Wilson R, Jitomir J, Willoughby D, Kreider RB. Effects of arachidonic acid supplementation on training adaptations in resistance-trained males. Journal of the International Society of Sports Nutrition. 2007;4:21.

[107] Ferrucci L, Cherubini A, Bandinelli S, Bartali B, Corsi A, Lauretani F, Martin A, Andres-Lacueva C, Senin U, Guralnik JM. Relationship of plasma polyunsaturated fatty acids to circulating inflammatory markers. The Journal of Clinical Endocrinology and Metabolism. 2006Feb;91(2):439-446.

[108] Harris WS, Mozaffarian D, Rimm E, Kris-Etherton P, Rudel LL, Appel LJ, Engler MM, Engler MB, Sacks F. Omega-6 fatty acids and risk for cardiovascular disease: a science advisory from the American Heart Association Nutrition Subcommittee of the Council on Nutrition, Physical Activity, and Metabolism; Council on Cardiovascular Nursing; and Council on Epidemiology and Prevention. Circulation. 2009;119(6):902-907.

[109] Seyberth HW, Oelz O, Kennedy T, Sweetman BJ, Danon A, Frölich JC, Heimberg M, Oates JA. Increased arachidonate in lipids after administration to man: effects on

prostaglandin biosynthesis. Clinical Pharmacology and Therapeutics. 1975;18(5 Pt 1): 521-529.

[110] Tallima H, Salah M, El-Ridi R. In vitro and in vivo effects of unsaturated fatty acids on *Schistosoma mansoni* and *S. haematobium* lung-stage larvae. Journal of Parasitology. 2005;91(5):1094-1102.

[111] El Ridi R, Aboueldahab M, Tallima H, Salah M, Mahana N, Fawzi S, Mohamed SH, Fahmy OM. In vitro and in vivo activities of arachidonic acid against *Schistosoma mansoni* and *Schistosoma haematobium*. Antimicrobial Agents and Chemotherapy. 2010;54(8):3383-3389.

[112] El Ridi R, Tallima H, Salah M, Aboueldahab M, Fahmy OM, Al-Halbosiy MF, Mahmoud SS. Efficacy and mechanism of action of arachidonic acid in the treatment of hamsters infected with *Schistosoma mansoni* or *Schistosoma haematobium*. International Journal of Antimicrobial Agents. 2012;39(3):232-239.

[113] Migliardo F, Tallima H, El Ridi R. Is there a sphingomyelin-based hydrogen bond barrier at the mammalian host-schistosome parasite interface? Cell Biochemistry and Biophysics. 2014;68(2):359-367.

[114] Migliardo F, Tallima H, El Ridi R. Rigidity and resistance of larval- and adult schistosomes-medium interface. Biochemical and Biophysical Research Communications. 2014;446(1):255-260.

[115] Berriman M, Haas BJ, LoVerde PT, Wilson RA, Dillon GP, Cerqueira GC, Mashiyama ST, Al-Lazikani B, Andrade LF, Ashton PD, Aslett MA, Bartholomeu DC, Blandin G, Caffrey CR, Coghlan A, Coulson R, Day TA, Delcher A, DeMarco R, Djikeng A, Eyre T, Gamble JA, Ghedin E, Gu Y, Hertz-Fowler C, Hirai H, Hirai Y, Houston R, Ivens A, Johnston DA, Lacerda D, Macedo CD, McVeigh P, Ning Z, Oliveira G, Overington JP, Parkhill J, Pertea M, Pierce RJ, Protasio AV, Quail MA, Rajandream MA, Rogers J, Sajid M, Salzberg SL, Stanke M, Tivey AR, White O, Williams DL, Wortman J, Wu W, Zamanian M, Zerlotini A, Fraser-Liggett CM, Barrell BG, El-Sayed NM. The genome of the blood fluke *Schistosoma mansoni*. Nature. 2009;460(7253):352-358.

[116] Protasio AV, Tsai IJ, Babbage A, Nichol S, Hunt M, Aslett MA, De Silva N, Velarde GS, Anderson TJ, Clark RC, Davidson C, Dillon GP, Holroyd NE, LoVerde PT, Lloyd C, McQuillan J, Oliveira G, Otto TD, Parker-Manuel SJ, Quail MA, Wilson RA, Zerlotini A, Dunne DW, Berriman M. A systematically improved high quality genome and transcriptome of the human blood fluke *Schistosoma mansoni*. PLoS Neglected Tropical Diseases. 2012;6(1):e1455.

[117] Tallima H, Al-Halbosiy MF, El Ridi R. Enzymatic activity and immunolocalization of *Schistosoma mansoni* and *Schistosoma haematobium* neutral sphingomyelinase. Molecular and Biochemical Parasitology. 2011;178(1-2):23-28.

[118] Young ND, Jex AR, Li B, Liu S, Yang L, Xiong Z, Li Y, Cantacessi C, Hall RS, Xu X, Chen F, Wu X, Zerlotini A, Oliveira G, Hofmann A, Zhang G, Fang X, Kang Y,

Campbell BE, Loukas A, Ranganathan S, Rollinson D, Rinaldi G, Brindley PJ, Yang H, Wang J, Wang J, Gasser RB. Whole-genome sequence of *Schistosoma haematobium*. Nature Genetics. 2012;44(2):221-225.

[119] Pugh RN, Teesdale CH. Synergy of concurrent low dose oxamniquine and praziquantel in schistosomiasis. British Medical Journal (Clinical Research Ed). 1983;287(6396): 877-878.

[120] Creasey AM, Taylor P, Thomas JE. Dosage trial of a combination of oxamniquine and praziquantel in the treatment of schistosomiasis in Zimbabwean schoolchildren. Central African Journal of Medicine. 1986;32(7):165-167.

[121] Utzinger J, Keiser J, Shuhua X, Tanner M, Singer BH. Combination chemotherapy of schistosomiasis in laboratory studies and clinical trials. Antimicrobial Agents and Chemotherapy. 2003;47(5):1487-1495.

[122] Borrmann S, Szlezák N, Faucher JF, Matsiegui PB, Neubauer R, Binder RK, Lell B, Kremsner PG. Artesunate and praziquantel for the treatment of *Schistosoma haematobium* infections: A double-blind, randomized, placebo-controlled study. Journal of Infectious Diseases. 2001;184(10):1363-1366.

[123] Liu R, Dong HF, Guo Y, Zhao QP, Jiang MS. Efficacy of praziquantel and artemisinin derivatives for the treatment and prevention of human schistosomiasis: A systematic review and meta-analysis. Parasites and Vectors. 2011;4:201.

[124] De Clercq D, Vercruysse J, Verlé P, Kongs A, Diop M. What is the effect of combining artesunate and praziquantel in the treatment of *Schistosoma mansoni* infections? Tropical Medicine and International Health. 2000;5(10):744-746.

[125] Ashley EA, Dhorda M, Fairhurst RM, Amaratunga C, Lim P, Suon S, et al. Spread of artemisinin resistance in *Plasmodium falciparum* malaria. New England Journal of Medicine. 2014;371(5):411-423.

[126] Wang W, Li TY, Ji Y, Qu GL, Qian YL, Li HJ, Dai JR, Liang YS. Efficacy of artemether and artesunate in mice infected with praziquantel non-susceptible isolate of Schistosoma japonicum. Parasitology Research. 2014;113(3):925-931.

# Chapter 9

# The Role of Chiggers as Human Pathogens

Paula Santibáñez, Ana M. Palomar, Aránzazu Portillo, Sonia Santibáñez and José A. Oteo

Additional information is available at the end of the chapter

http://dx.doi.org/10.5772/61978

**Abstract**

Trombiculid mites (Acari: Trombiculidae) are distributed worldwide ectoparasites of a wide range of vertebrates. More than 50 species are known to bite humans, and about 20 have medical importance. The larval stages (chiggers) of the genus *Leptotrombidium* are vectors of *Orientia tsutsugamushi*, causative agent of scrub typhus. This life-threatening disease is widely endemic in Asian Pacific regions where more than one billion people are at risk of acquiring the infection and around one million new cases are estimated to occur annually. In addition, although underreported and often misdiagnosed, trombiculiasis, defined as a dermatitis caused by the salivary secretion of biting chiggers, is present in America and Europe.

**Keywords:** Chiggers, Orientia tsutsugamushi, dermatitis, vectors

## 1. Introduction

This chapter includes a thorough description of the main characteristics, life cycle, and distribution of chiggers. Moreover, a comprehensive review of the responsibility of chiggers as infectious disease vectors and agents of troublesome dermatitis is given. The following pages cover, for the first time in a unique chapter, the current knowledge of chigger mites.

### 1.1. Taxonomy and distribution

Trombiculid mites (Acari: Trombiculidae) are widespread ectoparasites of a wide range of vertebrates. More than 50 species have been recorded attacking humans, and about 20 of them are considered to be medically important because they cause dermatitis or due to their role as vectors of human pathogens. The most relevant species are *Eutrombicula alfreddugesi* in North and South America, *Neotrombicula autumnalis* in Europe, and *Leptotrombidium* spp. in Asia [1].

Trombiculidae is one of the largest families in the Acari group, including more than 3,000 species [2]. Table 1 shows the taxonomic position of these mites.

| | |
|---|---|
| Phylum | Arthropoda |
| Subphylum | Chelicerata |
| Class | Arachnida |
| Subclass | Acari |
| Superorder | Acariformes |
| Order | Trombidiformes |
| Suborder | Prostigmata |
| Superfamily | Trombiculoidea |
| Family | Trombiculidae |

**Table 1.** Taxonomic classification of the family Trombiculidae.

Trombiculids are distributed worldwide, but they show their greatest diversity in the subtropical, tropical and southern temperate zones [3]. Table 2 shows the main trombiculid species and their geographical distribution.

| Species | Distribution | Disease |
|---|---|---|
| *Blankaartia acuscutellaris* | Hungary, Spain, Moldova, Ukraine, Russia, Sumatra, Malaysia, and Africa | Trombiculiasis |
| *Eushoengastia koreaensis* | Korea | Scrub typhus[a] |
| *Euschoengastia xerothermobia* | Europe | Trombiculiasis |
| *Eutrombicula alfreddugesi* | Canada, South of United States (except for the southwest), South and Central America (including West Indies) | Trombiculiasis |
| *Eutrombicula batatas* | Bolivia, Mexico, Central and South America, southwestern and southeastern United States | Trombiculiasis |
| *Eutrombicula lipovskyi* | United States: from Alabama and Tennessee West to Arkansas, Oklahoma and Kansas | Trombiculiasis |
| *Eutrombicula sarcina* | Southeast Asia, Australia and the Pacific Islands | Trombiculiasis |
| *Eutrombicula splendens* | Eastern United States (from the Gulf Coast North to Massachusetts, Minnesota) and Ontario | Trombiculiasis |

| Species | Distribution | Disease |
|---|---|---|
| *Eutrombicula wichmanni* | Japan, Southeast Asia, Australia, and Pacific Islands | Trombiculiasis |
| *Kepkatrombicula desaleri* | Italia, Austria, and Bulgaria | Trombiculiasis |
| *Leptotrombidium akamushi* | Japan, China, Southeast Asia, Indonesia, Philippines, and New Guinea | Scrub typhus |
| *Leptotrombidium arenicola* | Malaysia, Indonesia, and Thailand | Scrub typhus |
| *Leptotrombidium chiangraiensis* | Thailand | Scrub typhus |
| *Leptotrombidium deliense* | China, Taiwan, Sri Lanka, Nepal, Bangladesh, India, Myanmar, Vietnam, Cambodia, Thailand, Singapore, Brunei, Malaysia, Indonesia, Philippines, New Guinea, southwestern Pacific Islands, northern Australia, Pakistan, Kazakhstan, Uzbekistan, and Afghanistan | Scrub typhus |
| *Leptotrombidium fletcheri* | Southeast Asia, Malaysia, New Guinea, Philippines, Indonesia, and Melanesia | Scrub typhus |
| *Leptotrombidium fuji* | Japan | Scrub typhus[a] |
| *Leptotrombidium gaohuensis* | China | Scrub typhus |
| *Leptotrombidium imphalum* | Thailand | Scrub typhus |
| *Leptotrombidium intermedium* | Japan | Scrub typhus[a] |
| *Leptotrombidium kitasatoi* | Japan | Scrub typhus[a] |
| *Leptotrombidium orientale* | Japan, Korea, and Primorye region of Russia | Scrub typhus[a] |
| *Leptotrombidium pallidum* | Japan, Korea, and Primorye region of Russia | Scrub typhus |
| *Leptotrombidium palpale* | Japan, Korea, and Primorye region of Russia | Scrub typhus[a] |
| *Leptotrombidium pavlovsky* | Siberia and Primorye region of Russia | Scrub typhus |
| *Leptotrombidium scutellare* | Japan, northern China, Korea, Thailand, and Malaysia | Scrub typhus<br>Hantavirus[a] |
| *Leptotrombidium subquadratum* | South Africa | Trombiculiasis |
| *Neotrombicula autumnalis* | Europe (including British Isles, excluding Norway, Sweden, Finland, and northern Russia), Turkey, and Turkmenistan | Trombiculiasis |

| Species | Distribution | Disease |
|---|---|---|
| *Neotrombicula inopinata* | Spain, Czech Republic, England, Austria, Germany, Bulgaria, France, states of former Yugoslavia, Ukraine, Russia, Romania, Hungary, Slovakia, and Poland | Trombiculiasis |
| *Neotrombicula japonica* | Korea, Europe | Scrub typhus[a] Trombiculiasis |
| *Neotrombicula nagayoi* | Japan, China, and Russia | Trombiculiasis |
| *Neotrombicula zachvatkini* | Europe | Trombiculiasis |
| *Odontacarus* spp. | Southeast Asia, Australia, and the Pacific Islands | Trombiculiasis |
| *Shoengastia hanmyaensis* | Japan | Scrub typhus[a] |
| *Schoengastia* spp. | Southeast Asia, Australia, and the Pacific Islands | Trombiculiasis |
| *Trombicula toldti* | Austria | Trombiculiasis |

[a]Not confirmed.

**Table 2.** Distribution and diseases transmitted by the main trombiculid mite species [1,4–15].

Members of this family are known by several names depending on their distribution (Table 3). They are often confused with other mites or insects and are mistakenly named as Mower's mites [common name of *Leptus autumnalis* (Acari: Erythraeidae)] [16,17] or jigger, chigoe, and niguas [common names of *Tunga penetrans* (Insecta: Siphonaptera)] [18,19].

| Common names | Places |
|---|---|
| Harvest bug, harvest mite, harvest lice, red bug, red mite, berry mite, scrub-itch mite | North-America, Asia |
| Harvest mite | Europe |
| Aoutats, rouget, bête rouge | France |
| Orange tawny | Ireland |
| Augustelingen | Germany |
| Bicho colorado, coloradilla, ácaro rojo | South America |
| Isango | Peru |
| Tlazahuate | Mexico |
| Coloradita, chivacoa | Venezuela |

**Table 3.** Common names given to trombiculid mites worldwide. [2,4,10,16,17,20–22]

### 1.2. Life cycle

Trombiculid mites undergo seven stages in their life cycle: egg, deutovum, larva, protonymph, deutonymph, tritonymph, and adult (Figure 1). This cycle is characterized by alternating active and inactive instars, being the larva, deutonymph, and adult the active ones. Active postlarval stages are soil dwellers that prey on various arthropods and their eggs. Deutonymphs look almost identical to adult mites. Both present eight legs, but deutonymphs are slightly smaller. Sexual dimorphism is not apparently evident [23]. Larvae parasitize all groups of vertebrates, except fishes, whereas the small mammals and birds are the main hosts [1,5,19,24]. There are just a few reports of chiggers feeding on invertebrates [3]. Humans are only accidental hosts. However, the question of the host specificity of trombiculids still arises. Most likely, trombiculids are associated with specific habitats and attack and feed on the first available animal within their favorite habitat, although they can have preference for a particular host among the available ones [23,25].

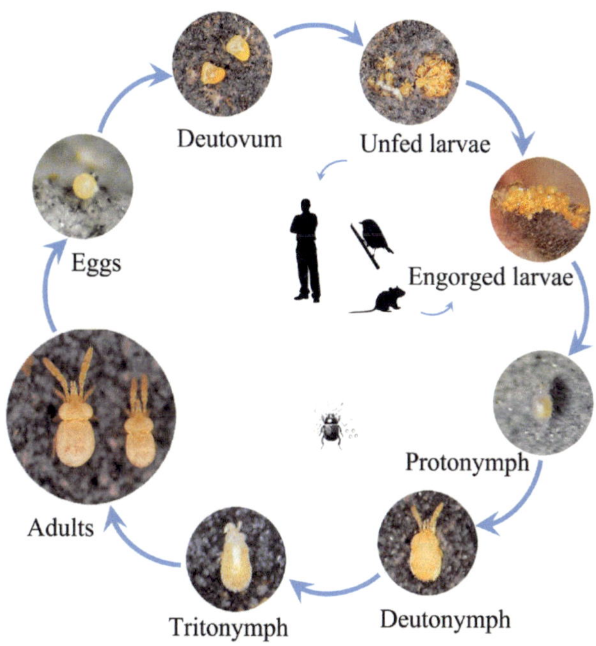


**Figure 1.** Schematic description of the trombiculids' life cycle. (Adapted from Takahashi *et al.*, 2003 with the permission of the author.)

During their life cycle, eggs are laid in well-drained soil, and six-legged larvae emerge from them. The general term "chigger" refers to the parasitic larval stage, and this is the name commonly given to trombiculid mites due to the importance of this instar. Chiggers are usually reddish but can vary between yellow and orange [1,26]. These tiny larvae (about 200 μm) climb onto low vegetation, where they aggregate into clusters to wait for a suitable host. On the host, chiggers mainly move to areas where the skin is especially thin and feed on lymph and tissue fluids of the dermal layer (but not blood). Ears, head, armpits, abdomen, genitalia, and the area around the tail are preferred in animals [4,27]. In humans, bites occur mainly in body exposed areas and at sites where the clothing constricts [17,28]. Once engorged (development to subsequent stage cannot take place unless larvae have fed on the host), larvae fall to the ground and develop to the nymphal stages and subsequently to adults (900–1,200 μm).

Trombiculid mites live in moist soil covered with vegetation such as grassy and weedy areas. In general, optimal living conditions require a relative air humidity of 80% (what explains that chiggers are not typically found on vegetation higher than 30 cm off the ground) and neutral to slightly alkaline soil. The optimum activity of chiggers occurs at temperatures of 25–30°C [26,29].

Trombiculid mites often form localized "mite islands" (or "mite focus", "larvae focus") in suitable areas inhabited by potential hosts [30]. Therefore, chiggers have a patchy distribution on the vegetation. Mite islands are quite clearly defined, and larvae could not be detected in their immediate vicinity [26,31]. A possible explanation for this focalization may be that chiggers apparently do not move more than a few meters from where they hatched. Chiggers would temporarily disperse if a host approached. On the contrary, if physical contact were not managed or if the host were not close enough for them to drop on it, chiggers would invariably and promptly return to the cluster and would continue waiting [32].

The life cycle of trombiculid mites has been mainly studied in the laboratory. The most outstanding feature of the life cycle is the constant duration of quiescent periods and the variable duration of active stages. Trombiculid mites usually have one generation per year, but with overlapping generations, each well synchronized with the seasons because they can overwinter in most stages (egg, larva, deutonynph, and adult) and because the adult mites have a long life span [33]. In boreal species, an egg-to-egg cycle ranges from 150 to 400 days, but it is shorter in tropical species [23]. In nature, the life cycle is supposed to be completed in 2–12 months or longer, depending on the species and environmental conditions. In temperate areas, there may be 1 to 3 generations per year, whereas in tropical regions the life cycle is shorter and continuous throughout the year [1]. In Europe, the duration has been estimated in five to seven months under favorable conditions [26].

As mentioned above, trombiculid mites only act as parasites during their larval stage. Thus, the greatest attention has been paid to chiggers. In addition, adults and deutonymphs of the majority of trombiculid species have never been observed on the soil surface (in fact, their habitats are mostly unknown). Therefore, the taxonomy of trombiculid mites is based solely on their larvae [34]. It is estimated that only the postlarval stage of less than 10% of the total of Trombiculidae species are known [7]. This is the case of some tropical species in contrast to the difficulty of finding active postlarval instars in northern countries [23].

### 1.3. Feeding process

It is well known that when feeding on hosts, chiggers develop a characteristic feeding tube (stylostome) in the host's skin. The stylostome is mostly formed of the larval salivary secretions solidifying in the host's epidermis [7]. Larva cuts the stratum corneum with its rather short chelicerae and stylostome allows chigger to reach the underlying connective tissue layer from which it obtains nutrients. The host's tissues around the stylostome are destroyed and necrotized. Beneath the distal end of the stylostome, an interstitial food cavity containing lymphoid and epithelioid cellular liquid elements is formed [23]. The feeding period in animal host, both in nature and reared in the laboratory, usually lasts 3–6 days [26,35]. However, feeding on humans may typically vary from 3 - 8 h to 1–2 days for most non-infectious chiggers, but 2–10 days for scrub typhus vectors [1,29,36,37]. It is supposed that more than 6 h are required for the transmission of the bacterium [14]. During this period, the larva remains on the skin surface. For this reason, most trombiculid larvae can be classified as ectoparasites. Larvae of some genera, however, can partly or even entirely embed within the skin of different body cavities frequently forming various types of capsules during feeding on amphibians and mammals [23]. In such cases, the feeding time is prolonged up to several weeks or even months. In lizards, specific adaptive structures of skin, known as "mite pockets", may evolve to decrease the possible damage from mite feeding [38]. It is generally thought that the organization and location of stylostome is species specific in trombiculid larvae, irrespectively of the host species and of the particular feeding site on the host, whereas the length of the stylostome is mostly a result of the width of the epidermal layer and the presence or absence of scabs at the attachment site [39].

## 2. Chiggers as vectors of infectious diseases

Although different microorganisms have been detected in different species of chiggers, their role as vectors of infectious diseases has been only demonstrated for scrub typhus.

### 2.1. Scrub typhus

Scrub typhus or tsutsugamushi disease [from Japanese words meaning disease (*tsutsuga*) mite (*mushi*) is a life-threatening arthropod-borne bacterial infection that presents as an acute undifferentiated febrile illness widely endemic in Asian Pacific regions. The disease is transmitted to humans by chiggers of *Leptotrombidium* spp. and is caused by the bacterium *Orientia tsutsugamushi*. Noteworthy are the reported cases that suggest other *Orientia* species as etiological agents of scrub typhus-like disease.

The disease was widely reported in soldiers during World War II [40] and now is an important illness for travelers to the endemic regions [41]. More than half (55%) of the world population lives in areas where scrub typhus is endemic, so over one billion people are at risk of acquiring the infection [42]. Approximately one million new cases have been estimated to occur annually [43]. However, this is surely an underestimation because recognition of the disease is difficult due to its overlapping clinical spectrum with other common causes of fever in this population, the lack of awareness among affected people, and the limitations of current diagnostic methods [44].

### *2.1.1. Etiology and epidemiology*

The etiological agent of scrub typhus, *O. tsutsugamushi* (previously known as *Rickettsia orientalis* or *Rickettsia tsutsugamushi*), is an $\alpha$-proteobacteria that was reclassified as a new genus separate from *Rickettsia* based on phenotypic and genotypic differences [45]. *Orientia* differs from *Rickettsia* in the structure of the cell wall, antigenic profile, and genome size, which is almost twice the size of the *Rickettsia* genome.

There are three prototype strains: Gilliam, Karp, and Kato; however, more than 20 antigenically distinct serotypes are present in endemic areas [46], and currently over 70 strains of *O. tsutsugamushi* are known [47]. As chigger mites are habitat specific, *O. tsutsugamushi* strains could have evolved mostly in separate biotopes, resulting in different serotypes depending on their location [48]. The general course and the prognosis of the disease is determined by the strain of *O. tsutsugamushi* implicated [49], although multiple factors such as the patient's age, genetic factors, and previous immunity are also involved [50]. It is very likely that chiggers, as it is assumed for ticks [51], have potential immunomodulatory effects in their saliva that could affect the pathogenesis, immunity, and outcome of the disease [47].

Chiggers act as reservoir and vector of *O. tsutsugamushi*, being wild rodents the main hosts. Infected mites maintain the infection through the trombiculids' life cycle by transstadial and transovarial transmission [52]. Reverse transfer from infected animals to chiggers occurs infrequently, and the bacteria transmitted in this manner are not usually passed on to the next generation [53]. Chiggers cofeeding on rodents seems to be more relevant for effective mouse-to-mite transmission of *Orientia* than feeding on rickettsemic hosts [54]. Nevertheless, the disease can only be transmitted to humans by chiggers already transovarially infected by *O. tsutsugamushi* [49].

Endemic regions are characterized by rice fields, scrubland, and the presence of primary deforestation [55,56]. Chiggers harboring the bacterium bite exposed individuals in vulnerable niches such as forests and infested undergrowth during occupational or recreational activities. *Leptotrombidium* chiggers feed on lymph and tissue fluids of the dermal layer for a period of 2–4 days [57]. Following the bite, the pathogen multiplies at the site of inoculation and subsequently induces local (eschar) and systemic manifestations of infection [58].

Several studies suggest the evidence of human infection with more than one strain of *O. tsutsugamushi* [59]. It could be explained by bites from different chiggers, each one infected with one strain or, alternatively, by the bite of individual chiggers infected with multiple strains [60].

Seasonal occurrence of scrub typhus is determined by the time of appearance of chiggers because humans are infected through bites of the larva. In temperate zones, scrub typhus season is observed mainly in the autumn but also in the spring [61]. More than 45 species of trombiculid mites are known to be infected with *O. tsutsugamushi* in nature, but only *Leptotrombidium pallidum, Leptotrombidium akamushi, Leptotrombidium scutellare, Leptotrombidium deliense, Leptotrombidium arenicola, Leptotrombidium imphalum, Leptotrombidium chiangraiensis, Leptotrombidium fletcheri, Leptotrombidium gaohuensis*, and *Leptotrombidium pavlovsky* are proven to transmit scrub typhus [1,13,14]. Principal vector species differ according to endemic areas

(Table 2): *L. akamushi, L. pallidum*, and *L. scutellare* mediate scrub typhus in temperate zones, such as Japan and Korea, whereas *L. deliense* and *L. arenicola* are the principal vectors in tropical and subtropical regions or Southeast Asia and the Southwest Pacific [49] (Figure 2).

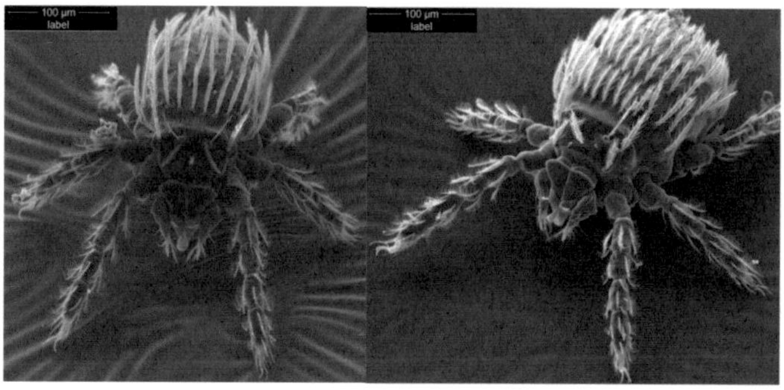

**Figure 2.** *Leptotrombidium intermedium* (left) and *Leptotrombidium pallidum* (right). Provided by Dr. Shatrov.

Scrub typhus is confined to a 13,000,000-km$^2$ definite geographic region, the "tsutsugamushi triangle," where it is widely distributed (Figure 3). It extends from northern Japan, Korea, and far-eastern Russia in the North, to northern Australia in the South and to Pakistan and Afghanistan in the West, as well as the islands of the western Pacific and Indian Oceans, including Taiwan, Philippines, New Guinea, Indonesia, and Sri Lanka [62].

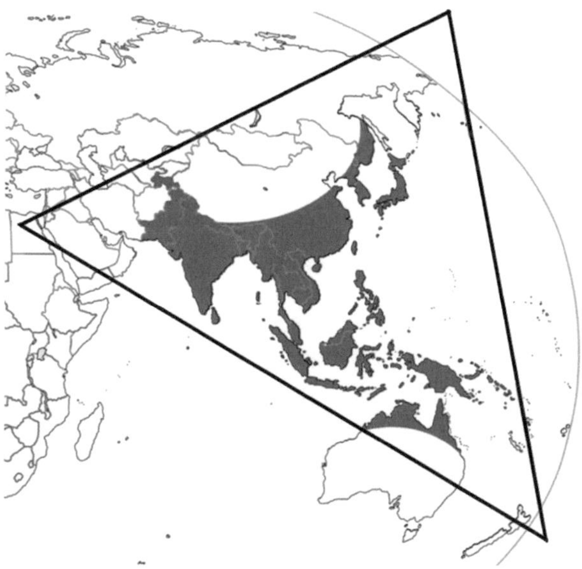

**Figure 3.** Tsutsugamushi triangle.

Several reports of scrub cases typhus-like infections have been described in unusual areas, indicating that a wider geographic distribution should be taken into account [47]. Thus, the recent isolation of *Orientia chuto* in a febrile patient who acquired the infection in the United Arab Emirates, the detection of another divergent *Orientia* sp. in a patient in Chile, and the serologic diagnoses of scrub typhus acquired in Africa reveal that the geographical range accepted until now may be an underrepresentation [63,64]. To date, the genetic diversity of the genus *Orientia* is being reviewed because until recently *O. tsutsugamushi* has been considered the sole species of the genus. Apart from *Leptotrombidium* spp., other trombiculid mites such as *Neotrombicula japonica* and *Eushoengastia koreaensis* have also been implicated as possible vectors of this disease [15,65].

The disease is considered rural, and the risk of infection is closely related to occupation. In areas where scrub typhus is prevalent, most cases are acquired through agricultural exposure. Most travel acquired cases of scrub typhus are associated with outdoor activities such as camping, rafting, or trekking in endemic areas [50]. Outbreaks related to military operations have been reported [66]. The impact of scrub typhus in pregnancy is less explored. Acute scrub typhus can be transmitted vertically but congenital malformation due to infection *per se* has not been demonstrated [67].

### 2.1.2. Clinical features and pathogenesis

Scrub typhus ranges in severity from mild and self-limiting to fatal depending on the duration of the illness, the strain of *O. tsutsugamushi*, the immune status, and other factors of the patients [14]. After an incubation period of 10–12 days (can vary between 5 and 20 days), the onset of the disease is characterized by an eschar and regional lymphadenopathy followed subsequently by fever, general malaise, headache, and myalgia. The disease is characterized by focal or disseminated vasculitis and perivasculitis, which may involve the lungs, heart, liver, spleen, and central nervous system [68]. Progression of scrub typhus is accompanied by generalized lymphadenopathy, rash, cough, and interstitial pneumonia, acute respiratory distress syndrome, gastrointestinal symptoms, meningoencephalomyelitis, myocarditis, acute renal failure, hypotensive shock, and disseminated intravascular coagulation may occur in severe cases [14,47,69].

The fever appears abruptly frequently accompanied by headache, myalgia, and malaise, with peaks on the 3rd–4th day of the disease and persists for more than 3 weeks in untreated cases. About a week after the onset of the symptoms, the eschar, which is not always present, is developed. It represents localized cutaneous necrosis at the site of mite feeding and is a typical scrub typhus marker, which is considered almost diagnostic [67]. It starts as a small papule that enlarges and subsequently undergoes central necrosis, and it eventually acquires a blackened crust with an erythematous halo that resembles a cigarette burn (Figure 4).

The common sites for finding an eschar are trunk, arms, and legs, but it also appears on the scalp, axilla, genitalia, waist, and other exposed parts of the body [14,49]. The prevalence of eschars in patients diagnosed by scrub typhus ranges from 7% to 97% [67,70]. These differences may be may be due to the difficulty in detecting small eschars in dark-skinned individuals and atypical appearance of eschars in areas of damp and moist skin. Multiple eschars have been

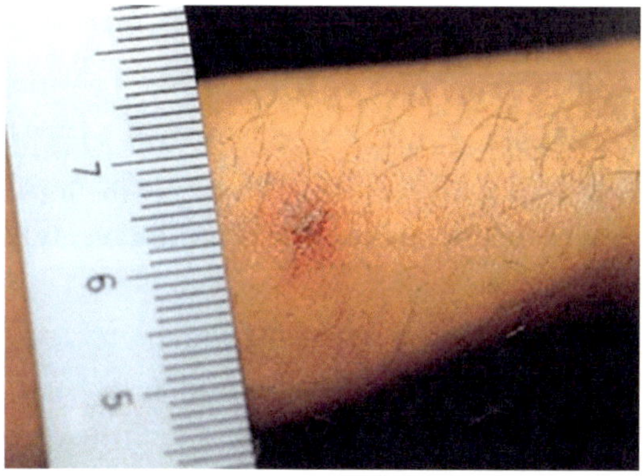

**Figure 4.** Eschar and erythema on the fifth day of illness in the left arm of a patient of a 36-year-old patient (photo provided by Dr. Takahashi).

reported in 0.6% to 2.2% of patients with confirmed scrub typhus [70]. Uncommonly, a maculopapular rash with centrifugal distribution may appear a week after the onset of these symptoms, starting on the chest, abdomen, or whole trunk and spreading to the limbs. Rash lasts a few days to a week [13,71]. Regional lymphadenopathy, characterized by tenderness and enlargement of the draining lymph node around the primary eschar, arises at the end of the first week after the disease onset [13]. Generalized lymphadenopathy appears 2–3 days later in some cases [72].

From the second week onwards, a proportion of patients (especially those untreated) will evidence of severe systemic infection. The extended vasculitis helps to explain the great diversity of clinical manifestations that have been described [49]. Respiratory symptoms, including interstitial pneumonia, acute respiratory distress, and pulmonary edema, are frequent. In fact, about 40% of scrub typhus patients complain of cough at the time of admission. Gastrointestinal symptoms comprise nausea, vomiting, abdominal pain, diarrhea, or gastrointestinal bleeding. Alterations in liver function and pancreatitis are also common. The central nervous system (CNS) is frequently affected. Indeed, *O. tsutsugamushi* is detected in the cerebrospinal fluid of 24% of the patients with no clinical signs of CNS involvement. Transient hearing loss, eye manifestations, confusion, neck stiffness, delirium, and mental changes occur frequently. Patients usually suffered from acute diffuse encephalomyelitis, encephalopathy, meningitis, or meningoencephalitis. Regarding the cardiovascular system, myocarditis, vasculitis, pericarditis, and rhythm abnormalities are often seen, but congestive heart failure is rare. Acute renal failure develops frequently in severe cases but may also occur in mild cases [13,14,61,62,67,69]. The case fatality rate in untreated patients is estimated in appropriately 10%, ranging from 0% to 30% [67].

At the beginning of the infection, *O. tsutsugamushi* mainly infects dendritic cells in the eschar [58]. The systemic dissemination of *O. tsutsugamushi* is suggested to be lymphogenous to the regional lymph nodes, followed by spread to target organs via the blood. This pathway was suggested based on the early development of lymphadenopathy in the regional drainage of the eschar as well as on animal experiments and clinical observations [14,47]. Once *O. tsutsu-*

*gamushi* infection progresses, the main target cells are vascular endothelial cells and macrophages of the reticuloendothelial system, although cardiac myocytes can also been infected [14]. The endothelial cells seem to have a central role in the systemic inflammation because *in vitro*-infected human dermal microvascular endothelial cells are activated to express interleukin (IL)-8 and monocyte chemoattractant protein just after the infection. Moreover, soluble endothelial cell-specific adhesion molecules (sE-selectin) are highly concentrated in serum at the early stage of the disease.

The basic histopathologic findings reveal multiplication of *O. tsutsugamushi* in the endothelial cells lining the small blood vessels, perivasculitis and focal interstitial mononuclear cell infiltrations, and edema. Perivasculitis may involve the lung, heart, brain, kidneys, gastrointestinal tract, liver, spleen, and lymph node [73].

### *2.1.3. Diagnosis and treatment*

Due to the severity of *Orientia* infection, treatment has to be started as soon as possible, even before having a conclusive microbiological diagnosis.

As in other infectious diseases, the gold standard of the diagnosis of scrub typhus is the isolation of the etiological agent by culture. Isolation of *O. tsutsugamushi* can be done in cell culture or in inoculated mice. Yolk sacs of 5- to 7-day-olds have been widely used in the past, but it was replaced by cell culture systems [74]. Currently, culture in HeLa, Vero, BHK, L929, ECV304, and HMEC-1 cell lines is the reference method for isolating *O. tsutsugamushi* from clinical samples [45,49,75,76]. These techniques are restricted to biosafety level 3 facilities and personnel with extensive experience. A positive result is given in an average time of 28 days, being inappropriate for the routine diagnosis of the disease. The shell-vial culture technique makes the detection of the microorganism possible in 48–72 h, allowing an early diagnosis before seroconversion [74,77]. *O. tsutsugamushi* can also be isolated by inoculating patient blood into mice, but results are not available in time to guide clinical management [78]. Mouse inoculation remains helpful when isolation of the organism from postmortem tissues is required [74].

The mainstay in scrub typhus diagnostics remains serology [79,80]. Nevertheless, despite their widespread use, all currently available serologic tests have limitations. The Weil–Felix OX-K agglutination reaction was the earliest serological tests used for clinical diagnosis of scrub typhus. It is inexpensive, easy to perform, and results are available overnight; however, it lacks specificity and sensitivity [46]. To date, the gold standard assay for the serologic detection of scrub typhus antibodies is the indirect immunofluorescence assay (IFA) [79]. Most frequently, IFA uses antigen from serotypes Karp, Kato, and Gilliam [46]. IFA is sensitive, and results are available in a couple of hours. Although it is accepted that a ≥4-fold increase in antibody titer between two consecutive samples (acute and convalescent-phase) is diagnostic, this is a retrospective diagnosis and cannot guide initial treatment [79]. Anyway, IFA is expensive and requires a level of technical expertise and equipment that may not be available in rural areas. Indirect immunoperoxidase is an alternative that eliminates the expense of a fluorescent microscope by substituting peroxidase for fluorescein [80].

The development of PCR amplification-based approaches have been incorporated to the diagnoses of infectious diseases even in nonreference laboratories. PCR has potential benefits in detecting *Orientia*-DNA before antibody response occurs. However, the high resource costs and training required for this technique make them impractical in many areas where scrub typhus is endemic. Moreover, the most appropriate specimen to use remains unclear. The PCR of eschar material yields more sensitive results than blood and remains positive even after the initiation of treatment. However, eschar-based PCR would diagnose a small amount of the cases in a scenario with a prevalence of eschars as few as 7%. Buffy coat could improve sensitivity compared with whole blood, but the use of blood-based assays is limited to the time window of rickettsemia [81,82]. Moreover, low copy numbers is an important handicap of DNA-based approaches. The optimal PCR target for diagnosing scrub typhus stays also uncertain. A target gene enabling specific but sensitive detection as well as sufficiently broad coverage of genotypes of *O. tsutsugamushi* is needed. A nested-PCR assay targeting the 56-kDa gene is highly specific, but sequence variability of this gene may affect primer annealing and, therefore, test sensitivity [83]. 16S rDNA-based *Orientia*-specific PCR may show a broader detection spectrum than an assay based on a more variable species-specific target, such as the 56-kDa gene [47]. Real-time PCR assays targeting the 47-kDa outer membrane protein and the *groEL* genes of *O. tsutsugamushi* are also very sensitive tools for the diagnosis of scrub typhus [78,84]. Recently, loop-mediated isothermal PCR assay (LAMP) targeting the *groEL* gene has shown diagnostic accuracy similar to real-time and nested conventional PCR assays [84]. This assay is simple and less expensive and can be considered a valid molecular method for the early diagnosis of scrub typhus.

The diagnosis and subsequently the antibiotic treatment are often missed or made late due to the lack of effective commercially available diagnostic tests and the lack of specificity of the early clinical presentation. It is important to remark that treatment must begin whenever scrub typhus is clinically suspected, without waiting for microbiological confirmation. It is well known that delayed treatment leads to complications such as adult respiratory distress syndrome, disseminated intravascular coagulation, acute renal failure, meningitis, meningoencephalitis, and gastrointestinal tract bleeding [57]. Bacterial proliferation and the time of antibiotic treatment are very important predictors of lethality.

The clinical discrimination of scrub typhus from other undifferentiated fevers is often very difficult because the clinical symptoms are similar. In patients presenting an eschar and/or rash, and generalized or regional lymphadenopathy in a endemic area, scrub typhus should be considered in the differential diagnosis along with rickettsialpox, Mediterranean spotted fever, dengue, leptospirosis, and murine typhus [55,71].

Mortality in the pre-antibiotic era was variable and in some series approached 60%, but specific and effective antimicrobial chemotherapy is now available [80]. Doxycycline and chloramphenicol are both effective oral or intravenous agents against scrub typhus, dissipating fever in 24 h in most patients [71]. Although the disease can be treated effectively with these antibiotics, reinfection and relapse frequently occur due to the wide variety of antigenically distinct serotypes [85]. Azithromycin and rifampicin are alternative drugs [61].

Currently, effective chemoprophylaxis or vaccination approaches for dealing with *O. tsutsugamushi* infection are still not available [42]. A prophylactic vaccine to scrub typhus is a public health priority because of its high incidence, high mortality, nonspecific clinical presentation, lack of sensitive diagnostic tests, and emergence of antibiotic resistance. The development of an effective and safe vaccine has to be strongly focused on T cell-mediated immunity, empirical testing of the immunogenicity of proteins encoded by conserved genes, and assessment of protection in relevant animal models that truly mimic human scrub typhus resistance [57]. Therefore, prevention of scrub typhus is based mainly on avoiding the chigger bites and the use of repellents during travel in rural areas of endemic countries [61]. Wearing protective clothing and self-examination after visiting arthropod-vector infested areas are also recommended [86].

### 2.2. Other chigger-borne infectious diseases

Nowadays, *O. tsutsugamushi* remains as the unique agent whose transmission by chigger bites has been confirmed. Nevertheless, trombiculid mites inhabit areas where the presence of several arthropod-borne microorganisms, their vectors, and reservoirs has been demonstrated. Thus, the vector competence of chiggers has long been investigated worldwide.

There are a lot of references in the old scientific literature that associate chiggers with the transmission of several pathogens, being *N. autumnalis* the most reported species. However, the majority of them correspond to secondary anecdotal information and present poor or no details [87]. In the 2000s, *Anaplasma phagocytophilum*-DNA was detected in unfed *N. autumnalis* chiggers collected on vegetation in a mountainous area from the North of Spain [88]. This finding remains doubtful taking into consideration that the infection occurred in unfed larvae, so chiggers are speculated to be true carriers of the bacteria and inherited it through transovarial transmission. The presence of rickettsiae was also investigated in chiggers of the same mountainous area of Spain. Amplicons compatible with infection by *Rickettsia* spp. were detected by molecular techniques in *Neotrombicula inopinata* collected over vegetation [89]. Up to date, these results remain unconfirmed. The vector competence of *N. autumnalis* chiggers for the transmission of *Borrelia burgdorferi* sensu lato (s.l.) has been also investigated. This bacterium was screened by PCR and further DNA hybridization in questing larvae collected on vegetation and feeding larvae removed from trapped micromammals in Germany [87]. Borrelial DNA was amplified in chiggers from 1 larva feeding on a white-toothed shrew (*Crocidura russula*), from a pool of 4 larvae feeding on a *Borrelia garinii*-infected laboratory mouse, and from 1 nymph that had previously fed as a larva on a *Borrelia afzelii*-positive laboratory gerbil. Therefore, the vector competence of *N. autumnalis* remains unclear. The presence of *B. burgdorferi* s.l. and *A. phagocytophilum* DNA was also been investigated by PCR and reverse line blotting in chiggers found on wild birds captured in the western Carpathian Mountains (Czech Republic) [24]. *B. garinii* and *B. valaisiana* were found in a pool of 5 chiggers from the genus *Neotrombicula* collected from a Eurasian Blackcap (*Sylvia atricapilla*). Regarding *A. phagocytophilum*, DNA was detected in none of the samples [87]. Trombiculid mites have also been associated to *Bartonella* spp. A new strain of *Bartonella* sp. was isolated from the gray squirrels *Sciurus carolinensis* in Georgia [90]. Then this bacterium was studied in ectoparasites removed from gray squirrels by PCR. None of the mites tested (*Eutrombicula splendens, Myiatrombicula cynos,* and *Neotrombicula whartoniy*) were positive, whereas 6 *Bartonella* spp. strains were detected, 2 in fleas and 4 in lice [91]. Furthermore, *Leptotrombidium* mites have been reported as carriers of *Bartonella tamiae* [92], species isolated from patients from Thailand [93].

Several rickettsiae previously found in humans as *Rickettsia akari, Rickettsia japonica, Rickettsia conorii, Rickettsia felis, Rickettsia typhi,* and *Rickettsia* sp. closely related to TwKM02, *Rickettsia australis,* and Cf15 were detected using molecular methods in trombiculid mites removed from wild rodents collected in Korea [94]. Although the rickettsial DNA was detected in mites, it has yet to be determined whether the DNA was amplified from the meal of an infected animal or from the mite tissue itself. Tsui *et al.*, (2007), identified TwKM02 and TwKM03 closely related to *R. australis* and *R. felis* URRWXCal2, respectively, in *Leptotrombidium* chiggers collected in Taiwan [95].

Chiggers are also suspected to be vectors of viral diseases [96]. The role of *L. scutellare* as possible vector of a Hantavirus causing epidemic hemorrhagic fever with renal syndrome (HFRS) in China was hypothesized [97]. The authors suggested that this mite could be naturally infected by HFRS virus and transmitted to vertebrates by biting and to its offspring via transovarian transmission. On the other hand, although the spread of Hantavirus had been thought to be exclusively by rodent excrement and urine, Hantavirus-RNA was detected in *Leptotrombidium* mites from Texas (2 larvae and 1 free-living predatory stage), suggesting a possible role in the transmission of Hantavirus pulmonary syndrome [98].

## 3. Chiggers and dermatitis

"Trombiculiasis," also called "trombiculosis," "trombidiosis," "chigger dermatitis," "scrub itch," or "seasonal dermatitis" is defined as an skin allergic reaction (dermatitis) caused by the salivary secretion of biting chiggers [1,99]. In our experience, as well as it is described in the literature, trombiculiasis is a common but underreported ectoparasitosis that is probably often misdiagnosed [100]. In many cases, trombiculiasis was primarily confused with a plant allergy [29], as it was the case in our country. The better understanding of trombiculid mites' life cycle and their interaction with humans have made possible a proper knowledge of this disease.

### 3.1. Etiology and epidemiology

Although not often reported in the literature, trombiculiasis is prevalent all over the world, except for the Arctic region [20]. However, it can be easily missed because it is normally transient and no systemic signs are present.

In nontropical areas, bites are particularly common in the late summer and early autumn, when outdoor activities are maximal and the peak of abundance of chiggers occurs [19,20,26,28,101]. Thus, trombiculiasis is also an important threat to travelers that visit infested areas being unaware of chiggers [37].

Mite islands are usually found in cleared land and scrub bush with grassy vegetation, warm soil temperatures, and high humidity. Suitable habitats also require the presence of potential hosts [31]. Trombiculids are also found in parks, gardens, lawns, and moist areas alongside lakes and streams [1]. Clusters of chiggers are usually waiting at elevated points of the ground-level vegetation, such as the end of grass stalk or on dried tree branches, until an animal or human passes by [8] (Figure 5).

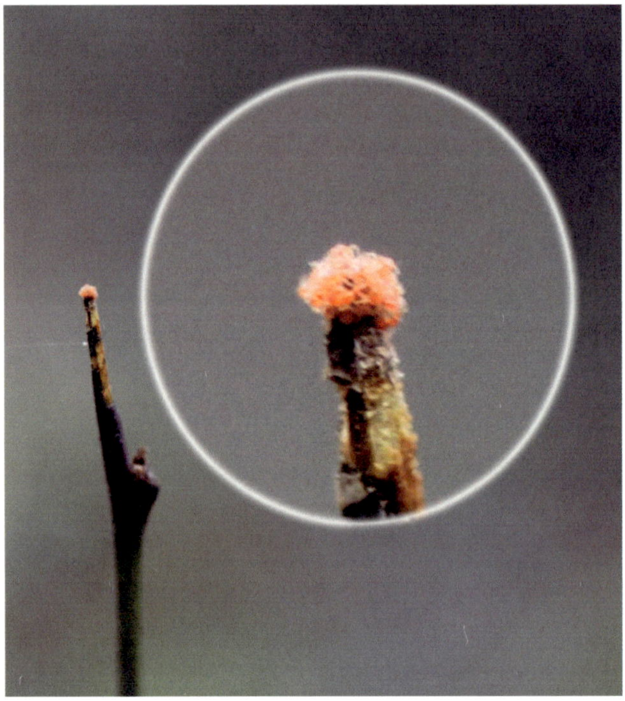

**Figure 5.** Cluster of unfed chiggers. Original contribution.

People are usually bitten during outdoor activities for recreational or professional purposes such as hunting, hiking, mushroom picking, forestry work, etc. [8,28,101]. Although the rate of people bitten is very high, apparently some persons are preferred by the chiggers, resulting in massive parasitization, while others remain unmolested even in highly infested areas [26,28].

More than 3,000 species of chiggers are known, but about 15 frequently bite humans and domestic animals causing cutaneous reactions [102] (Table 2). Species currently considered as the most frequent cause of trombiculiasis are *E. alfreddugesi* in the Americas, *N. autumnalis* in Europe, *Eutrombicula batatas* in South America, and *Eutrombicula wichmanni* in Southeast Asia, Australia, and the Pacific Islands [4,28,37,103].

*E. alfreddugesi* is the most common and widespread trombiculiasis-producing species in the New World. The larvae are present in the late summer and early autumn in temperate regions of its geographical range and throughout the year in the tropics and subtropics. It is particularly common in areas of secondary growth, along margins of swamps, and ecotones between woodlands and open fields or grasslands [1]. *E. splendens* is the second most common chigger attacking human in North America. This species is especially abundant in moist habitats such as swamps, bogs, and low-lying areas with rotting stumps and fallen trees. The seasonality is similar to *E. alfreddugesi* ones [1]. In addition, another mite causing trombiculiasis in the United States is *Eutrombicula lipovsky*. It is present in moist habitats, generally characterized by an abundance of decaying logs and stumps bordering swamps and streams [1].

*E. alfreddugesi* and *E. batatas* are the main species implicated in South-America. However, trombiculiasis attributed to *N. autumnalis* (isango) is well-known in Peru [21]. Recently, a "pest" called "Qhapa," with the same clinical features than trombiculiasis, has been associated with *E. batatas* in Bolivia [104]. In Venezuela, it is possible that a high percentage of the diagnosed scabies may actually be trombiculiasis [22]. Recently, *E. alfreddugesi* was implicated in a case of trombiculiasis in a tourist after a vacation in Brazil [20].

Seven chigger species are proven to cause trombiculiasis in Europe: *N. japonica, Neotrombicula zachvatkini, Euschoengastia xerothermobia, N. autumnalis, Kepkatrombicula desaleri, Blankaartia acuscutellaris,* and *Trombicula toldti* [6,29,105]. Recently, *N. inopinata* has been reported as a possible causative agent of trombiculiasis in Spain [8]. As stated above, it is generally accepted that *N. autumnalis* is the most common cause of trombiculiasis in Europe and the British Islands [1]. However, in many cases, the role of "harvest mite" has been attributed to *N. autumnalis* without enough taxonomic criteria. Therefore, other species may be causative agents of trombiculiasis, as occurred with *N. inopinata* in Spain [8] (Figure 6).

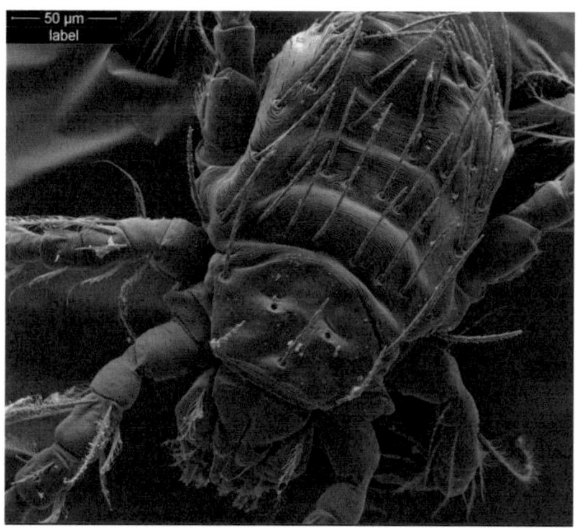


**Figure 6.** *Neotrombicula inopinata* (photo provided by Dr. Stekolnikov).

Although well known in many European regions, the scientific description of trombiculiasis cases have been only reported from Italy [36] and Spain [28]. Moreover, four different cases suspected of trombiculiasis caused by *N. autumnalis* were described in Croatia [106], and one case attributed to harvest mites was informed in the United Kingdom [107]. In Europe, trombiculiasis is associated with the late summer and early autumn [26,28,36,101]. In fact, *N. autumnalis* is known as the "European harvest mite" due to the seasonality of the disease [87]. Nevertheless, in the last years, trombiculiasis-like skin reactions have been reported in Germany not only in summer and autumn but also in early spring and in winter [31].

In Southeast Asia, Australia, and the Pacific Islands, the main involved mite is *E. wichmanni*. Nevertheless, *E. sarcina* and species of genera *Odontacarus* and *Schoengastia* are also causative agents of trombiculiasis [4]. In addition, *Neotrombicula nagayoi* was involved in human trombiculiasis in Japan [5].

A single case of trombiculiasis has been reported in Africa. *L. subquadratum* was described as a cause of severe itching and dermatitis in humans and dogs in South Africa [108].

It is generally accepted that to suffer from trombiculiasis, the antecedent of direct contact with vegetation is required. Nevertheless, it is important to remark that one of the patients reported in Guarneri *et al.*, 2005 [36] was not in contact with vegetation but presented similar clinical features than the one that was hunting with the dogs. The authors speculated that trombiculiasis was transmitted by direct contact with the infected dogs. The hypothesis is supported in the fact that the dogs were frequently allowed to sit on the legs of the patients, and the patient's lesions were concentrated on the abdomen and thighs. Dogs can be affected by chigger bites and suffer neurological and digestive forms that may be fatal. In our experience, massive infections are more frequents, and untreated dogs finally die. Dogs usually began with diarrhea, irritation, and ataxia. The precedent of visiting infested areas and the presence of "red points" in the dog's eyes are essential clues to guide the diagnosis [25]

Another example of disease caused by chiggers but without direct contact to vegetation is also a case of conjunctivitis induced by *N. autumnalis*, reported in a patient with no history of travelling, hill walking, gardening, or contact with vegetation [109]. There, the authors suggested mite infestation occurred by direct contact with the patient's cat. Nevertheless, there is no data about the cat in the manuscript. These cases suggested that close human contact with infected pets should be considered as an unusual route of trombiculiasis, so chigger transmission is possible without direct contact with infested soil or vegetation [36,109].

Previously, patients were rarely referred for dermatologist review unless symptoms were severe. Over the last 15 years, cases of severe trombiculiasis have increased in western Germany and in the United Kingdom [31,107]. The influence of climate and environmental variations, changes in leisure habits, and broader environmental awareness in the population have been speculated as possible explanations of this increase [26].

### 3.2. Clinical manifestation

Chigger bites are initially painless, and frequently the only sign of exposure is a severe itching. Then small, red bite like lesions appears on the skin [1,19]. Typical 1–2 mm diameter, pruritic, erythematous papules appear at the sites of the bites 3–24 h after exposure (Figure 7). [10,28,37,101,103].

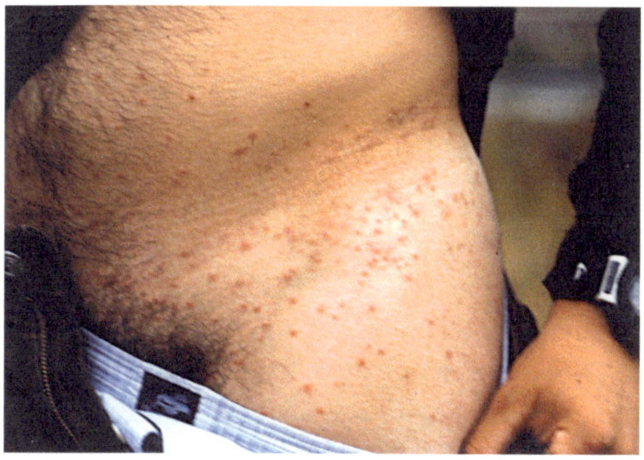

**Figure 7.** Typical papules of trombiculiasis in a patient bitten in La Rioja, Spain. Original contribution.

The presence of papulovesicles, which may gradually progress to pustules, crusty, scabby, eczematous, and ulcerated confluent forms of skin lesions, has also been described [17,26,103]. The pruritus is very intense, especially at night in bed. Although the chigger is not present, the papules and discomfort may persist up to 2–3 weeks, but regression of localized itching is generally observed in 1 week [26]. Since trombiculid mites share habitat with hard ticks, people may result coinfested. In fact, a patient suffering from trombiculiasis and having an "erythema migrans" (related to Lyme disease) was treated in our hospital. Furthermore, during an episode of trombiculiasis, two affected people and their dog had *R. felis* infection, possibly transmitted by fleas [110].

Chiggers usually "attack" in large numbers due to the clustering phenomenon, resulting in multiple grouped bites on infested hosts [32]. Given their preference for attaching where the skin is thin or in tighter contact with clothes, the bites tend to be concentrated around the knees, antecubital fossae, and ankles, thighs, axillary region, groins and genitalia, and wrists, and in areas constricted by clothing, such as along the belt line or the elastic borders or undergarments [1,17,26,28,101].

Trombiculiasis-causing chiggers do not survive more than 1–2 days feeding on humans due to the adverse host reaction and because they are remove by scratching [1,23]. The irritant effect of chiggers' saliva seems to induce both dermal inflammatory reaction of moderate intensity and an adaptive immune response. These salivary components generally reveal relatively moderate lytic properties and weak immunological characters [111]. The type of skin inflammatory response during the feeding of trombiculid larvae is determined by concomitant factors such as the site of the parasite localization, condition of the host's skin, among others [39]. Repeated exposures result in a more rapid and intense adaptive immune response [102]. Anyway, permanent or long-term human residents in an infested area increase their immunity as a result of continued bites, and some people can develop a high degree of tolerance to the antigenic substances injected by chiggers. However, the occurrence of unusual outbreaks of urticaria, increasingly severe pruritus or bulla formation, are indications of hypersensitivity to such antigenic substances [5]. It is clear that the natural hosts of trombiculids have to be sensitized with respect to parasites that may lead the development of the strong specific inflammatory response [39, 111].

### 3.3. Diagnosis and treatment

Diagnosis is based on the clinical manifestations, taking into consideration the history of being in contact with vegetation and the seasonality. As the etiological agent of the trombiculiasis is rarely found in the skin of the patients, these reactions are often misinterpreted and has been wrongly associated to plant allergies, flea or mosquito bites, or even scabies [26]. Cutaneous findings are nonspecific, so clinical examination would probably lead to a wrong diagnosis of a nonspecific itchy dermatitis, leading to use inadequate or needless medications. Then an accurate anamnesis is essential for making such challenging diagnosis. Chigger bites should be considered whenever any unexplained skin eruption is presented to the physician.

Chiggers are not easily seen on human's skin with the naked eye, and common magnification lenses and even dermoscopy (×10 magnifications) have some limitations. Recently, videodermatoscopy (×150 magnification) has been used to diagnose trombiculiasis caused by *N. autumnalis* in a man with a well-documented diagnosis of scabies [100].

Differential diagnosis includes infestations with other mite species (e.g., the itch mite *Sarcoptes scabiei*), or blood-sucking ectoparasites, such as bed bugs, fleas, ticks, and mosquitoes. Also, hypersensitivity to chemical substances or photoallergic skin reaction to contact with a plant (*Meadow dermatitis*) should be taken into consideration [26].

Treatment is primarily symptomatic and consists of antipruritics, antihistamines, and topical corticosteroids [112]. In our medical consultation, supportive measures such as oatmeal baths are also highly recommended. Antibiotics might be needed in case bacterial superinfection resulting from repeated scratching occurs.

After being in known areas of chigger activity, the dermatitis can be minimized, and the recovery time can be significantly shortened, by taking a hot soapy shower or bath and washing clothes with soap and hot water. These good practices are recommended immediately after exposure, in order to remove both unattached and attached chiggers, before they have firmly anchored to the skin (generally within 3–6 h following attachment) [1,26]. Once the papules are present, scratching should be avoided in order to prevent to excoriate the lesions and the infection.

Patients should be advised on preventive measures, including avoidance of high-risk areas when larvae are active. Since in many cases these results are unreasonable and contact with trombiculid mites is unavoidable, chigger infestation may be minimized by wearing protective clothing and soaking socks and trouser legs with insect repellents [112]. Usually, the use of repellent sprays and lotions containing benzyl benzoate or diethyltoluamide has been recommended [29]. Permethrin was successfully used as a clothing treatment for personal protection against chigger mites [113]. However, the active ingredient is no longer available for this purpose in the European Union [10,26].

Although better than before, our contemporary knowledge on the biology and ecology of these mites is still extremely limited. Currently, no reliable recommendations for the control of mites, except from personal protection, can be given [26].

## 4. Other human diseases associated to chiggers

Apart from trombiculiasis, chiggers are responsible for other less frequent conditions. The summer penile syndrome is a seasonal acute hypersensitivity reaction attributed to chigger bites [114,115]. It occurs in young boys with a history of bites or outdoor exposure, and it is characterized by the rapid onset of edema and pruritus of the penile skin. It has been described most commonly in the spring and summer in different regions of United States [114,115]. Another example is the unique case of conjunctivitis induced by *N. autumnalis*, reported in United Kingdom [109]. The patient had a 2-week history of a painful, gritty, red left eye, which failed to improve with a liquid paraffin eye ointment. On examination, her conjunctiva was found to be mildly red and she had normal visual acuity. On close inspection, a live mite was identified in contact with the left upper eyelid margin.

## 5. Conclusions

Chiggers are worldwide distributed ectoparasites that have to be taken into account as human pathogens. Their medical importance is based on their role as vectors of scrub typhus and as causative agents of trombiculiasis.

Scrub typhus remains as one of the most life-threatening infection in Asian Pacific regions. The development of a prophylactic vaccine against *O. tsutsugamushi* is of great interest in endemic regions. In addition, special attention should be paid on recent reports of scrub cases typhus-like infections in unusual areas, and on reviewing the genetic diversity of the genus *Orientia*.

More research studies are necessary in order to clarify the relationship of chiggers with other bacterial or viral infections.

Trombiculiasis is an extended but underreported condition that should be considered when pruritic dermatitis in people exposed to vegetation occurs. In risky areas, personal protection is the unique recommendation to reduce the parasitation. A deeper understanding of chiggers' life cycle, epidemiology and seasonality of trombiculiasis is required for a correct management of this annoying dermatitis.

## Acknowledgements

We are grateful to all members from the Centre of Rickettsiosis and Arthropod-Borne Diseases, Hospital San Pedro-Centre of Biomedical Research (CIBIR), Logroño (La Rioja), Spain. We also thank to Dr. Shatrov and Dr. Stekolnikov from the Zoological Institute of the Russian Academy of Science, St.-Petersburg, Russia, and Dr. Takahashi from the Saitama Medical University, Saitama, Japan, for providing us the pictures and for their invaluable help. Financial support was provided in part by two grants (FOMENTA 2007/14 and PREDOC 2008/29) from "Consejería de Educación, Cultura y Deporte del Gobierno de La Rioja", Spain.

## Author details

Paula Santibáñez*, Ana M. Palomar, Aránzazu Portillo, Sonia Santibáñez and José A. Oteo

*Address all correspondence to: psantibanez@riojasalud.es

Department of Infectious Diseases, Center of Rickettsioses and Arthropod-Borne Diseases, Hospital San Pedro-CIBIR, Logroño, La Rioja, Spain

## References

[1] Mullen G, O'Connor B. Mites (Acari). In: Durden L, Mullen G (ed.). Medical and Veterinary Entomology. Academic Press. 2002. p449–516.

[2] Brennan J, Goff M. Keys to the genera of chiggers of western hemisphere (Acarina: Trombiculidae. J Parasitol. 1977; 77(3):554–566.

[3] Moniuszko H, Mąkol J. Chigger mites (Actinotrichida: Parasitengona, Trombiculidae) of Poland. An updated distribution and hosts. Ann Parasitol. 2014; 60(2):103–117.

[4] Burns D. Diseases caused by arthropods and othernoxious animals. In: Burns DA, Breathnach SM, Cox NH GC (ed.). Rook's Textbook of Dermatology. 8th Edition. Blackwell Publishing. 2009.

[5] Takahashi M, Misumi H, Urakami H, Saito T, Misumi M, Matsumoto I, Suzuki H. A new member of the trombiculid mite family Neotrombicula nagayoi (Acari: Trombiculidae) induces human dermatitis. Southeast Asian J Trop Med Public Health. 2004; 35: 113–118.

[6] Ripka G, Stekolnikov A. First finding of the chigger Blankaartia acuscutellaris on a human host in Europe. Belgian J Entomol. 2006; 8: 147–151.

[7] ]Shatrov AB. Comparative and functional morphology of the mouthparts in larvae of Parasitengona (Acariformes). Zoosymposia. 2011; 6: 14–23.

[8] Stekolnikov A, Santibáñez P, Palomar AM, Oteo JA. Neotrombicula inopinata (Acari: Trombiculidae)—a possible causative agent of trombiculiasis in Europe. Parasit Vectors. 2014;7:90.

[9] Stekolnikov AA, Daniel M. Chigger mites (Acari: Trombiculidae) of Turkey. Zootaxa. 2012. 3216: 1–104.

[10] White G. Medical acarology and entomology. In: Gordon CC, Zumla AI (ed.). Manson's Tropical Diseases. 2003. p1717–1720.

[11] Kim JH, Roh JY, Kwon DH, Kim YH, Yoon KA, Yoo S, Noh SJ, Park J, Shin EH, Park MY, Lee SH. Estimation of the genome sizes of the chigger mites Leptotrombidium pallidum and Leptotrombidium scutellare based on quantitative PCR and k-mer analysis. Parasit Vectors. 2014; 7(1): 279–288.

[12] Rozendaal JA. Bedbugs, fleas, lice, ticks and mites. In: World Health Organization. Vector control: methods for use by individuals and communities. 1997. 236–283.

[13] Faccini-Martínez A, García-Álvarez L, Hidalgo M, Oteo JA. Syndromic classification of rickettsioses: an approach for clinical practice. Int J Infect Dis. 2014; 28: 126–139.

[14] Kim IS, Walker DH. Scrub Typhus. In: Guerrant RL, Walker DH, Peter WF (ed.). Tropical infectious diseases. Principles, pathogens and practice. 3th edition. Elsevier; 2011. p334–338.

[15] Lee H, Shim S, Song B, Choi E, Hwang K, Park M, et al. Detection of Orientia tsutsugamushi, the causative agent of scrub typhus, in a novel mite species, Eushoengastia koreaensis, in Korea. Vector Borne Zoonotic Dis. 2011; 11(3):209–214.

[16] Ken KM, Shockman SC, Sirichotiratana M, Lent MP, Wilson ML. Dermatoses associated with mites other than Sarcoptes. Semin Cutan Med Surg. 2014; 33:110–115.

[17] McClain D, Dana AN, Goldenberg G. Mite infestations. Dermatol Ther. 2009; 22:327–346.

[18] Witt LH, Linardi PM, Meckes O, Schwalfenberg S, Ribeiro RA, Feldmeier H, Heukelbach J. Blood-feeding of Tunga penetrans males. Med Vet Entomol. 2004; 18:439–441.

[19] Elston D. What's eating you? Chiggers. Cutis. 2006; 77(6): 350–352.

[20] Martens H, Melo MDM, Bosch W Van Den, Genderen PJJ van. A 'chigsaw' puzzle after a vacation in Brazil. Neth J Med. 2012; 70(7): 321–325.

[21] Beltrán M, Valdivia C, Ponce-Ramírez R, Chambergo M. Trombicula autumnalis (isangos) en un jardín de niños de la selva peruana. Rev Peru Med Exp Salud Publica. 2009; 26(1):58–60.

[22] Chaccour CJ. Trombiculiasis: reporte de dos casos y revisión de la literatura. Dermatologia Venez. 2005; 43(2):18–21.

[23] Shatrov AB, Kudryashova NI. Taxonomy, life cycles and the origin of parasitism in trombiculid mites. In: Morand S, Krasnov BR, Poulin R (ed.). Micromammals and Macroparasites Part II. Springer. 2006. p119–140.

[24] Literak I, Stekolnikov AA, Sychra O, Dubska L, Taragelova V. Larvae of chigger mites Neotrombicula spp. (Acari: Trombiculidae) exhibited Borrelia but no Anaplas-

ma infections: a field study including birds from the Czech Carpathians as hosts of chiggers. Exp Appl Acarol. 2008; 44: 307–314.

[25] Cakiroglu D, Pekmezci D, Meral Y, Gokalp G, Acici M. Trombiculidae larvae (Neotrombicula autumnalis) infestation in a Little Bittern (Ixobrychus minutus) in Turkey. Parasitol Res. 2008; 102:1077–1079.

[26] Kampen H. Die Herbstmilbe Neotrombicula autumnalis und andere parasitische Laufmilben (Acari, Trombiculidae) als Verursacher von Hauterkrankungen in Mitteleuropa. Biol Linz/Austria. 2002; 184:461–476.

[27] Nutall T. Pruritic dermatoses. In: Nutall T, Harvey RG, McKeever PJ (ed.). A colour handbook of skin diseases of the dog and cat. Manson Publishing; 2009. p51–52.

[28] Santibáñez-Sáenz P, Palomar-Urbina AM, Imaña-Rodríguez E, Oteo-Revuelta JA. Pruritic dermatitis after hiking in the mountains. Enferm Infecc Microbiol Clin. 2014; 32(9): 610–611.

[29] Kampen H. Trombiculiden und Trombidiose. Z Allg Med. 2000; 76:392–396.

[30] Moss P, Beeching NJ. Arthropods and ectoparasites. In: Cohen J, Powderly WG (ed.). Infectious Diseases. 2nd edition. Mosby-Elsevier; 2003. p.128–139.

[31] Schöler A, Maier WA, Kampen H. Multiple environmental factor analysis in habitats of the harvest mite Neotrombicula autumnalis (Acari: Trombiculidae) suggests extraordinarily high euryoecious biology. Exp Appl Acarol. 2006; 39:41–62.

[32] Traub BR, Wissernan CL. The ecology of chigger-borne rickettsiosis (Scrub Typhus). J Med Entomol. 1974; 11:237–303.

[33] Belozerov V. Seasonal adaptations in the life cycles of mites and ticks: comparative and evolutionary aspects. Trends in Acarology: Proceedings of the 12th International Congress. 2010. p.319–326.

[34] Mąkol J, Cichocki J, Felska M, Kłosińska A, Łaydanowicz J, Łupicki D, Gabryś G. A new data on biology and taxonomy of Neotrombicula inopinata (Oudemans, 1909) and Leptotrombidium russicum (Oudemans, 1902) (Acari: Actinotrichida: Trombiculidae). Ann Zool. 2010; 60:419–427.

[35] Shatrov AB. Some peculiarities of the life cycle and biology of chiggers in laboratory. Entomol Rev. 1996; 76:1197–1208.

[36] Guarneri F, Pugliese A, Giudice E, Guarneri C, Giannetto S, Guarneri B. Trombiculiasis: clinical contribution. Eur J Dermatology. 2005; 15:495–496.

[37] Díaz JH. Mite-transmitted dermatoses and infectious diseases in returning travelers. J Travel Med. 2010; 17(1): 21–31.

[38] ]Goldberg SR, Holshuh HJ. Ectoparasite-induced lesions in mite pockets of the Yarrow's spiny lizard, Sceloporus jarrovii (Phrynosomatidae). J Wildl Dis. 1992; 28:537–541.

[39] Shatrov AB, Takahashi M, Noda S, Misumi H. Stylostome organization in feeding Leptotrombidium larvae (Acariformes: Trombiculidae). Exp Appl Acarol. 2014; 64:33–47.

[40] Walker DH. Rickettsiae. In: Baron S (ed.). Medical Microbiology. 4th edition. University of Texas Medical Branch at Galveston. 1996; chapter 38.

[41] Portillo A, Oteo JA. Rickettsiosis as threat for the traveller. In: Rodriguez-Morales AJ (ed.). Current Topics in Tropical Medicine. 2012.

[42] Li T, Yang Z, Dong Z, Wang M. Meteorological factors and risk of scrub typhus in Guangzhou, Southern China, 2006–2012. BMC Infect Dis. 2014;14(1):139.

[43] Watt G, Parola P. Scrub typhus and tropical rickettsioses. Curr Opin Infect Dis. 2003; 16(5):429–436.

[44] Paris DH, Chansamouth V, Nawtaisong P, Löwenberg EC, Phetsouvanh R, Blacksell SD, Lee SJ, Dondorp AM, van der Poll T, Newton PN, Levi M, Day NP. Coagulation and inflammation in scrub typhus and murine typhus—a prospective comparative study from Laos. Clin Microbiol Infect. 2012; 18:1221–1228.

[45] Tamura A, Ohashi N, Urakami H, Miyamura S. Classification of Rickettsia tsutsugamushi in a new genus, Orientia gen. nov., as Orientia tsutsugamushi comb. nov. Int J Syst Bacteriol. 1995; 45(3):589–591.

[46] Kelly DJ, Fuerst PA, Ching W-M, Richards AL. Scrub typhus: the geographic distribution of phenotypic and genotypic variants of Orientia tsutsugamushi. Clin Infect Dis. 2009; 48(3):203–230.

[47] Paris DH, Shelite TR, Day NP, Walker DH. Unresolved problems related to scrub typhus: a seriously neglected life-threatening disease. Am J Trop Med Hyg. 2013; 89(2): 301–307.

[48] Fournier PE, Siritantikorn S, Rolain JM, Suputtamongkol Y, Hoontrakul S, Charoenwat S, Losuwanaluk K, Parola P, Raoult D. Detection of new genotypes of Orientia tsutsugamushi infecting humans in Thailand. Clin Microbiol Infect. 2008; 14:168–173.

[49] Seong SY, Choi MS, Kim IS. Orientia tsutsugamushi infection: overview and immune responses. Microbes Infect. 2001; 3:11–21.

[50] Panpanich R, Garner P. Antibiotics for treating scrub typhus. Cochrane Database Syst Rev. 2002; (3):CD002150.

[51] Francischetti IMB, Anderson SN, Mans BJ, Santos IM, Ribeiro JMC. The role of saliva in tick feeding. Front Biosci. 2010; 14:2051–2088.

[52] Traub R, Wisseman CL, Jones MR, O'Keefe JJ. The acquisition of Rickettsia tsutsugamushi by chiggers (trombiculid mites) during the feeding process. Ann NY Acad Sci. 1975; 266:91–114.

[53] Nakayama K, Kurokawa K, Fukuhara M, Urakami H, Yamamoto S, Yamazaki K, Ogura Y, Ooka T, Hayashi T. Genome comparison and phylogenetic analysis of Orientia tsutsugamushi strains. DNA Res. 2010; 17:281–291.

[54] Frances SP, Watcharapichat P, Phulsuksombati D TP. Transmission of Orientia tsutsugamushi, the aetiological agent for Scrub Typhus, to co-feeding mites. Parasitology. 2000; 120:601–607.

[55] Dhiman RC. Emerging vector-borne zoonoses: eco-epidemiology and public health implications in India. Front Public Heal. 2014; 2:1–6.

[56] Rodkvamtook W, Gaywee J, Kanjanavanit S, Ruangareerate T, Richards AL, Sangjun N, Jeamwattanalert P, Sirisopana N. Scrub typhus outbreak, Northern Thailand, 2006–2007. Emerg Infect Dis. 2013; 19(5):774–777.

[57] Valbuena G, Walker DH. Approaches to vaccines against Orientia tsutsugamushi. Front Cell Infect Microbiol. 2012; 2:170.

[58] Paris DH, Phetsouvanh R, Tanganuchitcharnchai A, Jones M, Jenjaroen K, Vongsouvath M, Ferguson DP, Blacksell SD, Newton PN, Day NP, Turner GD. Orientia tsutsugamushi in human scrub typhus eschars shows tropism for dendritic cells and monocytes rather than endothelium. PLoS Negl Trop Dis. 2012; 6(1).

[59] Sonthayanon P, Peacock SJ, Chierakul W, Wuthiekanun V, Blacksell SD, Holden MT, Bentley SD, Feil EJ, Day NP. High rates of homologous recombination in the mite endosymbiont and opportunistic human pathogen Orientia tsutsugamushi. PLoS Negl Trop Dis. 2010; 4(7).

[60] Chung MH, Lee JS, Baek JH, Kim M, Kang JS. Persistence of Orientia tsutsugamushi in humans. J Korean Med Sci. 2012; 27:231–235.

[61] Raoult D. Orientia tsutsugamushi (Scrub Typhus). In: Mandell GL, Bennett JE, Dolin R (ed.). Mandell, Douglas, and Bennett's Principles and Practice of Infectious Diseases. 7th edition. Elsevier; 2010. p.2529–2530.

[62] Jensenius M, Fournier PE, Raoult D. Rickettsioses and the international traveler. Clin Infect Dis. 2004; 39:1493–1499.

[63] Osuga K, Kimura M, Goto H, Shimada K, Suto T. A case of Tsutsugamushi disease probably contracted in Africa. Eur J Clin Microbiol Infect Dis. 1991; 10:95–96.

[64] Ghorbani RP, Ghorbani AJ, Jain MK, Walker DH. A case of scrub typhus probably acquired in Africa. Clin Infect Dis. 1997; 25:1473–1474.

[65] Pham X, Otsuka Y, Suzuki H, Takaoka H. Detection of Orientia tsutsugamushi (Rickettsiales: rickettsiaceae) in unengorged chiggers (Acari: Trombiculidae) from Oita

Prefecture, Japan, by nested polymerase chain reaction. J Med Entomol. 2001; 38(2): 308–311.

[66] Pages F, Faulde M, Orlandi-Pradines E, Parola P. The past and present threat of vector-borne diseases in deployed troops. Clin Microbiol Infect. 2010; 16(3):209–224.

[67] Rajapakse S, Rodrigo C, Fernando D. Scrub typhus: pathophysiology, clinical manifestations and prognosis. Asian Pac J Trop Med. Hainan Medical College; 2011; 5(4): 261–264.

[68] Raj S, Krishnamoorthy A, Jagannati M, Abhilash K. Splenic infarct due to Scrub Typhus. J Glob Infect Dis. 2014; 6(2):86–88.

[69] Rungta N. Scrub Typhus: emerging cause of multiorgan dysfunction. Indian J Crit Care Med. 2014; 18(8):489–491.

[70] Kim DM, Kyung JW, Chi YP, Ki DY, Hyong SK, Tae YY, et al. Distribution of eschars on the body of scrub typhus patients: a prospective study. Am J Trop Med Hyg. 2007; 76(5):806–809.

[71] Jeong YJ, Kim S, Wook YD, Lee JW, Kim K-I, Lee SH. Scrub typhus: clinical, pathologic, and imaging findings. Radiographics. 2007; 27:161–172.

[72] Kim DM, Kim SW, Choi SH Y. Clinical and laboratory findings associated with severe scrub typhus. BMC Infect Dis. 2010; 10(108).

[73] Lee JS, Park MY, Kim YJ, Kil H Il, Choi YH, Kim YC. Histopathological features in both the eschar and erythematous lesions of Tsutsugamushi Disease: identification of CD30+ cell infiltration in Tsutsugamushi disease. Am J Dermatopathol. 2009; 31(6): 551–556.

[74] La Scola B, Raoult D. Laboratory diagnosis of rickettsioses: current approaches to diagnosis of old and new rickettsial diseases. J Clin Microbiol. 1997; 35(11):2715–2727.

[75] Kim MK, Kee SH, Cho KA, Chung MH, Lim BU, Chang WH KJ. Apoptosis of endothelial cell line ECV304 persistently infected with Orientia tsutsugamushi. Microbiol Immunol. 1999; 43(8):751–757.

[76] Cho N, Seong S, Choi M, Kim I. Expression of Chemokine Genes in Human Dermal Microvascular Endothelial Cell Lines Infected with Orientia tsutsugamushi. 2001; 69(3):1265–1272.

[77] Lu HY, Tsai KH, Yu SK, Cheng CH, Yang JS, Su CL, Hu HC, Wang HC, Huang JH, Shu PY. Phylogenetic analysis of 56-kDa type-specific antigen gene of Orientia tsutsugamushi isolates in Taiwan. Am J Trop Med Hyg. 2010; 83(3):658–663.

[78] Singhsilarak T, Leowattana W, Looareesuwan S, Wongchotigul V, Jiang J, Richards AL, Watt G. Short report: detection of Orientia tsutsugamushi in clinical samples by quantitative real-time polymerase chain reaction. Am J Trop Med Hyg. 2005; 72(5): 640–641.

[79] Blacksell SD, Bryant NJ, Paris DH, Doust JA, Sakoda Y, Day NPJ. Scrub typhus serologic testing with the indirect immunofluorescence method as a diagnostic gold standard: a lack of consensus leads to a lot of confusion. Clin Infect Dis. 2007; 44:391–401.

[80] Koh GCKW, Maude RJ, Paris DH, Newton PN, Blacksell SD. Diagnosis of scrub typhus. Am J Trop Med Hyg. 2010; 82(3):368–370.

[81] Lee YS, Wang PH, Tseng SJ, Ko CF, Teng HJ. Epidemiology of scrub typhus in eastern Taiwan, 2000–2004. Jpn J Infect Dis. 2006; 59:235–238.

[82] Liu YX, Cao WC, Gao Y, Zhang JL, Yang ZQ, Zhao ZT, Foley JE. Orientia tsutsugamushi in Eschars from scrub typhus patients. Emerg Infect Dis. 2006; 12(7):1109–1112.

[83] Furuya Y, Yoshida Y, Katayama T, Yamamoto S, Kawamura A. Serotype-specific amplification of Rickettsia tsutsugamushi DNA by nested polymerase chain reaction. J Clin Microbiol. 1993; 31(6):1637–1640.

[84] Paris DH, Blacksell SD, Nawtaisong P, Jenjaroen K, Teeraratkul A, Chierakul W, Wuthiekanun V, Kantipong P, Day NP. Diagnostic accuracy of a loop-mediated isothermal PCR assay for detection of Orientia tsutsugamushi during acute scrub typhus infection. PLoS Negl Trop Dis. 2011; 5(9):1–7.

[85] Min CK, Yang JS, Kim S, Choi MS, Kim IS, Cho NH. Genome-based construction of the metabolic pathways of Orientia tsutsugamushi and comparative analysis within the Rickettsiales order. Comp Funct Genomics. 2008: 623145.

[86] García-Álvarez L, Palomar A, Oteo J. Prevention and prophylaxis of tick bites and tick-borne related diseases. Am J Infect Dis. 2013; 9(3):104–116.

[87] Kampen H1, Schöler A, Metzen M, Oehme R, Hartelt K, Kimmig P, Maier WA. Neotrombicula autumnalis (Acari, Trombiculidae) as a vector for Borrelia burgdorferi s.l. Exp Appl Acarol. 2004; 33:93–102.

[88] Fernández-Soto P, Pérez-Sánchez R, Encinas-Grandes A. Molecular detection of Ehrlichia phagocytophila genogroup organisms in larvae of Neotrombicula autumnalis (Acari: Trombiculidae) captured in Spain. J Parasitol. 2001; 87(6):1482–1483.

[89] Santibáñez P, Palomar AM, Santibáñez S PA and OJ. Chiggers (Acari: Trombiculidae) infected with rickettsiae in Spain: preliminary data. 6th International Meeting on Rickettsiae and Rickettsial diseases. 2011.

[90] Bown KJ, Ellis BA, Birtles RJ, Durden LA, Lello J, Begon M, Bennett M. New world origins for haemoparasites infecting United Kingdom grey squirrels (Sciurus carolinensis), as revealed by phylogenetic analysis of Bartonella infecting squirrel populations in England and the United States. Epidemiol Infect. 2002; 129:647–653.

[91] Durden LA, Ellis BA, Banks CW, Crowe JD, Oliver JH. Ectoparasites of gray squirrels in two different habitats and screening of selected ectoparasites for Bartonellae. J Parasitol. 2004; 90(3):485–489.

[92] Kabeya H, Colborn JM, Bai Y, Lerdthusnee K, Richardson JH, Maruyama S, Kosoy MY. Detection of Bartonella tamiae DNA in ectoparasites from rodents in Thailand and their sequence similarity with bacterial cultures from Thai patients. Vector borne Zoonotic Dis. 2010; 10(5):429–434.

[93] Kosoy M, Morway C, Sheff KW, Bai Y, Colborn J, Chalcraft L, Dowell SF, Peruski LF, Maloney SA, Baggett H, Sutthirattana S, Sidhirat A, Maruyama S, Kabeya H, Chomel BB, Kasten R, Popov V, Robinson J, Kruglov A, Petersen LR. Bartonella tamiae sp. nov., a newly recognized pathogen isolated from three human patients from Thailand. J Clin Microbiol. 2008; 46(2):772–775.

[94] Choi YJ1, Lee EM, Park JM, Lee KM, Han SH, Kim JK, Lee SH, Song HJ, Choi MS, Kim IS, Park KH, Jang WJ. Molecular detection of various rickettsiae in mites (Acari: Trombiculidae) in southern Jeolla Province, Korea. Microbiol Immunol. 2007; 51(3): 307–312.

[95] Tsui PY, Tsai KH, Weng MH, Hung YW, Liu YT, Hu KY, Lien JC, Lin PR, Shaio MF, Wang HC, Ji DD. Molecular detection and characterization of spotted fever group rickettsiae in Taiwan. Am J Trop Med Hyg. 2007; 77(161):883–890.

[96] Song G. Epidemiological progresses of hemorrhagic fever with renal syndrome in China. Chin Med J (Engl). 1999; 112(5):472–477.

[97] Wu G, Zhang Y, Guo H, Jiang K, Zhang J, Gan Y. The role of Leptotrombidium scutellare in the transmission of human diseases. Chin Med J (Engl). 1996; 109(9):670–673.

[98] Houck M, Qin H, Roberts H. Hantavirus transmission: potential role of ectoparasites. Vector Borne Zoonotic Dis. 2001; 1(1):75–79.

[99] Goff ML, Loomis RB, Welbourn WC, Wrenn WJ. A Glossary of Chigger Terminology (Acari: Trombiculidae). J Med Entomol. 1982; 19(3):221–238.

[100] Nasca MR, Lacarrubba F MG. Diagnosis of Trombiculosis by videodermatoscopy. Emerg Infect Dis. 2014; 20(6):1059–1060.

[101] Jiménez S, Gastón I, Pérez A, Oteo JA. A seasonal outbreak of human parasitation by chiggers in La Rioja (Northern Spain). Clin Microbiol Infect. 2001; Abstract: p16051.

[102] Arlian LG. Chiggers and Other Disease-Causing Mites. In: Resh VH, Cardé RT (ed.). Encyclopedia of Insects. Second edition. Elsevier; 2009. p152–156.

[103] Steen CJ, Carbonaro PA, Schwartz RA. Arthropods in dermatology. J Am Acad Dermatol. 2004; 50:819–844.

[104] ]Tweeten K, Muñoz-Bravo J. Qhapa, a pest causing skin irritations in nor Yungas region of Bolivia, identified as a chigger mite, Eutrombicula batatas. Trop Doct. 2008; 38(1):63–64.

[105] Shatrov AB, Stekolnikov AA. Redescription of a human-infesting European trombiculid mite Kepkatrombicula desaleri (Acari: Trombiculidae) with data on its mouthparts and stylostome. Int J Acarol. 2011; 37:176–193.

[106] Landeka N, Valic' J. Description of four different cases suspected on trombidiasis. In: Zbornik Radova 24 Znanstveno Stručno Edukativni Seminar, 2011; Split; 2012. p185–91.

[107] Yates V. Harvest mites-a present from the Lake District. Clin Exp Dermatol. 1991; 16(4):277–278.

[108] Heyne H, Ueckermann EA, Coetzee L. First report of a parasitic mite, Leptotrombidium (Hypotrombidium) subquadratum (Lawerence) (Acari: Trombiculidae: Trombiculinae), from dogs and children in the Bloemfontein area, South Africa. J S Afr Vet Assoc. 2001; 72(2):105–106.

[109] Parcell BJ, Sharpe G, Jones B, Alexander CL. Conjunctivitis induced by a red bodied mite, Neotrombicula autumnalis. Parasite 2013; 20(25).

[110] Oteo JA, Portillo A, Santibáñez S, Blanco JR, Pérez-Martínez L, Ibarra V. Cluster of cases of human Rickettsia felis infection from Southern Europe (Spain) diagnosed by PCR. J Clin Microbiol. 2006; 44(7):2669–2671.

[111] Shatrov AB. Stylostome formation in trombiculid mites (Acariformes: Trombiculidae). Exp Appl Acarol. 2009; 49:261–280.

[112] Jones J. Chiggers. Am Fam Physician. 1987; 36(2):149–155.

[113] Breeden G, Schreck C, Sorensen A. Permethrin as a clothing treatment for personal protection against chigger mites (Acarina: Trombiculidae). Am J Trop Med Hyg. 1982; 31(3):589–592.

[114] Smith G, Sharma V, Knapp J, Shields B. The summer penile syndrome: seasonal acute hypersensitivity reaction caused by chigger bites on the penis. Pediatr Emerg Care. 1998; 14(2):116–118.

[115] Schulert G, Gigante J. Summer penile syndrome: an acute hypersensitivity reaction. J Emerg Med. 2014; 46(1).